Assessing Individual Differences in Human Behavior

Assessing
Individual
Differences
in Human
Behavior

New Concepts,
Methods, and Findings

David Lubinski & René V. Dawis
Editors
Foreword by Lloyd G. Humphreys

Davies-Black Publishing
Palo Alto, California
A Division of Consulting Psychologists Press, Inc.

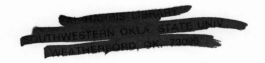

*This Festschrift is dedicated to
Lloyd H. Lofquist, Minnesota psychologist, educator,
mentor, counselor, administrator, researcher, theorist,
and unflagging advocate of individual differences.*

Published by Davies-Black, a division of Consulting Psychologists Press, Inc.,
3803 E. Bayshore Road, Palo Alto, CA 94303; 1-800-624-1765.

99 98 97 96 95   10 9 8 7 6 5 4 3 2 1
Printed in the United States of America

Library of Congress Cataloging-in-Publication Data
    Assessing individual differences in human behavior : new concepts,
    methods, and findings / David Lubinski & René V. Dawis, editors ;
    foreword by Lloyd G. Humphreys -- 1st ed.
        p.   cm.
    Includes bibliographical references and index.
    ISBN 0-89106-072-3
    1. Individual differences.   I. Lubinski, David John.   II. Dawis,
    René V.
    BF697.A78   1995
    155.2'2—dc20   95–11398
                                                               CIP

First edition
    First printing 1995

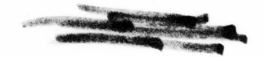

Contents

Foreword   ix
Introduction   xiii

Part 1   Historical Antecedents, Current Status, and New Directions   xxi

Chapter 1   The Challenge of Diversity   1
Leona E. Tyler, University of Oregon

Part 2   New Methodological Concepts   15

Chapter 2   Developments Toward a Cognitive Design System for Psychological Tests   17
Susan E. Embretson, University of Kansas

Chapter 3   Improving Individual Differences Measurement With Item Response Theory and Computerized Adaptive Testing   49
David J. Weiss, University of Minnesota

Chapter 4   Extension of the MAXCOV-HITMAX Taxometric Procedure to Situations of Sizable Nuisance Covariance   81
Paul E. Meehl, University of Minnesota

Chapter 5   Peaked Indicators: A Source of Pseudotaxonicity of a Latent Trait   93
Robert R. Golden and Mary J. Mayer, Albert Einstein College of Medicine

**Part 3   New Findings on Traditional Individual
             Differences Variables   117**

Chapter 6   Gender-Related Individual Differences
             Variables: New Concepts, Methods,
             and Measures   119
             Nancy E. Betz, Ohio State University

Chapter 7   The Psychological Test Profiles of Brigadier Generals:
             Warmongers or Decisive Warriors?   145
             David P. Campbell, Center for Creative Leadership

Chapter 8   Vocational Interests: Evaluating
             Structural Hypotheses   177
             James Rounds, University of Illinois
             at Urbana-Champaign

Chapter 9   Occupational Interests, Leisure Time Interests, and
             Personality: Three Domains or One? Findings From
             the Minnesota Twin Registry   233
             Niels G. Waller, University of California at Davis
             David T. Lykken and Auke Tellegen, University
             of Minnesota

Part 4   New Areas of Research   261

Chapter 10   Interpersonal Influence Theory: The Situational
             and Individual Determinants of Interpersonal
             Behavior   263
             Stanley R. Strong, Virginia Commonwealth
             University

Chapter 11   Not Everyone Can Tell a "Rock" From a "Lock":
             Assessing Individual Differences
             in Speech Perception   297
             James J. Jenkins and Winifred Strange,
             University of South Florida
             Linda Polka, McGill University, Montreal

Part 5   Commentaries   327

Chapter 12   On the Control of Human
Individual Differences   329
David Premack, University of Pennsylvania and
Laboratoire de Psycho-biologie de l'Enfant, Paris

Chapter 13   The Minnesota Counseling Psychologist as
a Broadly Trained Applied Psychologist   341
Howard E. A. Tinsley, Southern Illinois University

Chapter 14   My Life With a Theory   357
John L. Holland, Professor Emeritus,
Johns Hopkins University

Contributors   365
Index   371

Foreword

It is altogether fitting that a book reporting research on individual differences in human attributes be edited by two psychologists with ties to the University of Minnesota and contain chapters written by authors who also have ties to that same university. Interest in and support of research in this area has a long history at Minnesota. In the beginning and for many years thereafter, Donald Paterson was the primary person responsible, and he had the support of the department's chair, Richard Elliott. For many years, they *were* Minnesota in the eyes of fellow psychologists.

Research in individual differences at Minnesota from the start emphasized applications to the real world. The *Journal of Applied Psychology* originated in that department while several industrial selection tests bear the Minnesota name.

Interest in individual differences at Minnesota was not restricted to the industrial area, however. John Anderson, who directed the Institute for Child Welfare, brought Florence Goodenough from Stanford and Merrill Ruff from his participation in the Army Air Forces Aviation Psychology Program. Starke Hathaway of the clinical faculty was largely responsible for the development of the *Minnesota Multiphasic Personality Inventory* (MMPI). Fundamental principles in the use of tests for predictive purposes, such as the importance of base rate in real-world phenomena and the superiority of actuarial versus clinical prediction, are associated with Paul Meehl and the University of Minnesota. Leona Tyler, a Minnesota graduate, wrote one of the best and most influential books concerned with individual differences that appeared in my lifetime (Tyler, 1965).

Research at Minnesota became described very early on as "dustbowl empiricism." A bit later, Fred Skinner added grist to the critics' mill. Make no mistake, the phrase was used demeaningly. The attitudes revealed by its users were detrimental to the development of our discipline. What passed for theory in the time of William James is still all too popular today. Change in our discipline from philosophy to science has been slow. Unfortunately, few test theorists accept data on predictive validity as a critical ingredient of construct validity.

This topic could lead to a long discussion of the philosophy of science, but I am not qualified for that task. As a fellow "dust-bowl empiricist," I believe strongly in the importance of the following propositions: Scientific theory largely evolves from dependable data. The theory that is developed must be vulnerable to a reasonable standard of statistical disproof. Our discipline requires more dependable data in many areas, so sophisticated use of meta-analysis has been a welcome development. An indirect source of support for these propositions is furnished by the substantial negative correlation one observes between the success of a discipline as a science and the degree of ferment within the discipline about philosophical issues. (I was pleased to see that many of these sentiments were reinforced in John Holland's chapter in this book.)

A largely overlooked attribute of scientific theory that Paul Meehl has described should be added. Theory should become more vulnerable as research progresses. Predictions made early in the development of a theory may be quite gross, but finer distinctions should gradually emerge. Psychological research that follows the pattern of simplistic hypothesis testing follows the opposite course. Ability to reject the hypothesis of a zero difference in means or a correlation of zero in the population becomes easier as research proceeds. A p-value of .05 provides a modest degree of confidence in only the *sign* of a difference or correlation. Reporting an effect size provides a small amount of additional information. In contrast, a developing science needs to predict the *size* of differences and correlations.

It is altogether proper that Minnesotans take a contemporary leadership role in research on individual differences. As one surveys the entire discipline of psychology, the dependable data and scientific theory from research on individual differences have more to offer in the solution of present-day social problems than any other subarea of psychology. Both the data and the theory behind individual differences are a critical, though typically rejected, component of the data based on socially defined groups that the social sciences frequently apply to the same problems (Humphreys, 1991). The magnitude of individual and group differences on measures of human attributes and the real-world performances that measures of these attributes are able to forecast are responsible for the underappreciation or outright rejection of the psychology of individual differences and its quantitative methods. This is unfortunate from a scientific point of view, because an objective appreciation of these methods and the data that they produce is sorely needed across all of the social sciences.

One drawback I see to the rational discussion of the conclusions from research on individual differences and their implications for important social issues is the continuing controversy over genetics and the rejection of generic contributions to individual differences in important human attributes (cf. Waller, Lykken, & Tellegen, this volume). The idea that there is a genetic *contribution* and *not* determination, to individual differences in measured intelligence has been criticized as implausible to impossible. I maintain that the only basis for such criticism is a conception of mind as an immaterial entity independent of the physical body. There is no basis for such conclusions in biology. And this is not the consensus among a number of psychology's mainstream empirical scientists on the topic of intelligence (Arvey, Bouchard, Carroll, Cattell, Cohen, Dawis et al., 1994).

This volume underscores the importance of assessing individual differences in human behavior across multiple psychological contexts: clinical, counseling, and experimental (including psycholinguistics), along with new methods for assessing both traits *and* types. Behavioral as well as social scientists who choose not to assess parameters of individual differences might consider the possibility that assessing traditional dimensions of individual differences could very well provide clarification to the behavioral domains that they are currently examining, and which are in need of intensive scientific study.

This book should contribute to a revival of interest in research on individual differences. A renewed interest in individual differences has surfaced, offering possible insight into addressing the pressing social problems facing us. Whatever our society ultimately adopts as solutions to problems such as crime, education, and poverty, the psychology of individual differences will factor prominently in the most effective ones.

Lloyd G. Humphreys
University of Illinois-Champaign

REFERENCES

Arvey, R. D., Bouchard,T. J., Jr., Carroll, J. B., Cattell, R. B., Cohen, D. B., Dawis, R. V., et al. Mainstream science on intelligence. (1994, December 13). *Wall Street Journal.*
Humphreys, L. G. (1991). Limited vision in the social sciences. *American Journal of Psychology, 104,* 333–353.
Tyler, L. E. (1965). *The psychology of individual differences* (3d ed.). Englewood Cliffs, NJ: Prentice-Hall.

Introduction

Psychology, in Cronbach's 1957 phrase, is two disciplines: experimental and correlational. The first, which exists in the service of psychological theory, attends to means and functions; the second, which provides the basis for most of psychology's applications, attends to variances and covariances, that is, to individual differences. Indeed, the second discipline of psychology is, or should be, better known as the psychology of individual differences.

It was the study of individual differences that provided the occasion for the discovery/invention of *co-relation*. Galton, of course, was the discoverer/inventor of this concept, but it was his supporter and admirer, Karl Pearson, who almost single-handedly developed the mathematics of correlation. Starting with his introduction of the standard deviation (defined with respect to the normal curve of error), Pearson developed, in fairly rapid succession, the product-moment method of calculating correlation, partial correlation, multiple correlation, tetrachoric correlation, biserial correlation, correlation ratio or nonlinear correlation, chi square (which has turned out to be invaluable to statisticians and psychometricians), and even the "method of principal axes" (which, published in 1901, anticipated Spearman, the acknowledged founder of factor analysis, by three years).

To Karl Pearson (E. S. Pearson, 1938), correlation was a

> category broader than causation,...of which causation was only the limit.... Galton...freed me from the prejudice that sound mathematics could only be applied to natural phenomena under the category of causation. Here...was a possibility...of reaching knowledge—as valid as physical knowledge...in the field of human conduct. (p. 19)

Correlation is a different mode of explanation. Where causation relies on functional relations, that is, one-to-one mappings, correlation encompasses one-to-many and many-to-one mappings (and, therefore, one-to-one mappings as well). Correlation, unlike causation, is symmetrical and thus can look backward ("postdiction") as well as forward (prediction). Unlike causation, it is not bound to the arrow of time. As Pearson pointed out, causation is only a special case of correlation. Yet students of psychology are routinely taught that causation is superior to correlation.

Also unappreciated by most people is the fact that much of scientific psychology's contribution to everyday life results from correlational psychology. Much of applied psychology is the application of the psychology of individual differences—witness educational psychology, industrial and organizational psychology, and counseling psychology. The single most socially significant psychological invention is the psychological test, an invention originally intended to aid the first psychologists in their observations (thus filling the same function as the telescope to astronomer-physicists and the microscope to biologists). The psychological test has since evolved into an instrument for mapping the domains of human skills, abilities, achievements, aptitudes, attitudes, preferences, interests, values, needs, and personality traits. As such, the psychological test has found great use in the assessment and evaluation of individuals and, hence, in the selection and placement of people in school and in the workplace.

Even applications that originated from experimental psychology (e.g., conditioning and human factors engineering) or from the other major contemporary fields of psychology, such as social psychology, developmental psychology, and clinical psychology, have dealt with individual differences. This is because human variability and human variation are ubiquitous and inevitable characteristics of human behavior. If variance is the phenomenon to be explained, then accounting for variance is the name of the psychologist's game. If individual differences are to be accounted for, then correlation is the way—perhaps the only way—to do it. Thus, the psychology of individual differences lies at the very foundation of the science of psychology. And yet not too many psychologists would be willing to acknowledge this.

At least one group of psychologists are invested in individual differences. Since Donald G. Paterson joined the University of Minnesota's Department of Psychology in 1921, Minnesota graduates have been steeped in the individual differences point of view and have been major contributors to the individual differences research literature. This book, written by Minnesota graduates, aspires to be one such contribution, occasioned as it is to honor one of Minnesota's own: Lloyd H. Lofquist, founder of the university's Counseling Psychology Program.

In a larger sense, this volume is intended to underscore the vital but relatively unnoticed role that the psychology of individual differences plays in our current understanding of human behavior. It is intended to showcase the wide range of issues—theoretical as well as practical, substantive as well as methodological—that are addressed by individual differences psychology. It is intended to rekindle interest in what is possibly the fundamental puzzle of human behavior—its variability or, put another way, its inconsistency.

This volume is organized into five parts. Part 1 is given over to one of the last pieces of writing by the late Leona Tyler, for years the elder stateswoman of counseling psychology and author of one of the most widely read texts on the psychology of individual differences. In this remarkably wide-ranging chapter, Tyler surveys the high points in the evolution of the psychology of individual differences, making numerous pithy observations, pointing out the relevance of individual differences to the cultural diversity controversies of our time, and arguing one more time for her favorite cause, that of individuality.

Part 2 focuses on method. In Chapter 2, Susan Embretson writes about *construct representation* in the measurement of individual differences. She bridges the gap between cognitive psychology and individual differences psychology, a current version of the experimental versus correlational disjunction. She demonstrates how cognitive theory (and findings) can be used to drive test design and, in particular, item writing. Embretson's unique contribution vividly illustrates how construct representation can be accomplished in methodical fashion, given theory. With her approach, test constructors need no longer rely solely on *nomothetic span* to demonstrate construct validity for their measures.

In Chapter 3, David Weiss writes about a paradigm revolution of sorts in psychometrics, which is essentially the measurement of individual differences. He shows in reasoned detail how the "new" paradigm—item response theory—in conjunction with adaptive testing, improves on the "old" paradigm of Spearman and Pearson—classical test theory—the paradigm on which the first generation of individual differences psychologists essentially "cut their teeth." Weiss provides a welcome integration of material widely scattered in the literature and shows how computerized psychological testing can realize Binet's dream of truly individualized psychological assessment. Weiss goes farther and sketches out new directions for individual differences research to pursue, taking off on the potentialities offered by item response theory.

Chapters 4 and 5 are about a basic question in individual differences research: the problem of distinguishing between variables that are quantitative or dimensional—those reflecting differences in degree—and variables that are qualitative or categorical—those reflecting differences in kind. The dimensional trait model has so dominated the discipline that few psychologists have paid attention to the possibility of identifying truly qualitative traits. Paul Meehl is one of the few who has done so. Since the 1960s, he has intensively studied the question of inferring the existence of a taxon from quantitative indicators when an acceptable criterion is unavailable. Meehl, with the help of his student, Robert Golden, has developed a number of search procedures called *maximum covariance methods,* so called because they take advantage of the statistical truism that variance and, therefore, covariance, are at a potential maximum when $p = q = .50$. These methods are premised on the assumption that the indicators are uncorrelated both within the taxon and within its complement, a situation not usually found in practice. In Chapter 4, Meehl proposes a method that gets around this limitation by making use of the extremes of the distribution where the proportion of taxon members or complement members presumably approaches 1.0.

In Chapter 5, Robert Golden and Mary Mayer revisit the question of inferring taxonicity from quantitative indicators. They show that if the indicators used are *peaked*—which occurs when the several indicators maximally discriminate at about the same level of the trait, as they often do when rating scales or psychometric scales are used—there is a high risk of identifying spurious taxons. With peaked indicators, even if all the tests for taxonicity required by current methods can be met, there is no guarantee that the trait is truly taxonic. What is more, pseudotaxons can have face validity, appear cohesive, and even make good intuitive sense. Only by using indicators with truly interval scale properties (e.g., time, weight, distance) can we avoid this problem.

Part 3 focuses on what might be considered traditional individual differences variables, the variables of original concern to the psychology of individual differences. In Chapter 6, Nancy Betz deals with the "first variable" of individual differences research: gender differences (or what was once called sex differences). Betz fills a gap by focusing on gender-related personality traits and, in particular, on so-called "masculinity" and "femininity." (The topic of gender differences in ability has been amply discussed in the literature.) She reviews the research and the controversies, showing how the terms masculinity and femininity have outlived their use (to many, they couldn't be called useful). She criticizes the proliferation of concepts and measures, the impoverishment of method, and the paucity of integration and theory and suggests a different tack for researchers to take.

David Campbell, in Chapter 7, reports on psychological test data compiled on a relatively underreported but societally vital occupational group: U.S. military leaders. He reviews a variety of data sets— ability, behavioral assessment, personality, and interest—on a large group of brigadier generals. These data paint a clearly delineated psychological portrait of what Campbell terms the "decisive warrior," whose (modal) personality pattern if it lacks the "softening patina of education and democracy," could be that of the "aggressive warmonger."

Chapter 8 by James Rounds is about one of the variables that individual differences psychology put on the map—vocational interests. Rounds uses a large collection of data (60 correlation matrices with large Ns) and complex data-analytic methodology (multidimensional scaling, among others) to examine and map the domain of vocational interests in meticulous detail. He reports confirmation of some old findings (Holland's order and calculus hypotheses, Prediger's two dimensions), disconfirmation of others (Holland's hexagon hypothesis, Roe's circular hypothesis), and new findings (gender differences at different levels of abstraction, failure of basic interest factors to map onto the Holland model). Rounds concludes by contending that circular (two-dimensional) structure-of-interest models do a poor job of mapping the domain of *basic* interest dimensions.

Niels Waller, David Lykken, and Auke Tellegen report in Chapter 9 on a large data set (occupational interests, leisure time interests, personality traits) on a large adult sample of same-sex twins (almost 800 pairs), including 67 pairs separated at infancy and reared apart. Their chapter includes original contributions in measurement and methodology (new methods for ipsative scaling and nonmetric multidimensional scaling), as well as new findings. They conclude that the three domains of occupational interests, leisure time interests, and personality traits, although related in meaningful ways, are essentially separate domains, psychometrically speaking. Along the way, they describe numerous interesting findings (e.g., the heritability and stability of interests, another fundamental interest dimension to add to Prediger's two, and the polarity of occupational and leisure time preferences).

Part 4 is about new areas in individual differences research, topics unexamined by the first generation of individual differences psychologists. One of these is interpersonal behavior. In Chapter 10, Stanley Strong presents an interpersonal influence theory based on his premise that "much of human behavior is intended to influence others to behave hospitably to one's needs." Strong constructs a classification of interpersonal behaviors based on the following: the two axes of emotional resources ("that I offer and need and that you offer and need") and material resources ("that I have or need and that you have or need"); the four poles of ingratiation versus intimidation, for the emotional resources axis, and self-promotion versus supplication, for the material resources axis; and, consequently, the eight major interpersonal behavior classes of nurturant, cooperative, docile, self-effacing, distrustful, critical, self-enhancing, and leading. Strong reviews research on the determinants of interpersonal behavior, focusing on three major sets: the other's interpersonal behavior, relationship dependence, and, of course, individual differences—gender, the traits of dominance and affiliation, and dissatisfaction with relationships.

Another new area for individual differences is language behavior. In Chapter 11, James Jenkins, Winifred Strange, and Linda Polka review the intriguing literature, which includes their own extensive studies, on speech perception of a foreign language. When we learn our native language, we also apparently foreclose our ability not only to say but also to hear certain sounds in a foreign language. Jenkins, Strange, and Polka dissect the seemingly simple but very complicated phenomenon that native Japanese speakers experience in discriminating between the American English /r/ and /l/ sounds. Their chapter points to our relative lack of knowledge about the speech perception problems of second-language learners (as opposed to their speech production problems, of which we know much more) and our need to learn more about the role of perceptual abilities in producing individual differences in speech perception.

We conclude with three commentaries in Part 5. In Chapter 12, David Premack advances the very interesting proposition that the vast range of individual differences in the human species would surely tend toward the fragmentation of the species were it not for centripetal factors that serve to control human individual differences. Premack identifies and discusses three of these factors: the art of pedagogy, the human disposition to share experience, and the relative lack of creativity in human beings. Pedagogy—a distinctively human invention that goes beyond learning and imitation—is a powerful producer of conformity. But pedagogy as well as language would not be possible without the human disposition to share experience. And, finally, the species does not fragment more because humans are not as creative as they think they are; in fact, their inventiveness is rather limited. Thus, despite individual differences, the human family remains together.

In Chapter 13, Howard Tinsley discusses what is good—and bad—about Minnesota training, illustrating his commentary with observations about the work of University of Minnesota graduates (Betz, Campbell, Rounds, and Waller et al.) and some of his own experiences as a Minnesota-trained counseling psychologist. To Tinsley, the four cornerstones of his Minnesota education were (a) an individual differences and developmental philosophy, (b) methodological rigor, (c) integration of arbitrarily bounded areas of psychological knowledge and theory, and (d) application of this knowledge to the amelioration of the problems of society. One danger of the Minnesota way is its fixation on method, because method can become rewarding unto itself—to the blurring of focus on the substantive issues. But the risk is worth the potential outcome: a scientist-practitioner (or, as Meehl would prefer, a "scientific practitioner") who is deeply interested in the discipline but is mindful of a responsibility to apply the science for the good of humanity.

The last chapter and final commentary is John Holland's address at the 40th anniversary celebration of counseling psychology at the University of Minnesota in April 1993. In quintessential Holland fashion, he fearlessly roils the waters of complacency and current fad. Holland questions the new philosophies of science and the new research agendas of fractious, fractionating groups; he attacks the excessive dependence of research on grant funding and the interlocking directorships of the peer review process; he defends the denigrated but necessary role of vocational counseling and suggests that the old Minnesota tradition of "dust-bowl empiricism" may not be so bad after all—a proposition with which the two Minnesota-trained editors can hardly disagree.

REFERENCES

Pearson, E. S. (1938). *Karl Pearson: An appreciation of some aspects of his life and work*. Cambridge, UK: Cambridge University Press.

Part One

Historical Antecedents, Current Status, and New Directions

Individual differences are a primary fact of psychology. People differ, and the range of differences among people is large—on just about any human attribute that can be measured or observed reliably. Individual differences were the bane of the early experimentalists of psychology, and they still are to some contemporary experimentalists. In the experimental paradigm, individual differences contribute to *error variance*, which often swamps the "main effects." Not until James McKeen Cattell doggedly pursued the idea was it accepted that individual differences could be systematic and significant and used as a foundational stone for psychological measurement. The evolution of the psychological test—with its means and standard deviations, its norms and standard scores, its correlations and factors—has more than justified Cattell's then-heretical idea. Today, the psychological test stands as the most important invention that psychological science has bequeathed to society.

But individual differences are more than a single fact or a set of facts. They represent the basis for a philosophy, or at least a point of view. The concept of freedom is founded on the fact of individual differences. If we were all alike in every respect, we would not feel the need to be free to "do our own thing." We would all be doing the same thing. The concept of tolerance—of "live and let live"—is necessary because of individual differences, because we can be so different in some respects, even if we are alike in others. The concept of individuality is most parsimoniously described with the language of individual differences. The fact that each of us is not exactly like any other person is most economically captured in a vector of individual differences scores. The concept of diversity cannot be made more concrete than in the phrase—and in the facts inherent in—individual differences.

Leona Tyler was, in her day, a leading spokesperson for individual differences, having written a definitive textbook on the subject. In what was probably her last piece of writing, Tyler traces the evolution of the field and elaborates on the ideas just discussed in Chapter 1 of this volume. She develops her favorite themes of individuality, choice, and possibility. She also makes the case for diversity. She is critical of the status quo in the psychology of individual differences and, wise counselor that she was, sketches directions that the field can progress toward.

Chapter 1

The Challenge of Diversity

Leona E. Tyler
University of Oregon

Scientists who study any aspect or fraction of the living world must come to terms with its most basic characteristic—diversity. There are, in the first place, the millions upon millions of species of plants and animals. But even more impressive is the fact that within each species—at least among those that reproduce sexually—each individual is unique. We plant what appear to be identical seeds, but the individual plants that grow from them differ from one another in size, shape, number of blossoms, and various other characteristics. Puppies in the same litter are not identical even at birth, and they grow up into dogs with distinct individualities.

As we have come to understand genetic processes, a major source of individuality has become apparent. In sexual reproduction, the chance pairing of chromosomes from the two parents results in a far larger number of genotypes than of individuals in the parent generation. Since Darwin, this realization has provided one of the essential foundations of evolutionary biology. Mayr (1976) discusses this aspect of evolutionary theory at some length.

The world we live in presents an inexhaustible variety of habitats for living creatures—arctic tundra, tropical rain forest, ocean depths, grasslands, desert, mountains. Because of diversity, some individuals are able to survive in an environmental niche in which others perish. Thus, new species arise. This is the principle of natural selection, Darwin's most significant contribution to the scientific thinking of our time.

Of course, natural selection based on genetic processes is not the only source of diversity in living creatures. Gene pools undergo spontaneous mutations. Habitats change over the years, and the inhabitants adapt variously to these changes. The sources of human

1

diversity are even more complex than those underlying diversity in life in general. As life proceeds, no two individuals undergo precisely the same sequence of experiences. This is true even for monozygotic twins, who begin life with identical gene assortments. Before these twins leave the womb, differences can develop, and, as life proceeds, they increasingly become separate individuals. We have come to realize that the old arguments about whether heredity or environment—nature or nurture—is the cause of human individuality are irrelevant. A human individual represents an interaction of unique genetic endowment with a unique course of development. It is a complex, nonadditive process.

MEASURING INDIVIDUAL DIFFERENCES

Down through the centuries, individual differences between human beings have been recognized and described. Novelists and poets, portrait painters and sculptors have portrayed human individuality in all its glory and its poignancy. Philosophers, physicians, and prescientific psychologists proposed typologies for the classification of persons, often based on anatomical or biochemical differences. After the opening of psychological laboratories during the latter part of the nineteenth century, scientific psychologists tended to reject such rough classifications and to concentrate on *measurement,* which they considered to be an essential aspect of science. While most of the early psychologists were seeking to discover general laws that would apply to all human beings, a few became interested in the differences between individual subjects in the experiments, rather than the conclusions being drawn about human nature in general. Thus, the mental testing movement was born.

The movement grew and flourished. The measurement of laboratory variables, such as reaction time, discrimination of weights and sizes, and numbers of nonsense syllables memorized in a given length of time, soon gave way to an all-out attempt to measure intelligence. Aptitudes and special talents, school achievement, and personality traits became foci of research that eventually led to published tests.

What is often not recognized by persons discussing mental testing—whether they are devising new instruments, interpreting individual scores, or criticizing the whole undertaking—is that psychological measurement differs from physical measurement in an important way: Scores do not represent *amounts* of anything. What they show is how the person tested compares with other people with regard to the trait under consideration. A child's IQ of 50 does not represent 50 units of anything. It does not tell us that this child is twice as intelligent as another child whose IQ is 25, nor does it indicate that the child is half as intelligent as a child whose IQ is 100. It indicates only that in the population providing the norms for the test, this person is considerably below average.

In order to be useful as psychological measures, raw scores in seconds or inches or number of questions answered correctly have to be transformed in some way that will give them meaning. This is usually accomplished by arranging to administer the test to a representative group of persons from the population with which the test taker might legitimately be compared. This produces a *distribution* of scores. The score each individual makes receives its meaning from the place it occupies in this distribution. As the years have passed, more and more sophisticated systems of "derived scores" have been invented. But basically, understanding what a single score means—one's own or someone else's—involves comparing the person tested with other people.

APPLIED INDIVIDUAL DIFFERENCES

At the beginning of the psychological testing era, psychologists anticipated that tests would serve two purposes in a complex society like ours. On the one hand, they would be useful tools for persons charged with the responsibility of *selecting* the best qualified persons for particular positions. They would make it easier to decide which applicant would get the job, which students would qualify for admission to select colleges, and which children would be chosen to participate in special school programs. On the other hand, they expected tests to be useful in helping *individuals* decide what to do with their lives and find the positions or roles in society that their unique combinations of abilities and personality characteristics would fit most closely, thus maximizing their productiveness and personal satisfaction. These two purposes can be labeled the *selection purpose* and the *counseling purpose*. As the years have passed, the former of these purposes has been achieved to a much greater extent than the latter. Tests have contributed much more to the task of finding a person to fit a slot than to the task of finding a slot to fit a person. The trait measurement approach is workable in selection because one needs to consider only a limited number of traits—those relevant to the position being selected for. These can be measured separately and combined through the use of appropriate statistical techniques. The situation is quite different in the case of a person asking the questions, What shall I do with my life? and Where do I belong? Everything about the person is relevant, but, obviously, everything cannot be tested.

The technique ordinarily utilized for portraying the uniqueness of a person who has been tested for a number of traits is the *profile* or *psychograph,* which has been widely used in vocational counseling.

An important study conducted under the auspices of the Employment Stabilization Research Institute at the University of Minnesota (Dvorak, 1935) showed that the average profiles of workers in different occupations differed markedly. In the early years of aptitude testing, the problem in the utilization of profiles was that different tests had been standardized on different norm groups, so that scores could not be considered strictly comparable. Factor analysis solved this problem. By administering a varied set of test materials to a large and appropriately selected group of subjects and analyzing the correlations between different subtests, it was possible to delineate special abilities for which individual scores would be strictly comparable. The *General Aptitude Test Battery* (GATB), developed over the years by the United States Employment Service, is an outstanding example of a test that has proved useful in both selection and counseling.

In considering how psychologists have dealt and might deal with individuality, it is convenient to distinguish between ability and personality tests. Ability tests are made up of items and questions that reveal what an individual knows or can do. The test results can be considered to represent a *sample* of what the person can do in the world outside the testing room. Personality tests, however—at least the most commonly used ones—consist of items that ask people to report on their behavior and feelings about various subjects and in various situations. There is no guarantee that the answers constitute a sample of what a person actually does or actually feels. Personality tests are more properly labeled questionnaires. But the scores, like those on ability tests, are derived from norm groups. They tell us whether the person's self-description registers more self-esteem or sociability than those of other people with whom one can legitimately be compared. Personality theorists and assessment specialists have, of course, been aware of this characteristic of so-called personality measurement and the possible biases to which it is subject and have worked out ingenious ways of controlling and compensating for response sets, such as social desirability or acquiescence. However, interpretation of scores on even the best of the personality measures contains a modicum of uncertainty that is not present in interpretations of ability test scores.

But differences in personality characteristics are fully as important in theoretical or practical problems involving individual differences as differences in abilities are. Over the years, since the idea of measuring human mental characteristics first took root in our culture early in the twentieth century, tests have proliferated to the point that measuring instruments have been published for hundreds of special abilities and personality traits. Especially in the realm of personality, there is no limit to the number of traits someone considers worthy of measurement. This state of affairs makes the possibility of portraying individuality by means of a profile or psychograph appear less and less promising. The profile method has been used to put together an individual's scores on a limited assortment of personality traits selected for a particular test, such as the *Minnesota Multiphasic Personality Inventory* (MMPI), and interpretations of profiles have even been programmed into computers. But no one claims that an MMPI profile or any other test profile depicts an individual in all of his or her complexity. There are too many other traits that could have been measured that were not, and to measure them all in any individual is an obviously impossible task. Psychologists attempting to conceptualize human diversity are facing the realization that the technology of trait measurement is not adequate for the undertaking.

Thus, as the years have passed, some psychologists have become increasingly doubtful about the adequacy of the quantitative-normative technology as the sole foundation for a science of human individuality. For one thing, considerable public criticism has been expressed in recent decades (Haney, 1981). Low-scoring individuals and groups object to the stigma they see these scores imposing on them and insist that the intelligence tests are biased against them. Even some who receive scores in the middle range of the distribution suffer loss of self-esteem, especially when such scores conflict with high family expectations. They find it easier to blame the tests than to accept the fact that there are individual differences in intellectual ability.

Especially since the beginning of the civil rights movement, arguments have raged over the possibility of test bias and the difficulty of reconciling employment testing with the goals of affirmative action. The outcomes of several major court cases as well as legislation have influenced both public policy and public opinion with regard to intelligence and other ability tests. Considerable evidence has accumulated indicating that the tests constructed according to the most advanced psychometric principles are *not* biased and predict performance equally well in all population groups (Tyler, 1980). But such evidence does little to diminish the hostility toward the whole testing enterprise in large sectors of the population.

Public hostility toward personality testing has another basis. Here, too, because of standardization requirements, value connotations accompany scores—higher-lower, better-worse, sound-unsound, and so forth—but because items often describe symptoms or difficulties, high scores tend to be bad, while low scores tend to be good. Especially since the practice of computer storing information has become universal, individuals worry over the possibility that personality test results casting doubt on their mental health may be used against them at some later time. The right to privacy has received increasing attention during recent years.

Psychologists engaged in research on individual differences and the application of its findings to human concerns have been able to counter these criticisms, and ability and personality testing continue to flourish. But some thinkers are troubled by a fundamental question: Should the psychology of individual differences be *solely* a psychology of trait measurement? Is analyzing traits the best or the only means for analyzing individuals?

There are, of course, different ways of thinking about traits. To statistically sophisticated professionals, traits are dimensions of individuality and measurements are distances along these dimensions. The layperson is more likely to regard a trait as either a possession or a capacity. Inherent in all these conceptions is an assumption that all human beings have the same assortment of traits and that they differ only in relative amounts of each that they possess.

In order for the accepted systems of derived scores to work properly and have the same meaning from place to place and from year to year, a test must be designed in such a way that the raw scores (the sum of the scores for answers to questions asked) will fall into a normal distribution, the familiar bell-shaped curve. This means that about half the derived scores (IQ, *t*-scores, etc.) will always be below average and that there will always be some very low scores as well as some very high ones. Taking standardized tests almost forces individuals to judge their own worth by comparing themselves with others—and self-esteem often suffers as a result. Again and again, critics of education report with shocked alarm that 50% of our sixth graders score below the sixth-grade reading norms!

The very success of the quantitative approach to understanding intelligence differences, the first area to be explored, may have misled us as we attempted to apply the same methods to a wider range of abilities and personality characteristics. It makes sense to assume that all human beings have some intelligence and that they differ mainly in how much they have to call upon. But is this a valid assumption for musical talent or scientific interests or schizophrenia?

As the years have passed, some concepts and movements have appeared that at least partially transcend the predominant normative approach to ability testing. This has happened especially in applied fields where the second purpose described above predominates, that of enabling individuals to find a place in society where they can lead productive and satisfying lives. In industry, assessment centers have been set up to make comprehensive studies of high-level individuals who may qualify for management positions (Bray & Moses, 1972). In rehabilitation services, especially those designed to place individuals with mental disabilities into niches that suit them, the shift of emphasis from normative measurement has also occurred. In education, dissatisfaction with ability and achievement tests has grown as evidence accumulates that they do not provide any guarantee that each individual leaves the school system equipped to find a place that fits him or her in our complex society. A demand has been created for a different kind of mental test. Counselors and others engaged in the effort to understand and assist individuals need tests of *competencies* rather than *abilities*. A competency is a developed skill, something an individual knows how to do. The important questions to ask are "Which competencies does the person have in his or her repertoire?" and "How can the person develop those one lacks but would like to possess?" (Tyler, 1978, chap. 6).

Although the branch of psychology we label individual differences still rests principally on an assumption that individuality consists of the relative amounts of various traits each person possesses, measurement theory and practice have been undergoing important changes during recent decades, many of them discussed in some detail in this book. Some thinkers have sought to find ways of making raw scores meaningful without the use of norm tables. *Criterion-referenced* tests have been proposed as an alternative to *norm-referenced* tests for some purposes. They have been especially useful in education because they are designed to show how far an individual has progressed along a series of graded steps in a particular learning process. Such designs have been facilitated by the shift in test theory and technology to a position emphasizing analysis of the characteristics of individual items rather than total scores. If items related to a given trait are put together in a graded, ladderlike sequence, the level at which an individual shifts from success to failure indicates where one stands with regard to the trait without the necessity of comparing the individual with others represented in the norm tables. This approach facilitates the *adaptive* individualized testing procedures that have come into use since the advent of computers.

INDIVIDUAL DIFFERENCES
IN PERSONALITY

New thinking about how individuals differ has been even more apparent in personality than in ability assessment. It has brought into question the adequacy of the trait concept itself. For years it has seemed to me that the basic aspects of individuality are *choice* and *organization*

(Tyler, 1959). Several largely unconnected developments have contributed to our understanding of these characteristics. The one with the longest history is the assessment of choices that delineate the *direction* in which an individual life is proceeding, the measurement of *interests*. The long series of research studies by E. K. Strong, Jr., and, since his death, by the Center for Interest Measurement Research, has shown that scores on the *Strong Interest Inventory (Strong)* have a different meaning from scores on most ability and personality tests. In 1927, Strong brought out the first version of an instrument constructed in a new way. It was an inventory of work-related items toward which respondents indicated their likes, dislikes, and preferences. Scoring keys for separate occupations were based on a comparison of the tabulations of responses for groups of successful men in the occupations with those of a group of "men in general." The score on one of these occupational scales did not represent the *amount* of interest the respondent showed in anything. What it did provide was a clear answer to the questions: Am I or am I not similar to people engaged in this occupation? Would I fit in? In what direction have my experiences and choices so far pointed me?

One important feature of the Strong assessment technique, not always recognized by those who use it, is that scores are based on one's rejections as well as one's positive choices. In fact, for some of the scoring keys, "Dislike" responses far outnumber "Like" responses. They indicate what one has ruled out in one's development of a unique individuality. Strong, in an informal discussion of what it is that interest tests measure, once explained that an individual's results showed the *direction* in which she or he was headed. Unfortunately, this interpretation of the meaning of interest measurement has never become widespread. New interest measures often consist of only items that respondents say they like or are interested in and do not reflect what they have ruled out of their lives. The interest score is thought to show *how much* of a hypothetical trait, such as artistic interest, the respondent possesses, rather than *which* of the possible directions life might take has been chosen.

Research on values also involves choices and directions. Smith's (1963, p. 332) definition of values was "conceptions of the possible that are relevant to selective behavior." A particular value orientation, such as "social" or "religious," can, of course, be regarded as a personality trait and be measured by an inventory in which the sum of one's responses to a number of items thought to be related to the value produces a score purporting to show *how much* of that value one possesses in comparison with others in the norm group. But other approaches have been tried—approaches revealing more about *which* possibilities one has incorporated in one's life and the direction one's life is now taking.

A large and comprehensive project was undertaken by Rokeach (1973). He distinguished between *terminal values*—representing end states of existence, such as peace, freedom, and security—and *instrumental values*—representing modes of conduct through which end states are attained, such as helpful, obedient, and responsible. He asked a large number of respondents representative of the U.S. population to rank 18 terminal values and 18 instrumental values in order of importance to them personally. There were very marked individual differences, and they were related to the political behavior, ideologies, and attitudes individuals manifested in their daily lives. In addition to the substantive knowledge it provides, this study demonstrates that the *ranking* of important concepts can be a methodological alternative to the usual trait measurement techniques in exploring individual differences.

MORE ENCOMPASSING FRAMEWORKS

To understand an individual, we need to know not only which of the many developmental possibilities have been chosen, but also how they have been *organized* into a coherent *structure*. A person's likes and dislikes, attitudes and opinions, and values and principles are not separate and independent of one another. The organizational process accompanies the selection process. By the time adulthood is reached, most of the choices made from the manifold possibilities that confront a person are controlled by these structures built of former choices.

The attempt to find some means of dealing with human diversity that would be more economical and workable than the measurement of an ever-increasing number of separate traits has involved a continuing interest in typologies. During the 1940s, a system developed by Sheldon was very popular. The major distinction was between three types of physique and their related temperaments. More recently, a system based on Carl Jung's psychological types is being widely used. The *Myers-Briggs Type Indicator*® (MBTI®) personality inventory is the instrument used in making this distinction.

But the problem of assessing the structure of individual personalities is not solved by defining types. Over the years, some psychologists have hoped to find other substitutes for the predominant trait measurement techniques. The most important of these was George Kelly (1955). For Kelly, the basic entity was not the trait, but the *construct*, by which he meant a transparent template that a person creates and then attempts to fit over the realities of which the world is composed. He invented a way to identify an individual's constructs without reference to the scores of other individuals and to describe the pattern of the individual's personality in terms of the construct system. Kelly's ideas have generated a considerable amount of research in psychiatry, education, psychology, and various other fields (Tyler, 1978, chap. 8).

The 1980s brought a revival and revitalization of a movement initiated by Henry Murray 50 years before (Murray, 1938). The objective of *personology* is intensive study of individuals by methods not limited to standardized tests—case studies, biographies and autobiographies, personal documents such as diaries and letters, and interviews. For the personologists, the basic unit is the person, not the trait, and in the course of their work, some promising new approaches to research have been developed as alternatives to trait measurement. It is not inconceivable that the nature of the psychological specialty of individual differences may be transformed by such research. New theoretical formulations have proposed concepts that may facilitate the study of the unique patterns or structures that constitute individuality.

One of Murray's basic concepts was that of *thema*. He considered it to be the pattern of thinking and behavior that an individual generates in dealing with internal *needs* and external *press*. *Script theory*, as developed by Tomkins (1979), is a current and influential attempt to describe personality structures in units more meaningful than trait measurements. The individual is thought of as a playwright constructing a personal drama as she or he passes through the successive stages of life. The raw material for scripts are *scenes*, affect-laden "happenings" as interpreted by the person. Scenes vary in their complexity—in how many characters, places, and actions they involve—but each must include at least one affect (excitement, fear, enjoyment, anger, etc.) and at least one object of that emotion. As life goes on, the person puts together sets of scenes that resemble one another in some way and develops rules, strategies, and the like for dealing with them. These are scripts. There are some scenes that are universal because of the biologically determined affects with which all human beings are endowed and the common experiences of infancy. But scripts are highly individual constructions because each person puts together a unique combination of scenes. They are entities *constructed* by the individual, not passively accepted. Tomkins has continued to develop script theory, making a major distinction between *humanistic* and *normative* scripts and identifying other script structures, such as *commitment* scripts, *nuclear* scripts, and *ideological* scripts. Eventually, it may be possible to sketch a rough outline of an individual personality by specifying which combination of these scripts is being followed, thus providing an assessment technique not dependent on the normative measurement of separate traits, but identifying structures directly.

Research by personologists like Tomkins is *idiographic* rather than *nomothetic*, to use terms popularized by Gordon Allport (1937) and widely discussed in later years. Nomothetic research seeks to discover principles and processes characteristic of humanity as a whole; idiographic research explores unique individual systems. The rise and growth of clinical psychology has made intensive study of individual lives legitimate; the controversy has centered on the question of whether such efforts are truly scientific.

A recent attempt to deal with this problem in research on individual differences was made by Lamiell (1987). He has been attempting to develop what he calls an *idiothetic* theory of personality, person-centered rather than variable-centered, utilizing measurement techniques but cutting them loose from their normative concomitants. Instead of comparing an individual's experiences, feelings, goals, and actions with those of other individuals, idiothetic techniques compare them with what, for the particular person in question, they are not but might have been. Although research under the idiothetic banner is still in an early stage, there have been attempts in this direction over the years by psychologists interested in individuality rather than normative measurement. Perhaps the Rokeach investigations of values could be considered examples of such efforts, in that each subject's ranking of the values is a measurement not based on norms.

A SUGGESTED APPROACH

In the approach to a scientific study of human diversity that I have been struggling to follow for a number of years (Tyler, 1978, 1992), the key word is *possibilities*. Knowing what we now know about the complex interaction between genetic determiners, nutritional and chemical influences before and after birth, socioeconomic factors, childrearing methods, and educational opportunities and techniques in the development of human individuals, we can see that human nature as a whole has a far wider scope than the personality of any one individual. The possibilities for development inherent in human nature are infinitely numerous. But an individual is faced with absolute limits as to how many of these possibilities can be actualized in his or her life. Each person has only 24 hours in each day and lives only a limited number of years. In every human life, some possibilities are selected to be actualized, while others are ruled out. Some of the selection is accomplished for the person by family and culture. For example, out of the several thousand languages one might learn, a human infant learns one, and possibly a few others. The process of selecting and ruling out possibilities also involves choices the individual makes as development proceeds. For example, currently, much is being said about the choice a young person makes about whether or not to experiment with drugs, partly because of a realization that this choice will strongly affect future individuality.

Human diversity constitutes a greater challenge in the complex societies of our time than it did in the simpler societies of the past. Our society could not function without the unique contributions of unique individuals. Its members cannot be considered to be identical, interchangeable parts. They do not just compete with one another; they complement one another.

Psychology, especially the psychology of individual differences, has a major part to play in helping societies meet this challenge. The technology of mental testing has become an essential component of programs for the utilization of human resources. But it has been more successful in assessing abilities than in assessing personality, and it has been more useful to the "gatekeepers"—those whose responsibility it is to select individuals for particular places—than to the individuals themselves, as they seek to find places to fill. I have become convinced that we need to realize the limitations of the prevailing trait measurement approach and develop other techniques for exploring human individuality. Some steps in this direction have been discussed in this chapter. As we make progress in these and in other as yet unseen directions, the psychology of individual differences may well become the basic science in humankind's attempt to meet the challenge of diversity.

REFERENCES

Allport, G. W. (1937). *Personality: A psychological interpretation*. New York: Holt, Rinehart and Winston.

Bray, D. W., & Moses, J. L. (1972). Personnel selection. *Annual Review of Psychology, 23,* 109–118.

Dvorak, B. J. (1935). *Differential occupational ability patterns*. Minneapolis: University of Minnesota Press.

Haney, W. (1981). Validity, vaudeville, and values: A short history of social concerns over standardized testing. *American Psychologist, 36,* 1021–1034.

Jung, C. G. (1923). *Psychological types*. London: Routledge & Kegan Paul.

Kelly, G. S. (1955). *The psychology of personal constructs*. New York: Norton.

Lamiell, J. T. (1987). *The psychology of personality: An epistomological inquiry*. New York: Columbia University Press.

Mayr, E. (1976). *Evolution and the diversity of life*. Cambridge, MA: Harvard University Press.

Murray, H. A. (1938). *Explorations in personality*. New York: Oxford University Press.

Rokeach, M. (1973). *The nature of human values*. New York: Free Press.

Smith, M. B. (1963). Personal values in the study of lives. In R. W. White (Ed.), *The study of lives*. New York: Atherton.

Tomkins, S. S. (1979). Script theory: Differential magnification of affects. In H. E. Howe, Jr., & R. A. Dienstbier (Eds.), *Nebraska Symposium on Motivation* (Vol. 21). Lincoln: University of Nebraska Press.

Tyler, L. E. (1959). Toward a workable psychology of individuality. *American Psychologist, 14*, 75–81.

Tyler, L. E. (1978). *Individuality*. San Francisco: Jossey-Bass.

Tyler, L. E. (1980). Tests are not to blame. *Behavioral and Brain Sciences, 3*, 354–355.

Tyler, L. E. (1992). Counseling psychology—Why? *Professional Psychology: Research and Practice, 23*, 342–344.

Part Two

New
Methodological
Concepts

Measurement is a hallmark of the psychology of individual differences. Edward Lee Thorndike, the pioneer individual differences psychologist, said, "Anything that exists, exists in some amount, and can be measured." The prolific growth of psychological testing has given ample substance to Thorndike's aphorism. The list of measured individual differences variables is long—abilities, skills, aptitudes, achievements, attitudes, opinions, preferences, interests, needs, values, satisfactions, temperaments, and personality traits. Along with this phenomenal growth came the development of psychometric theory, with its basic concepts of scale, reliability, and validity. The application of psychometric theory to test construction has progressed from dependable rules of thumb to sophisticated statistical models. But with these developments there came an unease in the larger society about the ways psychological testing had been used, culminating finally in an anti-testing movement. The status quo was challenged, the dialectic was joined, and measurement in individual differences had to move in new directions.

In Part 2 of this volume, we present three new directions in which the field has been moving—directions alluded to by Tyler in her opening piece. Susan Embretson, in Chapter 2, discusses the idea of constructing a test from theory, giving new meaning to "construct" validity. She shows how theory can be used to guide the generation of test items. Not only does this concept rationalize this aspect of test construction; it also binds psychological tests to psychological theory, bridging the chasm between the two disciplines of psychology—the experimental and the correlational.

In Chapter 3, David Weiss collects and compresses in one chapter much of what is known about *adaptive testing*, the idea of fitting the assessment to the individual. With adaptive testing, the individual is no longer compared with a norm group, with all the invidious implications such comparisons can trail in their wake. Yet adaptive testing is objective measurement, not unlike height or weight. It has been used effectively in the measurement of ability. The question now is, How many other human individual differences attributes can be successfully assessed through this method?

In Chapter 4, we touch on *taxometrics*, the new direction that Paul Meehl has pioneered. Tyler mentioned typology as an antidote for the excesses of trait measurement. Typologies have been invented and continue to be invented, but if the typologies do not "carve nature at its joints," they will collapse from their artificiality. It is to this problem of ascertaining "true types" that Meehl has devoted his not inconsiderable energies during the past two or three decades. In his chapter, Meehl discusses one of the difficult problems in taxometrics and proposes a solution. In Chapter 5, Robert Golden (Meehl's student) and Mary Mayer discuss another difficult problem—the issue of inferring taxonicity from quantitative indicators, with its ironic consequences, and show how the problem can be detected.

Chapter 2

Developments Toward a Cognitive Design System for Psychological Tests

Susan E. Embretson
University of Kansas

Lingering doubts about the theoretical status of cognitive tests contrast sharply with their practical success. Cognitive measurement, ranging from general intelligence tests to specific aptitude tests, is one of psychology's strongest contributions because predictive validity has supported applications in many diverse areas. Yet serious doubts about just what the tests measure have continued from the first conference on intelligence (1921) into contemporary research. Carroll and Maxwell (1979) noted in their *Annual Review of Psychology* chapter that the theoretical nature of cognitive tests was still controversial and, in fact, had progressed little since the first author had reviewed the field 25 years previously. Carroll and Maxwell were concerned not with the amount of research, but with the type of data that were available. That is, the supporting research typically consisted of correlations between test scores and other measures of individual differences, rather than studies that were more directly concerned with the theoretical mechanisms or entities that underlie successful test performance.

The type of supporting data also is related to methods for evaluating specific items. That is, including an item on a test is justified by the magnitude of its discrimination (typically a biserial correlation with total score) rather than by a description of how the item stimuli operationalize aspects of the theoretical constructs. Although using item discriminations to evaluate quality is consistent with the supporting data (i.e., the correlates of total score), the relevancy of item content to the construct is not addressed directly. Thus, questions about specific item content, such as sometimes arise in litigation on testing, must be addressed by referring to a chain of correlations; that is, the item correlates with total score, which, in turn, correlates with external criteria. Even if the chain contains high correlations, which often it does not, the data are not particularly compelling inasmuch as correlations can arise from many sources other than the hypothesized construct.

Carroll and Maxwell (1979) thought that cognitive psychology, merged with cognitive measurement, seemed promising as a new foundation for theories of aptitude and intelligence. Since their article appeared, many studies have sought to link cognitive theory to cognitive measurement. Two different contemporary approaches to studying aptitude are *cognitive correlate analysis* and *cognitive component analysis*. In cognitive correlate analysis (e.g., Hunt, Lunneborg, & Lewis, 1975), test scores are correlated with individual differences in basic cognitive processes, as operationalized by laboratory tasks. In cognitive component analysis (e.g., Sternberg, 1977), tasks that are similar to test items are decomposed to identify the processes that are involved in item solving. Recent books (e.g., Dillon, 1985; Embretson, 1985; Snow, Federico, & Montague, 1980; Sternberg, 1981, 1983, 1985) and numerous articles (e.g., Carroll, 1976; Egan, 1980; Hunt, 1978; Just & Carpenter, 1985; Pellegrino, 1985, 1988) have concerned this topic.

Although test developers are very interested in how cognitive psychology can contribute to building cognitive tests, actual test development procedures and test interpretation have not been influenced greatly. One explanation is that traditional test theory has neither the conceptual framework nor a procedural framework within which the potential of cognitive theory can be fully realized. Conceptually, although construct validity (Cronbach & Meehl, 1955) is the traditional framework for integrating theory and empirical results, it only partially incorporates the potential of the information processing paradigm of cognitive psychology. A reformulation of the construct validity concept should centralize the role of cognitive theory. Procedurally, although traditional test development is concerned with achieving optimal psychometric properties, particularly internal consistency, cognitive theory has no explicit role. The purpose of this chapter is to present some conceptual and procedural developments toward a cognitive design system that uses cognitive theory in the construction of cognitive tests.

CONSTRUCT VALIDITY
AND COGNITIVE PSYCHOLOGY

Construct validity (Cronbach & Meehl, 1955) was postulated as a conceptual framework to guide theoretical interpretations of test scores. Cronbach and Meehl emphasize elaborating the nomological network as the basis of establishing a test as a measure of a construct. A primary source of data for test meaning is the correlation of test scores with other measures, particularly other tests and criterion assessments. The nomological network can also include correlations of test scores with individual differences on more basic cognitive variables, such as processing on laboratory tasks derived from cognitive theory (e.g., Hunt et al., 1975) or processing components that are extracted from a simplified version of the measuring task (e.g., Sternberg, 1977). Furthermore, the information processing models that are developed from either approach also can be included in the nomological network to guide theoretical interpretation.

However, although cognitive psychology variables can be incorporated readily into the nomological network, this approach limits the potential of contemporary cognitive theory for cognitive measurement. When construct validity was first proposed, the functionalist paradigm was prevalent in psychology, along with a scientific philosophy of logical empiricism. Construct validity fit well with functionalism and logical empiricism because meaning was determined empirically from a network of relationships rather than rationally. That is, the "vague, avowedly incomplete network gives the constructs whatever meaning they do have" (Cronbach & Meehl, 1955, p. 289).

Even when first proposed, however, Bechtoldt (1959) criticized the construct validity concept as confounding the meaning of the test score (i.e., the theoretical construct that is measured) with the significance of the test score (i.e., the variables that the construct predicts). Using Bechtoldt's distinction, the original construct validity concept can be characterized as deriving meaning from significance.

Bechtoldt's critique had little impact, however, as his preferred measurement strategy, using operational definitions to provide meaning, offered no real alternative for interpreting test scores. Focusing on operational definition gives a primary role to the measuring task (i.e., scored items). However, the functionalist paradigm that guided psychological research during the 1950s did not provide theories that could categorize complex measuring tasks, such as intelligence or personality test items, or that could provide explanations of performance on these tasks. Thus, focusing on operational definition seemingly would remove theoretical meaning from test scores.

However, psychology has changed substantially since the construct validity paradigm was proposed. In a previous paper (Embretson, 1983), I proposed that the shift of psychology to a more rationalistic approach, such as that reflected by the information processing paradigm, provided an opportunity to reformulate the construct validity concept as well. That is, construct validity could be postulated to consist of two separate aspects: construct representation and nomothetic span. The distinction corresponds roughly to Bechtoldt's (1959) distinction between meaning and significance, respectively.

Construct representation is the meaning of the test score in terms of the processes, strategies, and knowledge structures that a person must apply to solve items. To assure relevancy to test performance, construct representation ultimately must be established on items that belong to the psychometric domain. As noted by Pellegrino and Lyons (1979), cognitive component studies that are limited to the simplified versions of items that are easy to study experimentally may not identify essential aspects of processing for aptitude. Nomothetic span, on the other hand, concerns the significance or usefulness of the test score for measuring individual differences. That is, nomothetic span concerns the relationships of test scores, say, ability scores, to other measures of individual differences, the traditional data given in support of test validity. However, although crucial for a test, nomothetic span is secondary to construct representation. That is, the significance of a test score derives from its meaning.

Distinguishing construct representation from nomothetic span centralizes cognitive theory in several ways. Test meaning is anchored to cognitive theory because construct representation depends on the mental processing operations that are employed to solve items. Furthermore, if the theory is empirically supported, tests can be designed for a specific meaning. That is, item stimuli can be manipulated to influence the processing operations that an examinee uses to solve items. Also, many experimental studies result in estimates of the impact of item content on performance, which is directly useful in designing items for a specified difficulty level. In contrast, traditional test development relies on heuristics for item content inasmuch as significance follows meaning. And if significance depends on meaning, tests can be designed for nomothetic span as well. Thus, test design can manipulate both construct representation and nomothetic span.

An Example of Cognitive Psychology

The Spatial Relations Test of the *Differential Aptitude Tests* (DAT), which is well established psychometrically, provides a good example of what cognitive psychology can add to understanding what the test measures and evaluating specific items. Spatial folding items that are

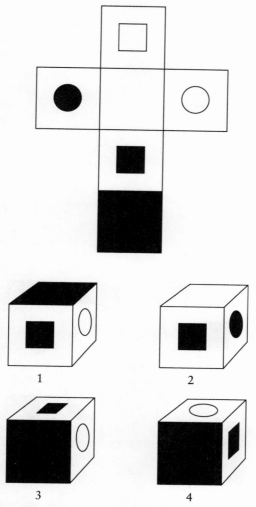

Figure 1 A spatial folding item with difficult distractors

similar to DAT items are presented in Figures 1 and 2. The Spatial Relations Test is typically interpreted as a measure of spatial aptitude, which involves the mental manipulation of objects. Supporting data include correlations with criteria that presumably involve mental manipulation (e.g., grades in shop or drawing courses) with other spatial tests and with tests of different traits, such as verbal reasoning. Although the Spatial Relations Test correlates somewhat too highly with verbal tests, the correlations primarily support labeling the test as involving the mental manipulation of objects.

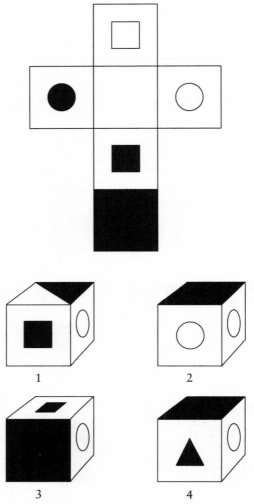

Figure 2   A spatial folding item with simple distractors

In contrast, a cognitive theory of the task would provide much greater detail about the strategies, processes, and knowledge structures that are involved in mental manipulation of objects. For example, in one theory of the spatial folding task (Embretson & Waxman, 1989), four independent stages in item solving—encoding, anchoring, folding, and confirming—are postulated. Empirical support for the theory has been obtained by independently manipulating the difficulty of the stages by different aspects of the item stimuli. This type of empirical support not only contributes to understanding the basis of item solving, but also enables specific items to be evaluated by how their stimulus properties influence the different stages.

Consider the items that are presented in Figures 1 and 2. The two items have the same stem and key (the third alternative) but seemingly different distractor sets. However, the traditional psychometric index, item discrimination, may not necessarily distinguish between these items. Even if the mental efforts involved in solving the items are quite different, both items, in fact, could correlate highly with total score if both kinds of items are well represented in the test.

However, cognitive theory provides a clear differentiation between the items in terms of their stimulus properties. Falsifying the distractors presented in Figure 1 involves folding the stem, whereas falsifying the distractors in Figure 2 clearly does not. That is, all distractors in Figure 2 can be falsified during encoding, an early stage in which the mismatching side markers are processed (i.e., the stem has no half-shaded side, only one white circle and no shaded triangle, as shown in alternatives 1, 2, and 4, respectively).

Differentiation between items by the impact of the item stimuli on processing requirements is central to cognitive psychology's potential for test design. In the spatial aptitude example, the encoding stage could be eliminated as a source of item solution by prohibiting distractors like those in Figure 2. As will be shown, more exacting specifications for items could concern the specific difficulty of the various stages and their interrelatedness in the item set. These specifications directly influence construct representation, but also will influence nomothetic span.

NATURE OF COGNITIVE DESIGN SYSTEMS

A cognitive design system can be used to influence construct validity by manipulating the cognitive complexity of items, which includes the components, strategies, and knowledge structures that are required for item solving. Manipulating the cognitive complexity of the items influences construct representation most directly. Nomothetic span is influenced indirectly, inasmuch as the correlations of test scores will depend on the external correlates of the mental operations that are entailed in item solution.

Influencing construct representation requires that performance in the psychometric item domain is well described by a cognitive model of the task. The model that is selected should not only meet ordinary criteria for theoretical adequacy but also reflect the intended measurement constructs. Items that do not fit the cognitive model should not be included in the test, as they reflect unintended cognitive constructs.

Several aspects of the test influence cognitive complexity. Most obviously, the specific stimuli in the item stem and the response alternatives influence the cognitive requirements for solution. However, cognitive complexity may also be manipulated by the conditions of

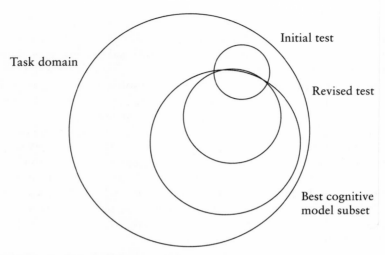

Figure 3   Goal for revising an existing test

item presentation. For example, the type and the amount of instruction preceding the items, or the amount of prior practice, also may impact substantially on cognitive complexity.

Figure 3 represents a schematic diagram that shows the relationship between the target test for the cognitive design system and a typical psychometric test in the same task domain. Existing tests have not been constructed by explicitly manipulating the stimuli that influence cognitive complexity. Thus, an existing test will not necessarily fit the cognitive model very well, as the items may contain stimuli that involve irrelevant or unintended sources of cognitive complexity. Thus, the existing test is shown in Figure 3 as only partially overlapping the set defined by the target cognitive model. The revised test, in contrast, is shown as completely contained by the target cognitive model. Thus, the goal of revising the existing test is to select and develop items in such a way that irrelevant and unintended sources of cognitive complexity no longer influence performance. A similar schematic can be specified for the development of new tests.

In summary, a cognitive design system is a framework for developing a test in which item performance is well described by a specific cognitive model. The cognitive model must be not only empirically plausible for actual test items, but it also must represent the intended theoretical constructs. Thus, the goal is a test in which performance is predictable from a cognitive model with sources of cognitive complexity that reflect the goals of measurement.

The cognitive design system consists of a series of steps, along with appropriate methods, to interface cognitive theory with ability measurement. The design system is general; it has been applied, at least partially, to influence construct validity on several popular item types, including verbal analogies (Embretson, 1985; Embretson & Schneider, 1989; Embretson, Schneider, & Roth, 1985), figural analogies (Whitely & Schneider, 1981), spatial folding (Embretson, 1987), verbal classification (Whitely, 1981), letter series (Embretson, 1985), paragraph comprehension (Embretson & Wetzel, 1987), and mathematical problem solving (Embretson, in press).

A major feature of the proposed design system is that an item's cognitive complexity is linked to its psychometric properties. Several measurement models have been proposed in which a psychometric model of item responses (i.e., latent trait models) contains parameters that characterize the cognitive complexity of items (Embretson, 1984; Fischer, 1973; Jannarone, 1986; Mislevy & Verhelst, 1990; Scheibelchner, 1985; Spada & McGaw, 1985; Stegelmann, 1983; Whitely, 1980). These models also specify how abilities and the item parameters combine to determine the probability of solving the item. Thus, abilities may be interpreted rather directly with respect to the cognitive complexity of the item.

A COGNITIVE DESIGN SYSTEM

Table 1 presents an outline of the stages in the proposed cognitive design system. As in traditional test development, the cognitive design system begins with a general specification of the goals of measurement and ends with empirical validation. However, the intermediate steps differ substantially from traditional test development. Construct representation is accomplished by item specifications that operationalize the intended sources of cognitive complexity on the test. The several steps leading to the calibration of item parameters—identifying task design features, developing a cognitive model, assessing the psychometric potential of the cognitive model, specifying item distributions on cognitive complexity factors, and generating items—are essential to construct representation. Because these steps differ from traditional test development procedures, they will be elaborated on here using the spatial folding task to illustrate the process. The remaining steps—banking items, assembling test forms, and validating the test—are familiar in the development of psychometric instruments. However, because these steps are related to construct representation, they also will differ from traditional test development procedures.

Table 1 Cognitive Design Systems

Specify general goals of measurement
      Construct representation (meaning)
      Nomothetic span (significance)
Identify design features in task domain
      Task-general features (mode, format, conditions)
      Task-specific features
Develop a cognitive model
      Review theories
      Select or develop model for psychometric domain
      Revise model
      Test model
Evaluate cognitive model for psychometric potential
      Evaluate cognitive model plausibility on current test
      Evaluate impact of complexity factors on psychometric
        properties
      Anticipate properties of new test
Specify item distributions on cognitive complexity
      Distribution of item complexity parameters
      Distribution of item features
Generate items to fit specifications
      Artificial intelligence?
Evaluate cognitive and psychometric properties for revised test domain
      Estimate component latent trait model parameters
      Evaluate plausibility of cognitive model
      Evaluate impact of complexity factors on psychometric
        properties
      Evaluate plausibility of the psychometric model
      Calibrate final item parameters and ability distributions
Bank items by cognitive complexity parameters
      $n_m q_{im}$ [weight x item score]
      b_{ik} [component subtask difficulty]
      $P_{strategy}$
Assemble test forms to represent specifications
      Fixed content test
      Adaptive test
Validate

SPECIFYING THE GOALS
OF MEASUREMENT

The measurement process should begin with an initial conceptualization of the intended theoretical meaning of the test score; that is, construct representation is anticipated in terms of the cognitive processes, strategies, and knowledge structures that the test developer intends to measure. The intended construct representation will guide the search for a more precise theoretical formulation, as well as guide decisions about item specification in the later stages of test development.

Of course, nomothetic span must also be considered; that is, the expected significance of the test score will also guide the specification of cognitive constructs. For the spatial folding task, the expected nomothetic span would probably include incremental validity over verbal ability for predicting achievement in areas involving mechanical, architectural, computer, or mathematical skills. Specifying the target nomothetic span guides construct representation because maximizing incremental validity over verbal tests implies that the items must be constructed to minimize the effectiveness of verbal processing strategies.

A major outcome of this stage is identifying the measuring task domain. Thus, for the intended construct of mentally manipulating three-dimensional objects, the spatial folding task defines a possible task domain with a satisfactory psychometric history. However, the goals of measurement also set some criteria for selecting appropriate subsets within the same task domain as the measuring task. That is, not all spatial folding items will represent mental manipulation processes.

IDENTIFYING DESIGN FEATURES
IN THE TASK DOMAIN

In this stage, both the general and the specific design features of items that may influence cognitive complexity are anticipated. These features may or may not be factors in the cognitive model to be developed. However, it is necessary to anticipate how some obvious surface features of the items may influence processing, especially so that various cognitive theories for the task domain can be compared. The cognitive literature on a task may involve theories with different constructs. The difference between theories may arise from applications to tasks that represent different subsets of features in the task domain.

Some general features that apply to most task domains are response format and the conditions of task presentation. General features can have broad effects on processing. For example, well-practiced tasks involve more automatic processing than unpracticed tasks (Ackerman, 1988). In addition, multiple-choice tasks require decision strategies, whereas completion tasks do not. Specific features apply to the particular task domain. These features may or may not have direct impact on cognitive processing. They may be related to, or may set constraints on, the variables that do influence processing.

Figure 4 presents some specific design features for the spatial folding task, namely, the shape of the unfolded stem and the type of marking for the side of the cube. All seven shapes presented in Figure 4 fold into a cube. Although Embretson and Waxman (1989) found that shape did predict processing difficulty for spatial folding items, shape was not included in any cognitive models because it had little unique contribution. Embretson and Waxman concluded that stem shape serves mainly to set constraints on the folding process. That is, a well-centered unfolded cube, such as shape 1 (forming a letter t) in Figure 4, will not require as many surfaces to be carried mentally in a single fold as shape 7. Similarly, the markings on the edge of the cube also may be related to item difficulty, but, again, by setting constraints. The directed markings, such as the diagonal shading, may influence the completeness of the folding process required to confirm an alternative.

DEVELOPING A COGNITIVE MODEL

The goal of this stage is to select or develop a cognitive model. In addition to the usual criteria for theoretical adequacy, such as empirical plausibility, parsimony, and so forth, cognitive models need to be evaluated for appropriateness to the goals of measurement and the selected measuring task. This critical stage may interact with the preceding stage in that either the goals of measurement are changed or a different subset of the task domain is selected. For example, perhaps the spatial folding task, as it appears on the DAT, involves mostly verbal-analytic processing. Thus, either the goals of measurement should be expanded to include verbal reasoning as an intended construct, or the task domain should be revised in order to eliminate the role of verbal-analytic processing.

Many item types that appear in cognitive tests have, in fact, been studied in cognitive psychology. Hence, this stage begins with a review of the theories and the empirical studies that are relevant to the task domain. This review needs to be broadly based, as the cognitive experiments are rarely performed on the same subset of the task domain that appears on a test. Furthermore, related item types may need to be reviewed as well. Thus, it is important to note both the general and specific features of the task domain to which a particular theory or study is applied.

Formal Domain

Stem shape: Designate the output that you want for the stem.

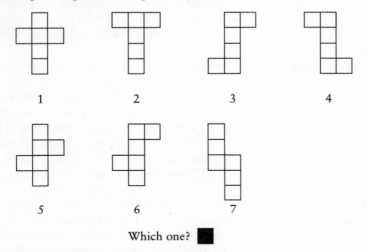

1   2   3   4

5   6   7

Which one? ■

Here are the possible markers for the sides of the cube.

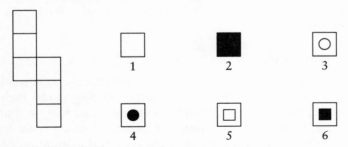

Figure 4   Specific task features for spatial folding items

The selected model is then tested for empirical adequacy on the psychometric task. If the subset of the task domain that contains the measuring task has not been studied, then the empirical adequacy of the cognitive model must be evaluated by standard experimental techniques involving response time and accuracy modeling. Response time is often a more meaningful dependent variable than accuracy for testing hypotheses about processing, as variations in the task stimuli are assumed to influence the duration, but not necessarily the outcome, of the various processing stages (Pachella, 1978). Accuracy, however, must also be modeled because not only is it an important task variable in its own right, but it is also the primary dependent variable in aptitude measurement.

This stage may involve more than one study because revisions of the model may be suggested by the data. Although this stage is not necessarily intended to constitute a major research program for the test developer, it obviously involves effort the test developer is unaccustomed to. However, this stage is essential to linking the test to cognitive theory.

Although the DAT spatial folding task has not been studied extensively, several empirically supported theories are relevant. Evidence from a variety of tasks (Cooper & Shepard, 1973; Just & Carpenter, 1985; Shepard & Metzler, 1971) supports mental rotation as the mental analogue of physical rotation because the angle of rotation is linearly related to response time. Spatial folding tasks are a relatively complex spatial task because folding, as well as rotation, may be required. Shepard and Feng (1972) found that number of surfaces carried mentally to fold an object also influences performance.

Recently, Embretson and Waxman (1989) developed models for three different processing strategies for DAT-type spatial folding items: (a) the attached folding model, (b) the verbal-analytic model, and (c) the direct folding model. The attached folding model is most directly related to the other spatial theories and models described earlier, and so it was examined as a possible guiding cognitive model for test development.

The Attached Folding Model

In the attached folding model, it is postulated that the stem is folded to fit a particular alternative. The attached folding model includes four major processes: (a) encoding, (b) attaching, (c) folding, and (d) confirming. In *encoding,* the stem and then the distractors are represented in short-term memory. Both the type and orientation of the markings (i.e., the circles, squares, or shading that appears on the sides) are noted. In *attaching,* two adjacent sides on the unfolded stem are mentally attached to the folded cube. This stage involves selecting the anchoring sides, rotating the stem (if necessary), and mentally attaching the stem to the alternative. In *folding,* the third side of the cube is mentally placed into position. In *confirming,* the third side that appears after folding is compared with the folded alternative. Figure 5 presents an illustration of the attaching and folding process.

The encoding process is probably influenced by the complexity of the markings on the cube, because encoding is largely a perceptual process in the spatial task. Confirming is probably also manipulated by the complexity of the marking, particularly if the marking appears differently from different sides, as in the half-shaded side in Figure 2. Attaching and folding, however, are more uniquely spatial processes;

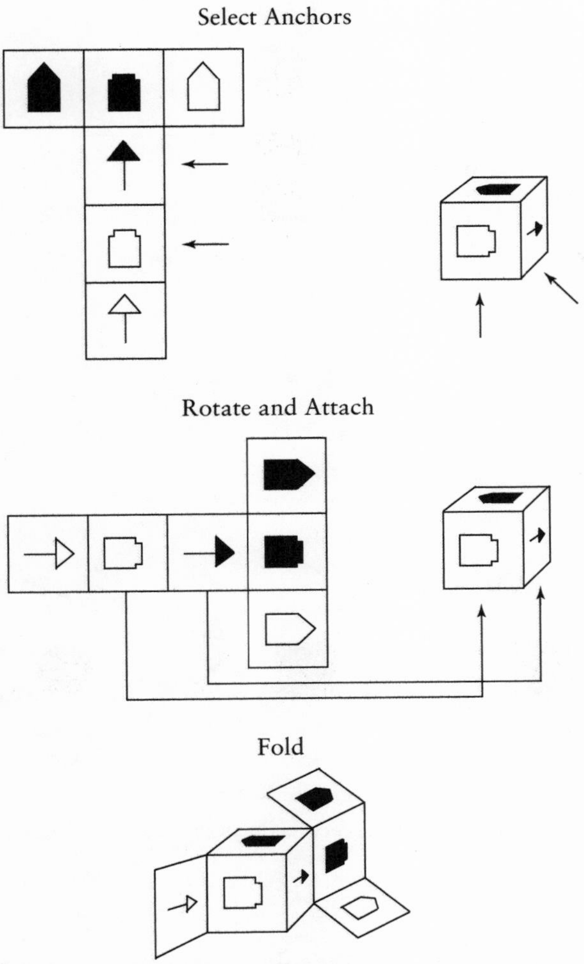

Select Anchors

Rotate and Attach

Fold

Figure 5   An illustration of attaching and folding

thus, the manipulation of their difficulty will be described more completely.

Figure 6 shows how the difficulty of attaching is varied by the degree of rotation of the stem to the alternative. An unfolded stem and three different correct alternatives that vary in attaching difficulty are presented. The stem can be directly overlaid on the first alternative without any rotation. The second and third alternatives, in contrast, require a 90-degree and 180-degree rotation of the stem, respectively.

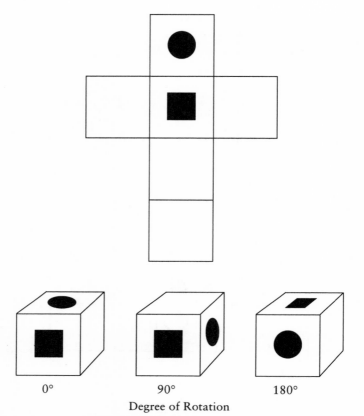

0°   90°   180°

Degree of Rotation

Figure 6   A stem and three correct answers that vary in attaching difficulty

Figure 7 shows how the difficulty of folding can be varied by the number of surfaces carried. Shown in Figure 7 are one correct alternative and three different stems. The first stem is the easiest to attach, because if the shaded circle and shaded square are attached, only one surface needs to be carried to complete the folding. However, if the sides that contain these two markings are attached for the second stem, two surfaces must be carried mentally to bring the third side into place. The last stem requires that three surfaces are carried.

Figure 8 shows the relationship between the processes of Embretson and Waxman's (1989) attached folding model. The model is applicable to multiple-choice formats as well as verification formats. Distractors that differ from the key in orientation or position must be more fully processed than distractors that match the key in every respect except the orientation of the marking on the third side.

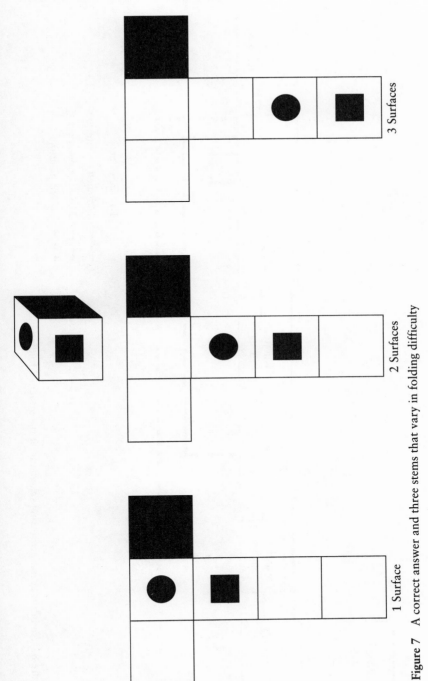

Figure 7 A correct answer and three stems that vary in folding difficulty

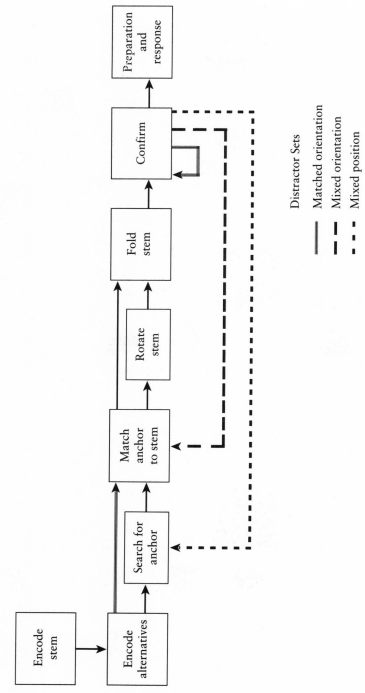

Figure 8   An information processing schematic of the attached folding model

Embretson and Waxman examined the empirical adequacy of the attached folding model in a series of studies. In an early study, verification items were developed to reflect variations in the attaching process and the folding process, in a degrees of rotation (3) × number of surfaces (3) × stem shape (4) × marker configuration (2) balanced design for the stimuli, which were varied within subjects. False problems were also constructed by a similar algorithm.

As was expected, the results indicated that both degrees of rotation and number of surfaces had significant main effects for both response time and accuracy on the tasks. However, number of surfaces and degrees of rotation interacted significantly, which did not support the independence of attaching and folding. The main violation of the model occurred for items with three surfaces carried and 0 degrees of rotation (i.e., they were too easy). However, despite this violation, the mathematical models indicated rather good prediction of response time ($R = .76$) and response accuracy ($R = .79$) from the variables of the attached folding model.

The experiment provided some support for the attached folding model, at least in the verification format. The processing difficulties are manipulated by easily controlled stimulus features that can be directly utilized in test development. However, the empirical departures from the model require further examination. The spatial folding task with three surfaces carried and 0 degrees of rotation may have been easy because subjects employ a verbal strategy for this condition; that is, the folding process may be unnecessary after the stem is attached because the subject could just note the position of the third side (right or left) on the stem and compare it to the alternative. In fact, model comparisons revealed that the verbal-analytic model had the same empirical plausibility as the attached folding model. Furthermore, the model also must show empirical plausibility when extrapolated to the DAT test items in which the response format is multiple choice rather than verification.

Another study presented by Embretson and Waxman (1989) supported the postulated independence of the attaching and folding stages in a revised variant of the spatial folding task. In the revised task, all sides had directed markings, as shown in the sample item in Figure 9. Here, the relative position of the markings on the sides cannot be confirmed unless the stem is fully folded. The study also examined the applicability of the model to the multiple-choice format. Mathematical modeling of response time and accuracy also indicated how the alternatives were processed; that is, the best model postulated that alternatives were processed in serial order and that processing terminated when the key was confirmed (i.e., the remaining alternatives beyond the key are not examined).

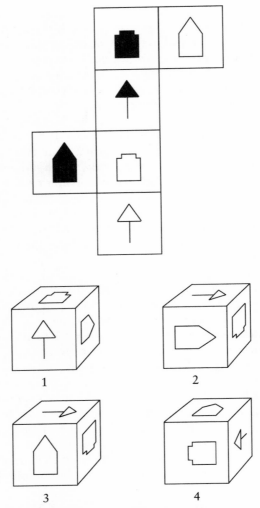

Figure 9 A spatial folding item with directed markings

To conclude this stage, the goals of measurement and the measuring task domain must be rectified with the empirical results. For the spatial folding example, the empirical findings indicate a potential conflict between the measuring task domain and the goals of measurement. If the measuring task domain is to include figures with nondirected markings on the sides, as in Figure 1, then the goals of measurement must be expanded; that is, the goal must be to measure competency in solving spatial tasks from effective application of either a spatial or a verbal-analytic processing strategy. If the goals of measurement are restricted to spatial processing, as initially formulated, then the measuring task must be limited to figures with directed markings so as to minimize verbal processing strategies.

In any case, the importance of this stage for test meaning cannot be overemphasized. Although the experiments described above are atypical in test development, they were not very costly or difficult to run. In comparison with empirical tryout of items, relatively few subjects (fewer than 100 subjects total) and little testing time (less than one hour for each subject) was required. The laboratory equipment consisted of ordinary personal microcomputers, with software readily available for item presentation (Vail, 1984).

EVALUATING THE COGNITIVE MODEL FOR PSYCHOMETRIC POTENTIAL

In this stage, the cognitive model is evaluated for psychometric potential for both the existing test and the new test. In both cases, parameters are estimated to reflect the impact of the cognitive complexity variables on the psychometric properties of the test. Ideally, parameters for the cognitive model are estimated from a component latent trait model (described below) applied to item response data. However, regression modeling of item difficulty may provide a good approximation. Data that have been collected in the previous stages, or archival data on the existing test, may be suitable for this stage.

The overall fit of the model, as well as the impact of the cognitive complexity factors on item difficulty and item fit, are the primary data. If possible, the impact of the cognitive complexity factors on differential item functioning (i.e., bias for different subpopulations) or item validity should also be studied.

To illustrate, regression models were fit to spatial folding items from both the DAT and a new test with the items taken from the cognitive modeling studies discussed earlier. The attached folding model was operationalized by scoring six complexity factors for each item. For encoding, unanchorable distractors (i.e., falsifiable perceptually) were scored as the number of distractors with markings that did not match the unfolded stem. For attaching, the degree of rotation to anchor the stem was scored for both the correct answer and the maximum distractor. For the folding process, the number of surfaces carried was scored for both the correct answer and the maximum distractor. Finally, confirming was scored by the existence of directed marking (i.e., half-shading, asymmetrical markings, etc.) on the sides of the cube. The DAT items varied on all six factors, but the new test varied only on four factors because the items had been constrained to include only directed markings and no unanchorable distractors.

Two different cognitive models were fit to item difficulties (p values were rescaled as $\ln(p/(1-p))$ to be comparable to latent trait model scales) for each test: (a) a full model that included all six complexity factors and (b) a reduced model that included only the two variables for the stem-to-key relationships (i.e., degrees of rotation and number of surfaces). Lower levels of prediction could be expected a priori for the new test because only four factors could be included in the full model. However, the results indicated that although the full model predicted the DAT item difficulties fairly well ($R = .63$), the difficulty of the new items was predicted even better ($R = .73$). Furthermore, the pattern of prediction varied between the DAT items and the new items. When only the stem-to-key relationships were included, prediction dropped substantially for the DAT items ($R = .23$) but not for the new items ($R = .69$). Thus, the distractor characteristics were very important for DAT item difficulty, whereas the stem-to-key relationships were very important for the difficulty of the new items.

These results suggest that the proposed cognitive model has good psychometric potential for two reasons. First, although far from perfect, the proposed cognitive model does predict performance on existing test items. Second, the proposed cognitive model will explain performance better on a revised version of the spatial folding task with directed markings and no unanchorable distractors.

Item fit must also be studied during this stage, but unlike in traditional test development, item fit can be related to specific complexity factors or to the whole model. For traditional test development, items with poor fit to the psychometric model (i.e., low discrimination) are discarded, but the specific source of misfit is unknown. If a specific factor is related to misfit, then selecting only items within certain levels on the factor can improve fit. For example, the spatial folding items fit poorly when the number of unmatched distractors is high. Eliminating items with one or more unmatched distractors would improve fit to the psychometric model.

SPECIFYING ITEM DISTRIBUTIONS
ON COGNITIVE COMPLEXITY

If the cognitive model has sufficient potential to describe performance on test items, the test developer can use the model to specify item distributions and to guide the construction of new items. In this stage, the test developer determines the target distribution of the cognitive complexity factors for the new test. The results from the preceding stages are considered in determining the complexity factor distributions as well as in setting constraints on specific or general task features that are not desirable in the cognitive model.

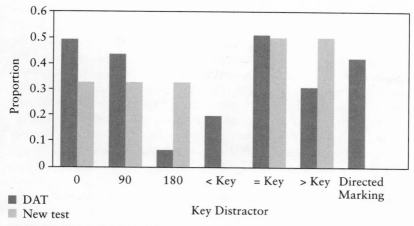

Figure 10   Distribution of degrees of rotation and directed markings in the items of two tests

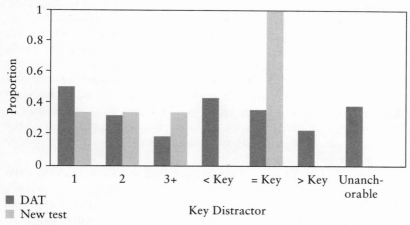

Figure 11   Distribution of number of surfaces carried and unanchorable distractors in the items of two tests

A useful starting point is to examine the current item bank. Figure 10 shows the proportions for the three degrees of rotation (0, 90, 180) to the key and to the maximum distractor relative to the key (degrees can be equal to, smaller than, or larger than the key). The proportion of items with directed markings is also shown in Figure 10. Figure 11 shows the proportions for the number of surfaces carried to the key (1, 2, 3+) and to the maximum distractor relative to the key (< key, = key, > key). Additionally, Figure 11 shows the proportion of items with unanchorable distractors.

An inspection of Figure 10 and Figure 11 suggests several explanations for the predictive power of the distractor characteristics in the DAT spatial items. First, many DAT items have unanchorable distractors that are easily falsifiable during the encoding stage. The inclusion of these distractors conflicts with the goals of measurement because they may be falsified without mental manipulation. Thus, they should be excluded. Second, many items have maximum distractors in which either the degrees of rotation or the number of surfaces carried is less than it is for the key. In such items, an effective strategy would be to falsify the distractors, which would be quite easy, and then the key can be selected by default (without processing it!). Thus, decision strategies for processing distractors can play a large role in responses to DAT test items. Although the impact of decision strategies does not conflict directly with the measurement goals, it is not specified by them, either. Thus, reducing the importance of decision strategies by decreasing items with easily falsifiable distractors would be desirable.

Figures 10 and 11 also show why the stem-to-key relationships contributed little to DAT item difficulty. The easier keys, requiring no rotation or only one surface carried, are overrepresented. Furthermore, many DAT items do not have directed markings. Because such items can be solved without fully folding the stem, spatial processing is not necessarily required. Finally, not shown in the figures, the stem-to-key variables are correlated with the distractor characteristics, which further weakens their unique contribution. Thus, it would be desirable to increase the number of difficult keys, use directed markings, and vary the distractors independently from the stem-to-key characteristics to increase spatial processing.

Figures 10 and 11 also show the specified proportions of the various complexity factors for a new test that is designed to maximize spatial processing from the stem-to-key relationships. In the new test, the number of surfaces carried to the key, the degrees of rotation to the key, and the distractor set type are counterbalanced in equal proportions. Two different types of distractor sets are included: (a) a set in which the distractors have the same relationship to the stem as the key (same number of surfaces carried and degrees of rotation) and (b) a set in which the distractors have the same number of surfaces carried to the stem as the key, but the degrees of rotation vary between the distractors (one each at 0, 90, and 180). Thus, a 3 (surfaces) × 3 (degrees) × 2 (distractor type) design yields 18 combinations that can be replicated with varying side markings or stem shapes. Two complexity factors are held constant, no items have unanchorable distractors, and all items have directed markings.

The relative proportions of values for the complexity factors that result from the crossed design also are shown in Figures 10 and 11.

The various levels of number of surfaces carried to the key and the degrees of rotation to the key are now equally represented on the test. Also, no distractors are easier than the key or are falsifiable during encoding (i.e., due to unanchorable distractors).

GENERATING ITEMS TO FIT SPECIFICATIONS

Once precise specifications are given, items may be generated. Furthermore, item difficulties may be anticipated from the design features by the regression modeling results obtained previously. If the cognitive model is sufficiently detailed, artificial intelligence may be used to write items to fit the specifications. Generating items by artificial intelligence is strong evidence that item control has been achieved, inasmuch as precise specifications are necessary. Of course, it also may have some practical advantages, such as the speed and cost with which new tests can be developed.

For the spatial task, for example, the impact of stimulus content on processing is quite clear, so that a computer program could be created to generate appropriate items to fill the specifications. The specific features of the items, such as shape and marking type, would be given a priori, then the program would find combinations of stem shapes and the marking configurations on the stem and the alternatives that fulfill a given specification. In theory, for complex verbal items, although the technology is certainly not currently adequate, artificial intelligence also could generate verbal items, even such complex items as paragraph comprehension. That is, if the cognitive model variables primarily concern semantic level and structure, a computer program could contain the lexical, syntactic, and other structural knowledge needed to generate items with differing complexity. For example, Schank and Abelson's (1977) prototypic program could generate text at varying levels of syntactic and semantic complexity, given a basic script and roles of actors and objects.

EVALUATING THE COGNITIVE
AND PSYCHOMETRIC PROPERTIES
OF THE REVISED TEST

This stage provides fundamental psychometric data for the new test. As in traditional test development, large-scale data are collected so that item difficulties and item fit may be calibrated, test properties (internal consistency or fit to a psychometric model) may be assessed, and ability norms may be prepared. Unlike traditional test development, this stage also provides three new types of data that are crucial to construct representation. First, the cognitive demands of the test, in terms of underlying processes, are assessed by fitting the cognitive model to the test. Second, individual items can be justified for test inclusion by the relative dependence on the processes and by the explanatory power of the cognitive model for item performance. Third, ability scores may be interpreted directly for potential for cognitive processing on particular items.

In this stage, the parameters of component latent trait models are estimated and both overall fit and individual item fit are evaluated. In component latent trait models, cognitive variables are linked to item responses by two mathematical models. One mathematical model relates the stimulus features or processing complexity of the item to performance. The other mathematical model predicts the encounter of an individual with a particular item. These mathematical models are known as latent trait models or as item response theory models.

The appropriate component latent trait model for the cognitive model developed for spatial folding example is the linear logistic latent trait model (LLTM; Fischer, 1973). Thus, LLTM will be described in detail here. In LLTM, item difficulties are modeled from variables that can be scored from each item (e.g., number of surfaces carried, degrees of rotation, etc.). However, it should be noted that the multicomponent latent trait model (MLTM; Whitely, 1980), in which the outcome of an item is predicted from the outcomes of the necessary processing components, and the general component latent trait model (GLTM; Embretson, 1984), which combines LLTM and MLTM, are appropriate for many other test items. MLTM and GLTM require cognitive models that relate component outcomes to the total item outcome.

The latent trait model in LLTM is a Rasch model, which is often used in test development. The Rasch model is the most simple traditional psychometric model in that it contains just one item parameter, item difficulty. The probability that an individual solves a particular item is given by an exponential model in which the individual's ability, θ_j, combines additively with the item's difficulty, b_i, as follows:

$$P(X_{ij} = 1) = \exp{(\theta_j - b_i)} / [1 + \exp(\theta_j - b_i)]. \qquad (1)$$

The major interest in testing is not the individual probabilities that are given in Equation 1, but the parameter estimates that give an individual's observed responses the highest likelihood; that is, the primary interest is estimating the individual's ability and the item's difficulty.

Component latent trait models can be viewed as extensions of the Rasch model that link response probabilities to cognitive processing variables. Fischer (1973) developed the linear logistic latent trait model (LLTM) to link item difficulty to a cognitive model of task complexity. Although Fischer's development preceded cognitive component analysis of test items (e.g., Sternberg, 1977), it is readily applicable to contemporary cognitive models. As in the Rasch model, LLTM models the probability that an individual *j* will pass item *i*, as follows:

$$P(X_{ij} = 1) = \exp(\theta_j - b_i) / [1 + \exp(\theta_j - b_i)]. \tag{2}$$

However, a second mathematical model is also contained implicitly in LLTM. That is, item difficulty is modeled from some factors that represent the cognitive complexity of the item as follows:

$$b^*_i = \Sigma_m n_m q_{im} + d \tag{3}$$

where

q_{im} = the complexity of item *i* on factor *m*

n_m = the weight of factor *m* in item difficulty

d = a normalization constant.

Equation 3 is analogous to a regression model of item difficulty.

Equation 2 and Equation 3 can be combined to give LLTM, eliminating b^*, as follows:

$$P(X_{ij} = 1) = \exp(\theta_j - \Sigma_m n_m q_{im} + d) / [1 + \exp(\theta_j - \Sigma_{mnm} q_{im} + {}_d)] \tag{4}$$

Thus, in LLTM, the item parameters to be estimated describe the complexity of the item on the cognitive factors. Ability combines additively with cognitive complexity to give the probability of response to an item with such a complexity pattern.

For the spatial folding example, items were generated by the design described above. LLTM parameters were estimated from large sample data on the new items for a model with three complexity factors: number of surfaces carried to key, degrees of rotation to key, and degrees rotation to the maximum distractor. (The number of surfaces carried to the maximum distractor always equals the key and, hence, is omitted.) Overall fit was quite good ($R = .81$), which indicates that test performance is well described by the attached folding model.

The relative contribution of attaching, folding, and confirming to a specific item may be evaluated by examining the LLTM equation for the item. For the spatial folding data, the following equation for item difficulty was calibrated:

$$b^*_i = .81q1 + .17q2 - .13q3 - 1.56 \tag{5}$$

where

$q1$ = surfaces carried to key

$q2$ = degrees rotation to key (/100)

$q3$ = degrees rotation to maximum distractor (/100).

Thus, the relative contribution of processes to item difficulty are given by the weights in Equation 5. Here, the number of surfaces carried to the key has the largest weight, so folding is the major process in the test items.

The specific sources of cognitive complexity can be given for each item. For example, the difficulty of the item in Figure 9 is explained by Equation 5. The correct answer (shape 3) involves 180-degree rotation and three surfaces carried. The maximum distractor (shape 2) involves a 180-degree rotation, and the number of surfaces carried (three) is equal to the key. Therefore, item difficulty is predicted as follows:

$$b^*_i = .81(3) + .17(1.80) - .13(1.80) - 1.56 \qquad (6)$$
$$= .942.$$

The item can be justified for test inclusion by its fit to the cognitive model. One index of item fit is the difference between the predicted and observed (i.e., Rasch model) item difficulty. In the item on Figure 9, the Rasch model item difficulty was 1.16, so the difference between the predicted value of .942 and observed value of 1.16 was quite small. Another index of item fit is a χ^2 test for each item, which was not significant for the item.

The meaning of an individual ability score can be interpreted in terms of potential to solve items with specified sources of cognitive complexity if the cognitive model fits well. Suppose that an individual has an ability of 1.7 (this is like a z-score of 1.0 in LLTM), which is high. The potential to solve the item in Figure 9 is given by the additive combination of ability and the sources of cognitive complexity, shown in Equation 7, as follows:

$$P(X_{ij} = 1) = \exp(1.7 - .942) / [1 + \exp(1.7 - .942)] \qquad (7)$$
$$= .68.$$

In contrast, this person would have a much higher probability of solving a similar item, but with only one surface carried to the key ($P = .92$). Thus, the relationship of ability to performance can be referenced to processing demands in particular items.

Another issue to be evaluated in this stage is differential item functioning (i.e., bias across subgroups, such as defined by race and gender). Although this is routinely evaluated in traditional testing, differential item functioning across populations can be interpreted in terms of processing by using a component latent trait model. For the spatial folding task, an important population comparison is males versus females, as prior research finds performance level differences that are attributed to processing differences (e.g., Bock & Kolakowski, 1973).

If LLTM is used, the weights of the cognitive complexity factors can be compared and interpreted for process differences between populations.

THE REMAINING STEPS

The last steps, banking items, assembling the tests, and validating abilities are also familiar problems in test development and will not be described in detail here. However, these steps will differ from traditional procedures because the item parameters now represent the impact of cognitive processing variables, rather than an atheoretical ordering of item difficulty. This difference will entail some changes in techniques in these stages, but these are beyond the scope of this chapter.

Test validation should be influenced by the preceding steps; that is, in terms of the construct validity framework, the altered construct representation of the test should influence nomothetic span. For example, a spatial aptitude test in which items have no unanchorable distractors should increase the role of spatial processing and, hence, give the test greater incremental validity for predicting criteria that involve spatial processing.

SUMMARY

Traditionally, cognitive tests have not been developed so that the meaning of the test score relies on the design of the measure. Instead, the construct validity of the scores has depended on the external relationships of the test score to other measures. Thus, the meaning of the test score is confounded with the significance of the test score. Consequently, cognitive tests are not attached to cognitive theory.

This chapter has presented a cognitive design system that uses mathematical models of cognitive processes to link cognitive tests to cognitive theory. The design system may be applied to either the item types that already appear on cognitive measures or new item types. The design system involves the cognitive theory of a task or item type to prescribe test content and appropriate test scores, as well as to guide test interpretation. That is, the meaning of the test score depends on construct representation, which is conceptually separate from its significance for predicting criteria and other measures.

A last issue to consider is the potential for theories of construct representation to guide score meaning. Can the full range of cognitive tests, or even personality and attitude measures, be understood in terms of theories about the processes that underlie performance? Obviously, theories with good explanatory power are needed. Such theories would be difficult or impossible to develop for many existing tests because the test items are constructed without detailed designs for stimulus content. Ambiguity in the item stimuli leads to variability in how individuals interpret the task and in what processes they choose to apply. Applying the proposed cognitive design system was shown in this chapter to reduce ambiguities in nonverbal aptitude items substantially. Similar applications to the verbal domain may be anticipated, due to the considerable experimental literature on verbal information processing. Even personality and attitude measurement may be amendable to a designed approach, inasmuch as the qualities of items that lead to reliable introspective reports (Ericsson & Simon, 1980) are becoming a major research agendum. In conclusion, the degree to which construct representation can guide score meaning in future tests will depend jointly on the design or redesign of the test stimuli and the extent to which a theory of performance on the designed task can be supported empirically. This could be considered a research agendum for psychological measurement.

REFERENCES

Ackerman, P. L. (1988). Determinants of individual differences during skill acquisition: Cognitive abilities and information processing. *Journal of Experimental Psychology: General, 117,* 288–318.

Bechtoldt, H. (1959). Construct validity: A critique. *American Psychologist, 14,* 619–629.

Bock, R. D., & Kolakowski, D. D. (1973). Further evidence of sex-linked major-gene influence on human spatial visualizing ability. *American Journal of Human Genetics, 25,* 1–4.

Carroll, J. B. (1976). Psychometric tests as cognitive tasks: A new "structure of intellect." In L. B. Resnick (Ed.), *The nature of intelligence.* Hillsdale, NJ: Erlbaum.

Carroll, J. B., & Maxwell, S. (1979). Individual differences in ability. *Annual Review of Psychology,* 603–640.

Cooper, L. A., & Shepard, R. N. (1973). Chronometric studies of the rotation of mental images. In W. G. Chase (Ed.), *Visual information processing* (pp. 141–163). New York: Academic Press.

Cronbach, L. J., & Meehl, P. E. (1955). Construct validity in psychological tests. *Psychological Bulletin, 52,* 281–302.

Dillon, R. F. (1985). *Individual differences in cognition* (Vol. 2). New York: Academic Press.

Egan, D. E. (1980). An analysis of spatial orientation tests. *Intelligence, 4,* 181–202.

Embretson, S. E. (1983). Construct validity: Construct representation versus nomothetic span. *Psychological Bulletin, 93,* 179–197.

Embretson, S. E. (1984). A general latent trait model for response processes. *Psychometrika, 49,* 175–186.

Embretson, S. E. (1985). *Test design: Developments in psychology and psychometrics.* New York: Academic Press.

Embretson, S. E. (1985). Studying intelligence with test theory models. In D. Detterman, *Current topics in human intelligence* (pp. 98–140). Norwood, NJ: Ablex

Embretson, S. E. (1987). Improving the measurement of spatial aptitude by a dynamic testing procedure. *Intelligence, 11,* 333–358.

Embretson, S. E. (in press). A measurement model for linking individual change to processes and knowledge: Application to mathematical learning. *Journal of Educational Measurement.*

Embretson, S. E., & Schneider, L. M. (1989). Cognitive models of analogical reasoning for psychometric tasks. *Learning and Individual Differences, 1,* 155–178.

Embretson, S. E., Schneider, L., & Roth, D. L. (1985). Multiple processing strategies and the construct validity of verbal reasoning tests. *Journal of Educational Measurement, 23,* 13–32.

Embretson, S. E., & Waxman, M. (1989). *Models for processing and individual differences in spatial folding.* Unpublished manuscript.

Embretson, S. E., & Wetzel, D. (1987). Component latent trait models for paragraph comprehension tests. *Applied Psychological Measurement, 11,* 333–358.

Ericsson, K. A., & Simon, H. A. (1980). Verbal reports as data. *Psychological Review, 87,* 215–251.

Fischer, G. (1973). Linear logistic test model as an instrument in educational research. *Acta Psychologica, 37,* 359–374.

Hunt, E. B. (1978). Mechanics of verbal ability. *Psychological Review, 85,* 109–130.

Hunt, E. B., Lunneborg, C., & Lewis, J. (1975). What does it mean to be high verbal? *Cognitive Psychology, 7,* 194–227.

Jannarone, R. J. (1986). Conjunctive item response theory kernels. *Psychometrika, 51,* 357–373.

Just, M., & Carpenter, P. (1985). Cognitive coordinate systems: Accounts of mental rotation and individual differences in spatial ability. *Psychological Review, 92,* 137–172.

Mislevy, R., & Verhelst, N. (1990). Modeling item responses when different subjects employ different solution strategies. *Psychometrika, 55,* 195–215.

Pachella, R. G. (1979). The interpretation of reaction time in information-processing research. In B. H. Kantowitz (Ed.), *Human information processing: Tutorials in performance and cognition.* Hillsdale, NJ: Erlbaum.

Pellegrino, J. W. (1985). Inductive reasoning ability. In R. J. Sternberg (Ed.), *Human abilities: An information processing approach* (pp. 195–225). New York: Freeman.

Pellegrino, J. W. (1988). Mental models and mental tests. In H. Wainer & H. I. Brown (Eds.), *Test validity* (pp. 78–89). Hillsdale, NJ: Erlbaum.

Pellegrino, J. W., & Lyons, D. W. (1979). The components of a componential analysis. *Intelligence, 3,* 169–186.

Schank, R. C., & Abelson, R. P. (1977). *Scripts, plans, goals and understanding.* Hillsdale, NJ: Erlbaum.

Scheibelchner, H. (1985). Psychometric models for speed-test construction: The linear exponential model. In S. Embretson (Ed.), *Test design: Developments in psychology and psychometrics* (pp. 219–244). New York: Academic Press.

Shepard, R. N., & Feng, C. (1972). A chronometric study of mental paper folding. *Cognitive Psychology, 3,* 228–243.

Shepard, R. N., & Metzler, J. (1971). Mental rotation of three-dimensional objects. *Science, 171*, 701–703.

Snow, R. E., Federico, P. A., & Montague, W. E. (1980). *Aptitude, learning and instruction, Volume 1: Cognitive process analysis of aptitude.*

Spada, H., & McGaw, B. (1985). The assessment of learning effects with linear logistic test models. In S. Embretson (Ed.), *Test design: New directions in psychology and psychometrics* (pp. 169–193). New York: Academic Press.

Stegelmann, W. (1983). Expanding the Rasch model to a general model having more than one dimension. *Psychometrika, 48*, 259–267.

Sternberg, R. J. (1977). Component processes in analogical reasoning. *Psychological Review, 31*, 356–378.

Sternberg, R. J. (1981). *Advances in the psychology of human intelligence* (Vol. 1). Hillsdale, NJ: Erlbaum.

Sternberg, R. J. (1983). *Advances in the psychology of human intelligence* (Vol. 2). Hillsdale, NJ: Erlbaum.

Sternberg, R. J. (1985). *Advances in the psychology of human intelligence* (Vol. 3). Hillsdale, NJ: Erlbaum.

Vail, D. (1984). *MICROCAT Testing System:* St. Paul, MN: Assessment Systems Corporation.

Whitely, S. E. (1980). Multicomponent latent trait models for ability tests. *Psychometrika, 45*, 479–494.

Whitely, S. E. (1981). Measuring aptitude processes with multicomponent latent trait models. *Journal of Educational Measurement, 18*, 67–84.

Whitely, S. E., & Schneider, L. M. (1981). Information structure on geometric analogies: A test theory approach. *Applied Psychological Measurement, 5*, 383–397.

Chapter 3

Improving Individual Differences Measurement With Item Response Theory and Computerized Adaptive Testing

David J. Weiss
University of Minnesota

Since the early days of the measurement of individual differences, classical test theory (e.g., Gulliksen, 1950) was the measurement model used to construct instruments for research and application in the measurement of individual differences. Classical test theory (CTT)—sometimes called true and error score theory or number-correct score theory—is based on the idea that each individual has some unobservable *true* score on a given trait, which is estimated by an *observed* score on a measuring instrument. CTT assumes that the observed score is an imperfect representation of true score and has developed concepts and procedures for determining reliability in an effort to quantify this difference. In addition to reliability, CTT provides instrument constructors with the concepts of item difficulty, item discrimination, and number-correct test scores.

Although CTT has provided researchers and practitioners of individual differences with instruments that have yielded useful research findings and applications, there are several technical problems with CTT that have limited research progress and impaired the usefulness of its instruments for some important applications.

SOME PROBLEMS
WITH CLASSICAL TEST THEORY

Item Statistics

One major problem with CTT results from its definitions of item difficulty and item discrimination. *Item difficulty* is defined as proportion correct—the proportion of examinees who answer an item correctly. *Item discrimination* is usually operationalized as the biserial or point-biserial correlation between a dichotomously coded item score (0 = incorrect, 1 = correct) and number-correct test score. An important problem with these CTT item parameters is that they are contingent on the sample of examinees to whom the items were administered. For example, if a set of test items is administered to a low-ability group of examinees, the item difficulties (and probably the item discriminations) are likely to be very different from those for the same items administered to a group of examinees of moderate or high ability. As a consequence, a test constructed on a group that has a certain ability (or other trait) level cannot be used directly on a group that has a different trait level, or on the same group at a later point in training or development if change has been assumed to have occurred. This makes it almost impossible to do meaningful research on change in test scores over time—including studies of development, growth, or decline—without elaborate and faulty procedures for "vertical equating." Nor is it feasible to measure individuals as they change over time on dynamic traits. Indeed, Cronbach and Furby (1970) concluded that the problem of measuring change with CTT was so complex that attempts to solve it should be abandoned. Although this conclusion was reached some years ago, no satisfactory procedures for measuring *individual* change have been proposed based on CTT.

The Number-Correct Score

The number-correct score in CTT is a second source of major technical problems. Because individuals' scores are based on the number of items they answer correctly (or in personality and other inventories, the number that are "keyed" for a given scale), test scores depend on the difficulty of the items used in the test selected: More difficult tests will result in lower average scores, while easier tests will result in higher scores. Because the item difficulties are group specific, it follows that the number-correct score is conditional on the group on which the test is normed. As a consequence, individuals could obtain different test scores if different items were used. This could then change the rank ordering of individuals, which would have undesirable implications for individual differences research and applications.

The number-correct score has other problems that limit its usefulness. First, it is artifactually limited to the number of questions or items in the instrument. Thus, in a test composed of 25 items, there are only 26 scores possible. Therefore, in a group of 10,000 individuals, only 26 differentiations can be made among those individuals, regardless of how many real differences there may be on the trait of interest. A closely related problem is that all items are treated equally in scoring. Therefore, a correct answer to an easy item is worth as much as a correct answer to a more difficult one. In fact, it is possible (albeit unlikely) for two individuals to obtain the same number-correct score on a test, with one person having correctly answered only the easy items and the other having answered only the difficult items. Obviously, the latter individual has more ability than the former, but the number-correct score cannot differentiate between them.

Reliability and the Standard Error of Measurement

Reliability is a pivotal concept in CTT, and it is the source of several problems. A number of theories of reliability have been developed, and numerous procedures are available to estimate reliability coefficients (Ghiselli, Campbell, & Zedeck, 1981). Without exception, however, these procedures produce reliability coefficients that are group specific. Thus, rather than there being one "reliability" for a specific measuring instrument, there are as many "reliabilities" as there are groups to which that instrument can be applied. Although this in itself might not be a serious problem, it results in some incongruous consequences.

Reliability in CTT is the basis for the calculation of the standard error of measurement (SEM), which is a confidence interval that can be placed around the estimate of a person's true score in order to help a test user locate that true score. As reliability increases, the confidence interval around the point estimate of true score (which itself is derived with the aid of the reliability coefficient) decreases, making the true score estimate more precise. But because reliability for a given measuring instrument will vary depending on the group with which the individual is measured, the precision of a person's true score estimate will also change, depending on the group. Consequently, it is possible in CTT for an individual to obtain a score that has different SEMs attached to it as a result of having taken the test with different groups. Even though the person's responses and score are the same, its "precision" can vary in CTT. This is an illogical and incongruous situation.

An additional problem with CTT's SEM is that it is computed as a constant value for a given test administered to a given group; that is, there is no provision for the SEM to vary as a function of trait level for a given test administration. As a consequence, everyone in the same group will receive the same SEM, and there is no satisfactory way to determine whether scores at different levels of the trait differ in their precision. When combined with the contingency of the SEM on the group to which the test is administered, these problems have led to the unfortunate result that the SEM has virtually been ignored in individual differences research and application, and most measurements have been considered essentially perfectly precise.

Instrument Development

A final major problem with CTT is that it provides little guidance for the development of measuring instruments for different purposes. Instrument construction procedures of CTT focus almost entirely on maximizing reliability. For example, CTT item analysis procedures (e.g., Crocker & Algina, 1986, chap. 14) suggest that instruments be constructed by first selecting items of .50 difficulty (proportion correct). This minimizes the sum of the item variances and serves to increase internal consistency reliability. The next step usually recommended is to do an item analysis by deleting items from the test that have low correlations with total score. This process is also designed to increase the internal consistency reliability of the measuring instrument.

The result of these procedures, however, is an instrument with all highly discriminating items of relatively equal difficulty. Instruments of this type are useful for certain measurement purposes but are inappropriate for other purposes. For example, CTT does not provide explicit guidance about how to construct a measuring instrument designed to select people for an occupation if there are both minimum and maximum cutoff scores to be used—that is, how to eliminate those that are both too high and too low on a trait. The procedures of CTT are inadequate for this task and result in only one restricted—and very limited—type of measuring instrument.

ITEM RESPONSE THEORY

Item response theory (IRT)—sometimes also called latent trait test theory, latent trait theory, or item characteristic curve theory—is a family of mathematical models that relates the performance of an individual on a test item to the underlying trait level of the individual. The fact that IRT is a family of test models is important because the basic concepts that pertain to the simplest IRT model also generalize to the more complex IRT models.

The IRT Family

The family of IRT models includes models that are useful for almost all types of data typically used in the measurement of individual differences. There are several IRT models for dichotomous test responses, such as those that result from the administration of a true-false personality inventory or a multiple-choice test scored as correct/incorrect. The equation below provides the mathematical model for the item response function (IRF) of the three-parameter logistic IRT model:

$$P_{ij}(1 \mid \theta_i) = c_j + (1 - c_j)/[1 + \exp[-1.7a_j(\theta_i - b_j)]].$$

This equation expresses the probability of a correct or keyed response to a dichotomously scored item (P_{ij}) as a function of the interaction between an individual with a specified trait level on a single underlying trait—represented by θ_i—and three parameters that describe the characteristics of a test item. These parameters are the item difficulty (b_j), the item discrimination (a_j), and the pseudoguessing parameter (c_j).

Figure 1 shows several item response functions for the three-parameter model for items that differ in terms of difficulty (their location along the difficulty/θ scale), the item discrimination (which is related to the slope of the IRF), and the pseudoguessing parameter (the lower asymptote of the IRF). A simplification of the three-parameter model that can be used for personality measurement (Reise & Waller, 1990) or for free-response ability or achievement test items is the two-parameter logistic model (Hambleton & Swaminathan, 1985, chap. 3). In this model, the c_j parameter is defined as zero; thus, test items differ only in terms of discrimination and difficulty. Finally, if all item discriminations can be assumed to be equal, the one-parameter logistic, or Rasch model (Rasch, 1980), is the result. These logistic models were developed as replacements for the mathematically more cumbersome normal ogive models originally developed for IRT (Lord, 1980, chap. 3), in order to simplify the process of estimating item parameters.

The concepts of item difficulty (interpreted as the location of the item on the difficulty/θ continuum) and item discrimination (interpreted as the slope of the IRF) carry over into the more complex models in the IRT family. Other members of the IRT family of mathematical models include models for so-called nominal, ordered, and continuous item responses. Models for nominal item responses (Baker, 1992, chap. 9; Bock, 1972) are useful for analyzing data from multiple-choice instruments in which there is more than one correct response to an item, or multiple-choice items in which the alternatives

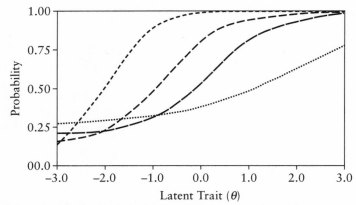

Figure 1   IRT item response functions (IRF) for the three-parameter model
for four items

---- $a_1 = 2.0$, $b_1 = -2.0$, $c_1 = 0.0$
— —· $a_2 = 1.5$, $b_2 = -.8$, $c_2 = .10$
——— $a_3 = 1.5$, $b_3 = .25$, $c_3 = .20$
········· $a_4 = .8$, $b_4 = 2.0$, $c_4 = .25$

are scored as partially correct (the partial credit model; Masters, 1982). In addition to the parameters of item location and item discrimination, these models include parameters for each item category that reflect the location on the trait and the discrimination of each item response category on the trait. In this way, all the responses provided by an individual to multiple-choice items are used directly in the scoring process to extract the maximum information from an individual's responses.

Models for ordered item responses (Andrich, 1978a, 1978b; Baker, 1992, chap. 8; Muraki, 1990; Samejima, 1969) are useful for the analysis of rating scale (e.g., Likert) data. In these models, the responses to each item are considered as separate categories, but as ordered categories on the trait continuum. Again, the concepts of category location and discrimination are added to the concepts of item difficulty and item discrimination.

Finally, among the unidimensional models, a model for continuous response data assumes that an individual responds on a rating scale by using a number in a range such as 0 to 100 to describe his or her status on a trait indicator (Samejima, 1972, 1973b). These numerical responses are treated as the generalization of a series of ordinal responses to a test item and are used relatively directly in the scoring of individual response data (Bejar, 1977), although the concepts of discrimination and difficulty still pertain to items and responses of this type.

Although the model presented in the equation shown earlier assumes that the item response space is unidimensional—that a person's response to a test item derives from a single underlying trait—multidimensional models for dichotomous items have been developed (Reckase, 1985; Reckase & McKinley, 1991), along with estimation procedures for these models (e.g., Carlson, 1987). These models represent a more realistic approach to instrument development and analysis for many dichotomously scored instruments because achieving strict unidimensionality in a measuring instrument is very difficult. Thus, in a multidimensional model, two or more dimensions are posited to account for the response data. As a consequence, the models allow the estimation of difficulty, discrimination, and pseudoguessing parameters for each of a number of independent dimensions to better account for the responses of real people to real test items.

A number of articles have demonstrated the relationships among IRT models, and between IRT models and other models of scaling psychometric data such as Guttman scaling (Mokken & Lewis, 1982), unfolding (Andrich, 1989), Likert scaling (Muraki, 1990), and Thurstonian scaling (Andrich, 1988; Jansen, 1984). Thus, IRT provides a comprehensive system of measurement for measuring a variety of psychological variables.

Characteristics of IRT Models

Following from the assumption of a particular mathematical form that describes the interaction between an individual and a test item are some important characteristics of IRT models. First, the parameters that describe an item—difficulty, discrimination, and other IRT parameters—are assumed to be sample independent within a linear transformation. This means that the item parameters are population parameters and that any differences (other than error) that occur among the samples on which item parameters are estimated can be corrected by a linear transformation, if appropriate data are available. This means that if item parameters are estimated on a low-level trait group, they can be transformed by a linear transformation to the parameters that would be appropriate for a middle or higher trait group and vice versa. This property of IRT parameters enables researchers to create a scale that cuts across trait levels through a process called linking.

Linking is the process of defining the transformation on a set of IRT item parameters that enables the parameters estimated on one sample from a population to be expressed on the same scale as the parameters on another sample from that population, even if the two samples differ in terms of trait level (Vale, 1986). An important property of the linking process is that item parameters are linked. However, because the item difficulty parameter and the θ parameter describing an individual's trait level are on the same scale (see earlier

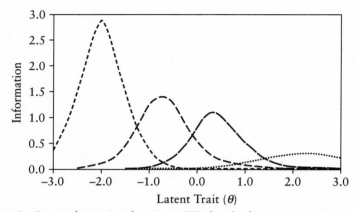

Figure 2   Item information functions (IIF) for the four items in Figure 1
- - - - $a_1 = 2.0$, $b_1 = -2.0$, $c_1 = 0.0$
— —· $a_2 = 1.5$, $b_2 = -.8$, $c_2 = .10$
—— $a_3 = 1.5$, $b_3 = .25$, $c_3 = .20$
········ $a_4 = .8$, $b_4 = 2.0$, $c_4 = .25$

equation), once the difficulty parameters are linked, the θ parameters of the two groups are expressed on the same scale or metric. Thus, from data on a low-level trait group, for example, the results of a linking study will permit the expression of that low-level trait group's θ estimates on the same scale as a higher-level trait group's estimates. This process is sometimes called preequating (Bejar & Wingersky, 1982) because it permits an individual's score to be equated to a score on the predefined scale without following the complicated procedures developed for CTT equating (e.g., Peterson, Kolen, & Hoover, 1989). As will be discussed below, this capability of IRT has important implications for the measurement of individual differences.

IRT has other characteristics that give it a level of applied utility well beyond that of CTT. The IRF in IRT can be transformed in a number of ways. One useful transformation of this kind is into item information functions (IIF). Figure 2 shows item information functions for the four items whose IRFs are shown in Figure 1. *Information* describes the precision of measurement for a given item as a function of the latent trait, θ. The IIF is a transformation of the IRF defined by dividing the squared slope of the IRF at each point on θ by the variance of the IRF at that level of θ. The higher the level of information, the greater the precision of measurement of that item at that point on the θ continuum. Thus, Item 1, which has the highest level of discrimination among those items portrayed in Figure 1 ($a_1 = 2.0$), also has the highest level of item information. *Precision*, in this case, refers to the capability of an item for differentiating among contiguous θ levels.

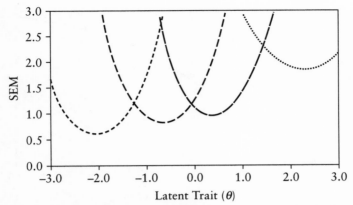

Figure 3 Standard error of measurement (SEM) functions for the four items of Figure 1

---- $a_1 = 2.0, b_1 = -2.0, c_1 = 0.0$
—–· $a_2 = 1.5, b_2 = -.8, c_2 = .10$
—— $a_3 = 1.5, b_3 = .25, c_3 = .20$
········ $a_4 = .8, b_4 = 2.0, c_4 = .25$

A second transformation of the IRF is derived by taking the reciprocal of the square root of the IIF. This results in an SEM function, as shown in Figure 3, which describes the conditional standard error of measurement for a given item at all levels along the θ continuum. It provides basically the same information as the IIF, but rather than displaying precision, it describes imprecision, or error of measurement. Thus, the items that have the highest levels of information at a given point on θ have the lowest levels of conditional standard error measurement.

Because IRT models assume that test items are locally independent—that is, the only relationship among the items that exists is the correlation among them that results from the common latent trait or traits that they measure—the IRFs, IIFs, and SEM functions are additive. A test is a collection of test items. Thus, adding the IRFs for a set of items results in the test response function (TRF) as shown in Figure 4. This function gives the sum of the probabilities of correct response to a group of test items (constituting a test) as a function of the latent trait. When this sum of probabilities is divided by the number of items, the TRF gives the average probability correct/keyed or the expected proportion correct/keyed.

The sum of a set of IIFs yields the test information function (TIF), which is shown in Figure 5 for the items of Figure 1. This also can be obtained by performing the same transformation of the TRF as is applied to the IRF to obtain the IIF. Thus, the TIF is the sum of the IIFs and is also the transformed TRF. The TRF shows how precisely the test measures at various levels of θ.

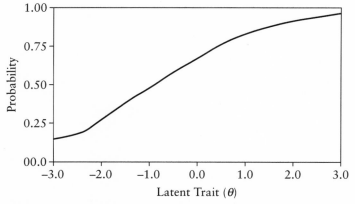

Figure 4   Test response function (TRF) for the four items of Figure 1

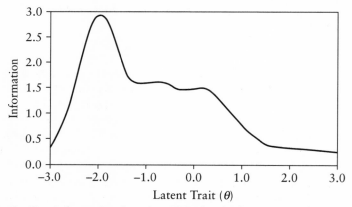

Figure 5   Test information function (TIF) for the four items of Figure 1

Finally, the reciprocal of the square root of the elements of the TRF results in the test SEM function, which describes the standard error of measurement that would result for various levels of θ, assuming the IRT model. Note that the test SEM function shown in Figure 6, which uses the items shown in Figure 1, indicates that—in contrast to CTT—the SEM for this test differs considerably at different levels of θ. Thus, IRT allows the test user to obtain estimated standard errors of measurement from the test SEM function for a set of test items at all levels of θ without administering those items as a test—all that is required is an IRF for each item.

The information/SEM functions of IRT permit a test constructor to design a test for a particular purpose. For example, a particular

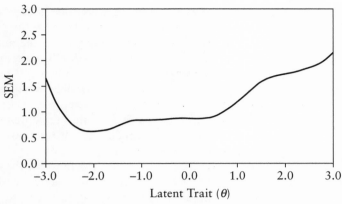

Figure 6 Test standard error of measurement (SEM) function for the four items of Figure 1

applied problem might require a test that screens out individuals whose scores are below a particular score level and simultaneously identifies individuals whose scores are above a different score level. Such a test might be used to identify those individuals who are underqualified or overqualified for a particular training program. Appropriate consideration of the measurement requirements of this situation would result in a test with an information function that peaks at both the lower and upper cutoff values on the trait continuum. Once the shape of the target information function is determined, the test constructor can use trial and error to select items from an item bank with estimated IRT item parameters to obtain the target information function. Alternatively, the test constructor might use one of an increasing number of computer-based procedures designed to select items algorithmically from an item bank in order to create a test with a specified information function (e.g., De Gruijter, 1990) while satisfying content and other considerations (e.g., Stocking, Swanson, & Pearlman, 1993; Swanson & Stocking, 1993). The result will be a test that is designed with its precision placed along the trait continuum at the point or points where maximum discrimination between individuals is required.

Estimating Trait Levels of Individuals

A major advantage of IRT over CTT is that it does not depend on the number-correct score. In its place, IRT uses trait-level estimation procedures that use all the information in each person's pattern of responses to the test items—that is, it takes into account which items were answered correctly and which were answered incorrectly—and considers the difficulties, discriminations, and guessing parameters of the items when estimating trait levels. As a consequence, the number of items in a test does not limit the range of test scores. Rather, in IRT, the number of possible test scores (i.e., trait-level estimates) is related to the number of *patterns* of responses that are possible in a given set of test items. Thus, for dichotomously scored items, the number of possible response *patterns* is 2^k, where k is the number of items in a test. As a consequence, IRT allows for much finer distinctions to be made in describing individual differences on a given trait.

Trait-level estimation using IRT begins with the IRFs for the items in the test. These IRFs are then considered in conjunction with the responses given by the examinee to the items. For example, suppose that Examinee A answered the four test items in Figure 1 with the response pattern 1, 1, 0, 0, where 1 indicates a correct answer and 0 an incorrect answer. To estimate this examinee's trait level using maximum likelihood estimation, the appropriate IRFs for this response pattern would be identified. Specifically, because the first and second items were answered correctly, the IRFs shown in Figure 1 for those items would be used. Because the examinee answered Items 3 and 4 incorrectly, however, the appropriate IRF is the probability of answering these items *incorrectly*. This probability is determined by subtracting the probabilities in Figure 1 from 1.0 for each of these two items. The result would be a "mirror-image" decreasing IRF that represents the probability of an incorrect response.

An assumption of IRT is that test items are *locally independent*. This means that the only correlation that exists among the test items is due to the latent trait(s) that they have in common—that is, that there are no extraneous factors affecting their intercorrelations. In the case of the unidimensional IRT models, local independence is usually assumed to hold if factor analysis of the test items results primarily in a single factor (Hambleton & Swaminathan, 1985, chap. 2). When test items are locally independent, their IRFs can be multiplied. Because IRFs are probability functions, their multiplicative product is a likelihood function.

Figure 7 shows the likelihood function that results from the response pattern 1, 1, 0, 0 to the four test items for Examinee A. Note that θ is on the horizontal axis of this function. The vertical axis is the likelihood of the response pattern. Thus, the values of the function for a specific value of θ indicate the likelihood that this response pattern to this particular set of items was the result of each value of θ. The question to be answered in estimating θ is, Which value of θ was *most likely* to have resulted in this pattern of response to this set of test

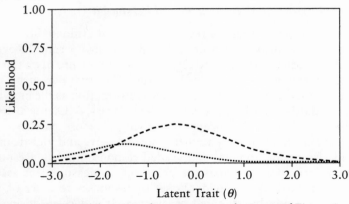

Figure 7 Likelihood functions for response to the items of Figure 1

- - - - Examinee A's response pattern of 1, 1, 0, 0
·········· Examinee B's response pattern of 1, 0, 0, 1

items? The statistical procedure that answers this question is called *maximum likelihood estimation*. Simply stated, the purpose of maximum likelihood estimation is to find the maximum of a likelihood function, such as that shown in Figure 7. Although the statistical procedures are complex (Baker, 1992, chaps. 3, 4), examination of Figure 7 shows that the maximum of the function for Examinee A is at approximately $\theta = -.4$. Thus, this value of θ represents the person's trait-level estimate because it is the most likely value of θ that would result in this response pattern, given the IRT model.

Figure 7 also shows the likelihood function for a different pattern of responses to the same four test items (i.e., 1, 0, 0, 1). Examinee B answered items 2 and 3 incorrectly, and items 1 and 4 correctly. Note that the likelihood function has its maximum at a different value of θ (−1.4), indicating that Examinee B's trait-level estimate is lower than Examinee A's (because B correctly answered one more difficult item), even though both obtained a number-correct score of 2 on the four items. Note also the differences in the peakedness of the two likelihood functions; this aspect of maximum likelihood estimation of θ is discussed below.

An additional advantage of maximum likelihood estimation in IRT is that it is *item independent*. This means that a person's trait level can, in principle, be estimated with any subset of items that are calibrated on the same scale, and the result will be essentially the same θ estimate (within sampling error). This property of IRT scoring procedures lays the groundwork for the fruitful marriage of IRT and adaptive testing procedures.

Individual Errors of Measurement and Person Fit

In addition to permitting the test constructor to evaluate how a test will measure at various levels of θ, IRT models also permit the evaluation of individualized standard errors of measurement after a test has been administered to a particular individual. The two-parameter normal ogive model defines response pattern information as the individualized standard error of measurement (Bejar, Weiss, & Gialluca, 1977; Samejima, 1973a). The concepts underlying response pattern information extend to the three-parameter normal ogive and logistic models, and also to the nominal and graded response models. Response pattern information describes the precision of measurement associated with a particular individual's set of responses to a set of IRT items with previously estimated parameters. It is derived during the process of maximum likelihood estimation of θ, and is related to the peakedness of the likelihood function. Because the reciprocal of the square root of information is expressible as a standard error of measurement, this permits individualized standard errors of measurement to be attached to a particular person's responses to a particular test instrument.

For the two likelihood functions in Figure 7, for example, there is a higher likelihood that Examinee A's θ level is between -1.5 and $+3$ than there is for Examinee B's to be in that θ interval. Throughout this range, Examinee A's θ estimates are, therefore, more likely, given the IRT model. Thus, because of the relationship between the height of the likelihood function and the precision of estimation, these two likelihood functions show that the confidence interval for estimating θ is smaller for Examinee A than it is for Examinee B. Therefore, Examinee A's θ estimate is more precise (i.e., has a lower observed SEM) than Examinee B's.

These standard errors of measurement, derivable from the likelihood function, are essentially independent of those for other individuals measured at the same time as a given individual because they depend solely on the individual's responses and the item parameter estimates that were derived previously from a reference group. Consequently, the result is a truly individualized standard error of measurement, in contrast to the group-dependent CTT SEM.

The idea of response pattern information is closely related to the concept of model fit. Response pattern information will be low if an individual's responses to a set of test items do not conform to the IRT model (e.g., Examinee B in Figure 7). Information will be high when the responses are consistent with the model (e.g., Examinee A). This concept of model fit has given rise in IRT to a subfield of research concerned with the fit of person data to a specified IRT model. This field has been referred to as *person fit* (Reise, 1990), *appropriateness measurement* (Drasgow, Levine, & McLaughlin, 1987), or *caution indexes* (Tatsuoka, 1984). All of these indexes are concerned with determining the fit of an individual's responses to an IRT model. They go well beyond the concept of response pattern information and should eventually, given a research base and development of appropriate indices, allow for the diagnosis of reasons that an individual does not respond in accordance with a specified model (e.g., Trabin & Weiss, 1983; Wright & Stone, 1979). Such reasons include cheating, malingering, warm-up effect, fatigue, and other currently unobservable influences on the precision of measurement.

The net effect of the further development of these person-fit indexes will be to allow users of psychological test data to identify individuals for whom the precision of measurement is higher (those with lower errors of measurement) and those for whom precision is lower (those with higher errors of measurement). Again, this has important practical implications for the use of psychological test data and individual differences research that will be discussed below.

The field of person-fit research has also led to an emphasis on the person in IRT that has not been a part of the historical development of either CTT or IRT. Since the mid-1950s, the emphasis in IRT has been on tests and test items, rather than on individuals. The new emphasis on person-fit has resulted in the development of models that add parameters for individuals, such as a person discrimination parameter, which is closely analogous to the idea of person-fit (e.g., Kiley, 1992; Strandmark & Linn, 1987). Eventually, these ideas will likely permit the estimation of a person guessing parameter for any responses in which guessing is possible.

ADAPTIVE TESTING

Basic Concepts

The field of psychological testing, the applied areas of individual differences, and research in individual differences have depended almost exclusively throughout the twentieth century on conventional psychological tests. In a conventional test, a set of test items is selected in advance to constitute a measuring instrument that will measure a particular psychological trait. All questions in that instrument are administered to every individual who takes that test. Only a few exceptions, such as the intelligence tests based on Alfred Binet's test model and a few other individually administered tests of that type, have not used the conventional testing approach.

In contrast, the Binet types of intelligence tests are *adaptive tests* (Weiss, 1985). In an adaptive test, test items are selected during the process of test administration for each individual being tested. Adaptive tests are designed to allow the test administrator to control the precision of a given measurement and to maximize the efficiency of the testing process. In the Binet test, items are classified during the process of development with respect to *mental age levels*. These levels correspond to increasing levels of item difficulty. When administering a Binet-type test, the test administrator begins test administration at whatever mental age level the examinee appears to be functioning. Items are scored as they are administered, and when all items at a given mental age level have been administered, the test administrator determines whether additional items are needed.

If the examinee answers some of the items at a given mental age level correctly, testing continues with items of either a higher or a lower mental age level. If none or only a few of the items are answered correctly, easier items are administered to that examinee. If all or most of the items have been answered correctly, more difficult items are administered. Test administration continues until two mental age levels are identified: one at which the examinee answers all items incorrectly (the ceiling level) and one at which the examinee answers all items correctly (the basal level). In between the ceiling and basal level is the effective range of measurement for that individual. The result of this adaptive item selection process is that individuals with different trait levels will be administered items at different difficulty levels. For example, consider the case of two children aged 10. One examinee may receive items ranging from mental age 10 to mental age 14. The other examinee may answer all items at age 10 incorrectly and, consequently, may receive test items ranging from mental age 10 to mental age 5.

The Binet tests have all the characteristics of an adaptive test. These include the following:

• *A previously calibrated pool of test items.* To create an adaptive test, test items must previously be administered to a group of individuals, and item difficulty and other data must be obtained on the items. An adaptive test based on IRT, for example, will use an item pool in which items have been previously calibrated for item difficulty, discrimination, and pseudoguessing parameters.

• *A procedure for item selection.* Because items are selected based on an examinee's answers to previous items, items must be scored as they are administered. Successive items to be administered are then based on how the examinee answered previously administered items.

- *A method of scoring the test.* Because the purpose of test adminis-̇ tration is to obtain a test score on an individual, the procedure for adaptive testing requires not only that items be scored as they are administered but also that a test score of some type be determined at multiple points during the process of test adminis- tration, or at least at the end of the test administration procedure.

- *A procedure for terminating the test.* In contrast to a conven- tional test, the number of test items is not fixed in an adaptive test. Thus, in a Binet-type test, an individual may receive test items from as few as two mental age levels to as many as eight or nine, depending on the individual's performance on the test.

IRT and Adaptive Testing

Research since the 1970s has shown that adaptive testing procedures are most effective when combined with IRT procedures (e.g., Kingsbury & Weiss, 1980, 1983; McBride & Martin, 1983). Thus, an item bank for use in adaptive testing can be calibrated according to an IRT model. The point at which a test is to be initiated, referred to as the *entry point*, can be determined by taking into account individual status vari- ables or other data about an individual (e.g., previous test scores, age, school grades). Explicit procedures for estimating an entry point for an adaptive test are available in conjunction with IRT, using Bayesian statistical methods (e.g., Baker, 1992, chap. 7; Weiss & McBride, 1984).

IRT procedures for estimating an individual's θ level are applicable to the adaptive testing process. Procedures of maximum likelihood or Bayesian estimation permit estimation of θ levels based on one or more responses made by a single individual in an adaptive test. Thus, a con- tinuous updating of θ can be accomplished after each item is adminis- tered in an adaptive test, and the successive items to be administered can be based on the θ estimate derived from all previous items administered.

Item selection rules derived from IRT and adaptive testing can ex- plicitly use the concept of item information (Hambleton & Swaminathan, 1985, chap. 6; Weiss, 1985). Thus, at a given current θ estimate, the most informative item not yet administered can be cho- sen for administration. When items are selected using this maximum information item-selection rule, the net effect is an extremely efficient procedure for reducing the error of measurement at each successive stage in the administration of an adaptive test (Weiss, 1985).

Finally, adaptive testing procedures developed in accordance with IRT can take advantage of a number of different procedures for termi- nating an adaptive test. Some of these procedures will be described below in the context of specific applied problems. One procedure frequently applied is to reduce the individualized SEM to a chosen level before a test is terminated. This may result in varying numbers of test items administered to different individuals, but it also can result in a uniform level of SEM for individuals tested. Thus, for the individual who responds essentially in accordance with the IRT model, a given level of SEM will be achieved more quickly than for the individual whose responses are not in accordance with the IRT model, thus resulting in a slower reduction of the SEM.

Computerized Adaptive Testing

Although individually administered tests are efficient and effective, they are labor intensive, requiring a highly trained test administrator to achieve necessary levels of standardization. When adaptive testing uses IRT, however, the calculations required at each stage of item selection would be impractical for a human test administrator to do. Under these circumstances, the adaptive test must be administered by interactive computers. Computerized adaptive testing, or CAT, provides the capability for administering items on an individual basis. Items are presented on the computer screen, and responses are entered on the keyboard or by a touch screen and are immediately scored by the computer. Various algorithms for selecting items according to maximum information or other criteria are then implemented using the computational capabilities of the computer (e.g., Vale & Weiss, 1977; Weiss, 1985), and, typically in less than a second, another item is then selected for administration and presented on the screen. Meanwhile, the computer continually updates the person's estimated θ level—again using IRT methods—and continually monitors the appropriate termination criterion. Once this criterion is reached, the test is terminated and appropriate messages to the examinee, including a score, if appropriate, are presented on the computer screen. The practicality of CAT for everyday testing applications has increased with the availability of fast microcomputers. Within the last 10 years, commercially available software for implementing IRT-based CAT has been developed and upgraded (Assessment Systems Corporation, 1987), and tests such as the Graduate Record Examination are now available as CATs.

Figures 8 and 9 show the record of two individuals proceeding through an IRT-based CAT. The X plotted for each individual is the individual's current θ estimate after each item is administered. The vertical bars above and below the X show the observed SEMs associated with the θ estimate. For Examinee A, shown in Figure 8, who responds in reasonable accordance with the IRT model, the test could

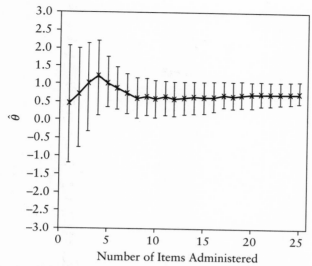

Figure 8   θ estimates and SEM bands from a CAT administered to Examinee A

be terminated after 25 items. Note that the change in successive θ estimates continues to reduce as each new item is administered, until the θ estimate stabilizes. In addition, the observed SEM continues to reduce as new items are administered until it, too, shows little change. Examinee B's responses, shown in Figure 9, are in less accordance with the IRT model for this set of items, so the reduction in the SEM is slower. For Examinee B, the SEM band at 25 items is approximately twice what it is for Examinee A. Assuming that the SEM observed for Examinee A was at the minimum level required to terminate the test, Examinee B might need an additional 15 or more items to reach the specified level of precision needed to terminate the test.

Research has shown that adaptive tests are more efficient than conventional tests (e.g., Brown & Weiss, 1977; McBride & Martin, 1983); that is, a given level of measurement precision can be reached much more quickly in an adaptive test than in a test in which all individuals are administered the same items. This is because the adaptive test selects the items that are most informative for each individual at each stage of test administration. Typical adaptive tests result in average reductions in number of items administered of 50%, and some reductions in the range of 80% to 90% have been reported, with no decrease in measurement quality (Brown & Weiss, 1977). In addition, adaptive tests allow control over measurement precision. Thus, adaptive tests result in measurements that are both efficient and effective.

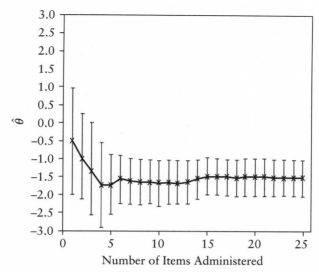

Figure 9   θ estimates and SEM bands for a CAT administered to Examinee B

SOLVING TWO IMPORTANT MEASUREMENT PROBLEMS WITH IRT AND CAT

Longitudinal Measurement

One of the most difficult problems in the measurement of individual differences is that of longitudinal measurement. This involves measuring individual change associated with growth, stability, or decline. In the context of CTT, the procedures available for measuring change result in paradoxes that essentially nullify efforts designed to do so.

Consider the problem of measuring growth using CTT. Assume that the growth occurs from Time 1 to Time 2 and that some level of change, on the average, is to be expected. Procedures of CTT require that a set of items be constructed to measure at a given level of difficulty. Thus, if the problem were to measure changes in spelling ability from fifth grade to eighth grade, for example, a set of test questions would be selected to measure at the level of fifth grade for the Time 1 measurements. At Time 2, most of the class would be expected to function at the level of eighth grade, so the items that constitute the Time 2 test should be those of approximately average difficulty for an eighth grader.

The measurement of individual change or growth, however, requires tests that are parallel. *Parallel tests* in CTT are defined as tests that have the same mean and standard deviation and are highly correlated

(Gulliksen, 1950). In the present example, if the tests have the same mean and standard deviation (on the underlying trait scale, not on the number-correct scale), they would both be measuring at either the fifth-grade level or at the eighth-grade level. Thus, for measuring change, it is not possible to have parallel tests with the same mean and standard deviation on the underlying trait.

To obtain reliable change scores in CTT, the two measurements must represent the same variable and at the same time be highly correlated (e.g., Feldt & Brennan, 1989, Equation 30). If the tests are highly correlated, this implies no change in individual differences from Time 1 to Time 2, although a mean difference is possible. Thus, individuals must retain their relative rank ordering in the two time periods in order for reliable individual change scores to be computed. As a consequence, the very process involved in the construction of tests using CTT in order to obtain reliable individual change scores negates the possibility of obtaining those change scores.

IRT, on the other hand, particularly when combined with CAT, permits a viable solution to the problem of measuring change, growth, or decline at the individual level. Recall that IRT assumes that item parameters are invariant within a linear transformation. By the process of linking, item parameters estimated on a group at one level of a given trait can be transformed to those of a group at another level of the trait. Thus, to create a scale that extends along the grade level continuum for spelling ability, for example, IRT parameter estimates on a set of items would be determined for the grade five group. Then, using an appropriate IRT linking procedure (Vale, 1986), parameter estimates on an eighth grade set of items, including an anchor test of the fifth grade items, would be estimated on an eighth grade group. Based on the difference observed on the common group of anchor items, the parameter estimates from one of the grade groups would be transformed onto the scale of the other grade group. If intermediate groups are included, such as grades six and seven, linking can be performed across each of the grade groups to develop a scale or metric that spans the range from grade five through grade eight.

Because the parameter estimates for each of the items included in both tests are now on the same scale, trait estimates derived from those items will also be on the same scale. For example, on the average, fifth graders will obtain ability estimates on spelling ability on the low end of the scale created by the linking. However, there may be some fifth graders who score as well as seventh or eighth graders. Conversely, eighth graders will obtain higher average scores on the scale, although individual differences can occur so that some eighth graders will score as low as the average level for fifth graders.

Once the linking has been completed, an efficient procedure for determining change or growth in spelling ability can be implemented using procedures of CAT. Because CAT recognizes and adapts to individual differences and trait levels during the process of item administration, testing would proceed on an individualized basis. In the absence of other information on their spelling ability, adaptive testing might start all fifth graders at the average difficulty level of items for fifth graders. However, during the process of test administration, the adaptive test would quickly adapt to the individual differences that exist among fifth graders. Thus, if a fifth grader answers all the items at the fifth-grade level correctly, she or he will rapidly begin to receive test items at levels between fifth grade and eighth grade. A very capable fifth grader will quickly be administered items increasing in difficulty through sixth-, seventh-, and eighth-grade levels. Conversely, a less able fifth grader who is operating essentially at the fifth grade level will receive items typically answered correctly by fifth graders. Using the termination criteria of adaptive testing, a test would be administered at Time 1 that measures each fifth grader to a prespecified level of precision.

As students proceed through sixth, seventh, and eighth grades, additional spelling tests can be administered and a profile of growth (or decline) in spelling ability can be developed for each student. IRT procedures make measurement on a common scale possible, and the CAT procedure makes test administration efficient. For example, at grade six, the same bank of precalibrated test items is available for the measurement of each student. But the computer will "remember" which questions each student has answered and what their final ability estimate and its standard error was. The adaptive item selection algorithm can be programmed to ignore items that were previously administered to a given examinee, and it also can use the point at which the individual terminated the test at the previous testing as the starting point for item selection.

The CAT procedure continues at each successive grade level, beginning each new adaptive test at the trait level previously exhibited by the student, ignoring previously administered items, and terminating when a measurement of sufficient precision has been reached. Alternatively, the procedure could be programmed to terminate when either one of two conditions has occurred: (a) a gain (or loss) in trait level has been noted or (b) no gain or loss can be detected. Although appropriate statistical theory has not yet been developed for making these decisions, a *significant* gain could be defined as a difference in two successive trait levels, taking into account their standard errors, that exceeds the two standard error bands placed around each θ estimate. No gain would be defined as a lack of difference after a sufficient number of items had been administered.

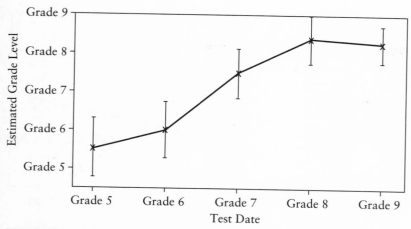

Figure 10 θ estimates and SEM bands on a five-occasion adaptive self-referenced test for Student A

For example, consider the student whose spelling level in fifth grade was at the average level of a seventh grader. When the sixth grade test is administered to that student, rather than starting at their current grade level of sixth grade, the test would start at their previously estimated seventh-grade ability level. If the student's spelling ability had not increased during the intervening year, the result will be a test score similar to what was obtained at the first testing, but based on a nonoverlapping set of items.

Figure 10 illustrates a testing sequence of this type for Student A; each plotted X and its standard error band represents the terminal θ estimate resulting from a CAT such as that illustrated in Figures 8 and 9. Note that the standard error of the ability estimate at the grade six testing for Student A is smaller than it was at grade five, indicating that there is greater certainty in that θ estimate when the student was in grade six than when she or he was in grade five. For Student A, who ended the grade five test with an ability estimate between the fifth-grade and sixth-grade levels, the sixth grade test would start at perhaps the upper range of the error band associated with the ability estimate obtained in fifth grade. For this student, a gain in spelling ability was noted and recognized by the adaptive testing procedure at the grade seven test administration; the result is an ability estimate for Student A that is between the seventh- and eighth-grade levels. A similar gain (but with an overlapping error band) is noted for Student A at the eighth grade testing, but no change was observed between the eighth and ninth grade testings. The tests administered to Examinee A required a total of only about 100 items across the five test administrations, or an average of 20 items per test, due to the efficiency of the CAT procedure.

New Methodological Concepts

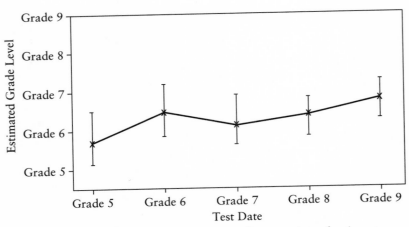

Figure 11   θ estimates and SEM bands on a five-occasion adaptive
self-referenced test for Student B

For Student B, as can be seen in Figure 11, no significant change in
estimated spelling ability was observed from grades five through nine.
Although there was an apparent increase in estimated ability between
grades five and nine—from slightly below grade six at the grade five
testing to about grade six and one-half at the grade nine testing—the
overlap of the SEM bands for these two θ estimates suggests that the
observed difference in the θ estimates was the result of chance measurement fluctuations and not real differences in ability levels for this
examinee.

This procedure for adaptively measuring change has been termed
adaptive self-referenced testing (Weiss & Kingsbury, 1984). Adaptive
self-referenced testing uses all the power of IRT and CAT to measure a
single individual efficiently and effectively. It is called *self-referenced*
to differentiate it from testing procedures that are *norm-referenced* or
criterion-referenced. As can be seen from the procedure, the measurement of change for an individual is determined with reference only to
that individual; hence, the measurements are self-referenced. The only
point at which data on other individuals is used, as in all aspects of
IRT, is in the procedure for estimating the item parameters and linking
those parameters to the common growth scale. The scoring procedure
at each measured time point is based on the individual's responses to
the items administered by the CAT procedure, in conjunction with the
item parameters. The measurement of change or growth, using the
individualized standard errors of measurement at each time point, can
be referenced only to a particular individual with the eventual development of appropriate statistical theory for making these decisions.

Thus, the procedure can, conceptually at least, identify people who have experienced growth or learning on a trait, no growth, or a pattern of decline.

This kind of measurement is not possible in CTT, yet it is characteristic of many research problems in the measurement of individual differences, particularly in developmental and educational areas. In developmental psychology, a variety of procedures has been proposed for measuring change as a developmental variable (Collins & Horn, 1991), but these are primarily concerned with group change rather than change at the individual level. By combining the power of IRT and CAT, adaptive self-referenced testing permits the measurement of growth without the problems and paradoxes that result from using CTT.

Determining Differences Between Individuals and Differences Within Individuals

For many applications in the measurement of individual differences, it is frequently important to determine if two or more individuals differ on a particular measurement. For example, in selecting individuals for a particular program or experience, it is important for an individual differences psychologist to know whether one individual has a higher score than another individual or individuals.

Using CTT, scores of two individuals can be compared to determine which is higher. But observed scores are imperfect indicators of true latent scores, even in CTT. Thus, procedures for estimating true scores in CTT, and associated standard errors, have been developed. However, as indicated earlier, the SEMs in CTT are group dependent. Thus, if one individual is measured in the context of one group and another individual is measured in the context of another group with a different trait level, the SEMs will not be comparable. In addition, CTT SEMs do not vary as a function of trait level, yet the information functions of IRT and their associated SEM functions show that a given test can measure with different precision at different trait levels (e.g., Figures 4, 5, and 6). Thus, with CTT, a psychologist can compare the number-correct (or estimated true) scores to determine which examinee has the higher score. But taking into account the SEMs associated with those scores will possibly result in erroneous conclusions.

IRT provides a procedure that could be used to determine whether two individuals differ on a given test and to make that determination more accurate. As indicated earlier, an individualized standard error of measurement is associated with an IRT trait estimate. Each individual measured will have a given trait estimate and his or her own standard error associated with it. CAT can be used to control the magnitudes of the standard errors for a given level of θ by varying the number of items administered to an individual.

One IRT-based procedure for determining whether two individuals differ on a given test would be to administer a test to the second individual using adaptive procedures designed explicitly to determine whether these two individuals differ. The procedure would be similar to administering a Time 2 test in adaptive self-referenced testing; that is, the adaptive test for the second (or succeeding) individuals would be designed to continue only as long as is necessary to determine whether the two individuals differ.

Two individuals can conceptually be said to differ when the two standard error bands surrounding their trait estimates do not overlap. In the case of two individuals whose trait levels are quite disparate, a decision of this type could be made rather quickly, because the SEM bands for the second individual will fall below those of the first individual quite rapidly. When two individuals are close in trait level, the testing time necessary to distinguish between them could be considerably longer. Again, appropriate statistical theory needs to be developed to determine when two individuals differ, taking into account the errors of measurement associated with their trait levels.

This process could even be extended to simultaneous testing of two individuals, where the adaptive testing procedure is designed to control test administration to two individuals simultaneously. In this procedure, the length of the tests for both individuals would be dynamically adjusted during the testing process as the computer program kept track of the trait levels and standard errors of each of the two individuals. Testing would terminate when it became clear that the two individuals differed in trait level, or when it became clear that they did not.

The procedures for determining whether two or more individuals differ are similar to procedures proposed earlier for what has been called *adaptive mastery testing* (Kingsbury & Weiss, 1983). In this procedure, an individual is tested against a fixed cutoff score. Testing for the individual continues only as long as is necessary to determine whether the individual is below or above the fixed cutoff. These procedures have been shown to be another important application of IRT and adaptive testing to the measurement of individual differences (Weiss & Kingsbury, 1984). The procedure for comparing two individuals is analogous, except that the cutoff score is considered to be measured with error and is operationalized as the first individual's score, against which the second individual's measurements are to be compared.

A similar application can be conceptualized for IRT and CAT for a single individual to answer the question of whether the individual significantly differs on elements of a profile of test scores. For example, consider the vocational counselor who has measured an individual on a multifactor ability battery. The measurements result in a profile on, say, nine traits. The counselor needs to know which is the examinee's highest trait and which traits differ from each other.

The current state of CTT does not permit a clear answer to this question. Although, again, CTT SEMs can be computed for each of the trait levels, these SEMs do not necessarily represent the correct SEMs for that individual. As a consequence, the counselor can simply interpret the observed differences on the profile with no statistical confidence.

IRT, possibly in conjunction with CAT, can provide a solution to this problem, again contingent on the development of appropriate statistical theory. This solution again uses the individualized SEMs available from IRT and perhaps the control of those SEMs derivable from CAT. CAT can be used in this case to make SEMs as small as possible so that confident conclusions can be drawn about the differences among elements of a multifactor profile for an individual. The sampling theory for these differences is more complex and may take longer to develop because it will need to take into account the intercorrelations among the profile variables. But at least for initial purposes, the profile of trait estimates with true individualized SEMs—and those SEMs made as small as possible by CAT—may facilitate the process of differentiating profile elements for a given individual. The result could be a much more useful set of multifactor measurements on a single individual for applied purposes.

SUMMARY

Although CTT has permitted the field of individual differences to develop greatly during the twentieth century, the combination of IRT and CAT will provide the impetus for a flourishing of the field during the twenty-first century. As described earlier, IRT and CAT permit solutions to a variety of important problems in the measurement of individual differences. As these technologies begin to be accepted by the measurement community and implemented by individual differences researchers, new applications of IRT and CAT will certainly develop, permitting solutions to other problems currently not fully addressed by classical test theory.

Research in individual differences is basic to the study of cognitive development. Thus, considerable effort is being expended in analyzing cognitive processes. IRT models for the analysis of response times, a variable frequently used in the field of cognitive processing, have been developed and will continue to be refined (e.g., Thissen, 1983).

These models are derivatives of the general IRT model and have all the power of their family relatives. Because cognitive process research is frequently done using computers, adaptive procedures will eventually be combined with IRT procedures to improve the measurement process and to make measurements more efficient.

One final area of application in the field of individual differences has to do with the apparent merger occurring between cognitive processing and IRT models. The area of person fit (e.g., Dragsow et al., 1987; Reise, 1990), which has developed during the last decade, holds promise for this merger. For example, one important question in the application of multidimensional IRT models is which multidimensional model is appropriate for a given application. Because procedures of model fit developed for dichotomous IRT models are generalizable to multidimensional models, it is possible to hypothesize various multidimensional models for IRT analysis that represent various cognitive processes. For example, multidimensional IRT models have been characterized as compensatory or noncompensatory (Sympson, 1978). Under a compensatory model, higher levels on one trait can compensate for lower levels on another trait. In a noncompensatory model, such compensation does not occur. For example, in an arithmetic story problem, a noncompensatory model appears to be more appropriate than a compensatory model, because no level of arithmetic ability will compensate for an inability to comprehend the verbal presentation of the problem.

The answer to the question of which model is more appropriate for a given set of abilities in the solution of a given problem is a question of cognitive processing. By hypothesizing compensatory and noncompensatory models at the individual level and analyzing model fit for individuals to these two competing models, conclusions could begin to be drawn about which cognitive processing model—compensatory or noncompensatory—is used by a particular individual in the solution of particular cognitive processing problems (i.e., ability tests). When combined with the procedures of adaptive testing to make the testing process more efficient, the use of such person-fit procedures could facilitate the understanding of how individuals respond to ability test items in terms of the cognitive processing model that underlies those responses.

IRT and CAT are fields of psychometric development that should greatly facilitate research in individual differences. As these models become further refined and applied in a variety of applications and research studies, new insights will emerge that were previously obfuscated by the earlier psychometric models and conventional testing procedures. Other applications and new models will also undoubtedly be developed over the next several decades.

REFERENCES

Andrich, D. (1978a). A rating formulation for ordered response categories. *Psychometrika, 43,* 561–571.

Andrich, D. (1978b). Application of a psychometric rating model to ordered categories which are scored with successive integers. *Applied Psychological Measurement, 2,* 581–594.

Andrich, D. (1988). The application of an unfolding model of the PIRT type to the measurement of attitude. *Applied Psychological Measurement, 12,* 33–51

Andrich, D. (1989). A probabilistic IRT model for unfolding preference data. *Applied Psychological Measurement, 13,* 193–216.

Assessment Systems Corporation. (1987). *Manual for the MicroCAT testing system* (3d ed.). St. Paul, MN: Author.

Baker, F. B. (1992). *Item response theory: Parameter estimation techniques.* New York: Marcel Dekker.

Bejar, I. I. (1977). An application of the continuous response level model to personality measurement. *Applied Psychological Measurement, 1,* 509–521.

Bejar, I. I., Weiss, D. J., & Gialluca, K. A. (1977). *An information comparison of conventional and adaptive tests in the measurement of classroom achievement* (Research Rep. No. 77–7). Minneapolis: University of Minnesota, Department of Psychology, Psychometric Methods Program, Computerized Adaptive Testing Laboratory.

Bejar, I. I., & Wingersky, M. S. (1982). A study of pre-equating based on item response theory. *Applied Psychological Measurement, 6,* 309–325.

Bock, R. D. (1972). Estimating item parameters and latent ability when responses are scored in two or more nominal categories. *Psychometrika, 37,* 29–51.

Brown, J. M, & Weiss, D. J. (1977). *An adaptive testing strategy for achievement test batteries.* (Research Rep. No. 77–6). Minneapolis: University of Minnesota, Department of Psychology, Psychometric Methods Program, Computerized Adaptive Testing Laboratory.

Carlson, J. E. (1987). *Multidimensional item response theory estimation: A computer program.* (Research Rep. No. 87–19). Iowa City, IA: American College Testing Program.

Collins, L. M., & Horn, J. L. (1991). *Best methods for the measurement of change: Recent advances, unanswered questions, future directions.* Washington, DC: American Psychological Association.

Crocker, L., & Algina, J. (1986). *Introduction to classical and modern test theory.* New York: Holt, Rinehart and Winston.

Cronbach, L. J., & Furby, L. (1970). How should we measure "change"—or should we? *Psychological Bulletin, 74,* 68–80. Errata, *Psychological Bulletin,* 1970, *74,* 218.

De Gruijter, D. N. M. (1990). Test construction by means of linear programming. *Applied Psychological Measurement, 14,* 175–181.

Drasgow, F., Levine, M. V., & McLaughlin, M. E. (1987). Detecting inappropriate test scores with optimal and practical appropriateness indices. *Applied Psychological Measurement, 11,* 59–79.

Feldt, L. S., & Brennan, R. L. (1989). Reliability. In R. L. Linn (Ed.), *Educational measurement* (pp. 105–146). New York: Macmillan.

Ghiselli, E. E., Campbell, J. P., & Zedeck, S. (1981). *Measurement theory for the behavioral sciences.* San Francisco: Freeman.

Gulliksen, H. (1950). *Theory of mental tests.* New York: Wiley.

Hambleton, R. K., & Swaminathan, H. (1985). *Item response theory: Principles and applications.* Boston: Kluwer-Nijhoff.

Jansen, P. G. W. (1984). Relationship between the Thurstone, Coombs, and Rasch approaches to item scaling. *Applied Psychological Measurement, 8,* 373–383.

Kiley, G. L. (1992). *The robustness of item and person parameter estimates to variation in person discrimination in the two-parameter logistic model.* Unpublished doctoral dissertation, University of Minnesota, Minneapolis.

Kingsbury, G. G., & Weiss, D. J. (1980). *An alternate-forms reliability and concurrent validity comparison of Bayesian adaptive and conventional ability tests* (Research Rep. No. 80–5). Minneapolis: University of Minnesota, Department of Psychology, Psychometric Methods Program, Computerized Adaptive Testing Laboratory.

Kingsbury, G. G., & Weiss, D. J. (1983). A comparison of IRT-based adaptive mastery testing and a sequential mastery testing procedure. In D. J. Weiss (Ed.), *New horizons in testing: Latent trait test theory and computerized adaptive testing* (pp. 257–283). New York: Academic Press.

Lord, F. M. (1980). *Applications of item response theory to practical testing problems.* Hillsdale, NJ: Erlbaum.

Masters, G. N. (1982). A Rasch model for partial credit scoring. *Psychometrika, 47,* 149–174.

McBride, J. R., & Martin, J. R. (1983). Reliability and validity of adaptive ability tests in a military setting. In D. J. Weiss (Ed.), *New horizons in testing: Latent trait test theory and computerized adaptive testing* (pp. 223–236). New York: Academic Press.

Mokken, R. J., & Lewis, C. (1982). A nonparametric approach to the analysis of dichotomous item responses. *Applied Psychological Measurement, 6,* 417–430.

Muraki, E. (1990). Fitting a polytomous item response model to Likert-type data. *Applied Psychological Measurement, 14,* 59–71.

Peterson, N. S., Kolen, M. J., & Hoover, H. D. (1989). Scaling, norming, and equating. In R. L. Linn (Ed.), *Educational measurement* (pp. 221–262). New York: Macmillan.

Rasch, G. (1980). *Probabilistic models for some intelligence and attainment tests.* Chicago: University of Chicago Press.

Reckase, M. D. (1985). The difficulty of test items that measure more than one dimension. *Applied Psychological Measurement, 9,* 401–412.

Reckase, M. D., & McKinley, R. L. (1991). The discriminating power of items that measure more than one dimension. *Applied Psychological Measurement, 15,* 361–373.

Reise, S. P. (1990). A comparison of person and item fit methods of assessing fit in IRT. *Applied Psychological Measurement, 14,* 127–137.

Reise, S. P., & Waller, N. G. (1990). Fitting the two-parameter model to personality data. *Applied Psychological Measurement, 14,* 45–58.

Samejima, F. (1969). Estimation of latent ability using a response pattern of graded scores. *Psychometrika Monograph* (No. 17).

Samejima, F. (1972). A general model for free-response data. *Psychometrika Monograph* (No. 18).

Samejima, F. (1973a). A comment on Birnbaum's three-parameter logistic model in the latent trait theory. *Psychometrika, 38,* 221–234.

Samejima, F. (1973b). Homogeneous case of the free-response model. *Psychometrika, 38,* 203–219.

Stocking, M. L., Swanson, L., & Pearlman, M. (1993). Application of an automated item selection method to real data. *Applied Psychological Measurement, 17,* 167–176.

Strandmark, N. L., & Linn, R. L. (1987). A generalized logistic item response model parameterizing test score inappropriateness. *Applied Psychological Measurement, 11,* 355–370.

Swanson, L., & Stocking, M. L. (1993). A model and heuristic for solving very large item selection problems. *Applied Psychological Measurement, 17,* 151–166.

Sympson, J. B. (1978). A model for testing with multidimensional items. In D. J. Weiss (Ed.), *Proceedings of the 1977 Computerized Adaptive Testing Conference* (pp. 82–98). Minneapolis: University of Minnesota, Department of Psychology, Psychometric Methods Program, Computerized Adaptive Testing Laboratory.

Tatsuoka, K. K. (1984). Caution indices based on item response theory. *Psychometrika, 49,* 95–110.

Thissen, D. (1983). Timed testing: An approach using item response theory. In D. J. Weiss (Ed.), *New horizons in testing: Latent trait test theory and computerized adaptive testing* (pp. 178–203). New York: Academic Press.

Trabin, T. E., & Weiss, D. J. (1983). The person response curve: Fit of individuals to item response theory models. In D. J. Weiss (Ed.), *New horizons in testing: Latent trait test theory and computerized adaptive testing* (pp. 83–108). New York: Academic Press.

Vale, C. D. (1986). Linking item parameters onto a common scale. *Applied Psychological Measurement, 10,* 333–344.

Vale, C. D., & Weiss, D. J. (1977). *A rapid item-search procedure for Bayesian adaptive testing* (Research Rep. No. 77–4). Minneapolis: University of Minnesota, Department of Psychology, Psychometric Methods Program, Computerized Adaptive Testing Laboratory.

Weiss, D. J. (1985). Adaptive testing by computer. *Journal of Consulting and Clinical Psychology, 53,* 774–789.

Weiss, D. J., & Kingsbury, G. G. (1984). Application of computerized adaptive testing to educational problems. *Journal of Educational Measurement, 21,* 361–375.

Weiss, D. J., & McBride, J. R. (1984). Bias and information of Bayesian adaptive testing. *Applied Psychological Measurement, 8,* 272–285.

Wright, B. D., & Stone, M. H. (1979). *Best test design.* Chicago: MESA Press.

Chapter 4

Extension of the MAXCOV-HITMAX Taxometric Procedure to Situations of Sizable Nuisance Covariance

Paul E. Meehl
University of Minnesota

THE PROBLEM OF MAXCOV-HITMAX IDEALIZATION

The MAXCOV-HITMAX taxometric procedure (Meehl, 1973; Meehl & Golden, 1982; Meehl & Yonce, 1995; various applications cited in Korfine & Lenzenweger, 1995; Lenzenweger, in press; Lenzenweger & Korfine, 1992; Meehl, 1992, p. 135; Nicholson & Neufeld, 1994; Waller, Putnam, & Carlson, 1994; and nonpsychopathology applications by Gangestad & Snyder, 1985; Strube, 1989) utilizes the manifest statistics among three fallible quantitative indicators to (a) infer latent taxonicity, (b) estimate latent parameters (e.g., taxon base rate, specificity and sensitivity at a cut), and (c) make Bayes-Theorem classifications of individuals, with corresponding diagnostic confidence statements. The procedure relies on a theorem that, absent nuisance correlation within the latent classes, the covariance $C_{yz}(x_i)$ of indicators y, z (*output pair*) computed on cases having a given score x_i on indicator x (*input indicator*) is a maximum when the x_i-interval is composed equally of taxon and complement (nontaxon) cases. This interval contains the x-value corresponding to the intersection of the two overlapping frequency functions, where ordinates $f_t(x)$ and $f_c(x)$ are equal; thus, it is the x-cut that minimizes misclassifications (= *hitmax cut* x_i locating the *hitmax interval* Δx_i); hence, the acronym MAXCOV-HITMAX. That is, we locate the hitmax cut on x by studying the behavior of the (yz)-covariance. While Monte Carlo runs and several real data studies show the procedure to be fairly robust under small or moderate departures from the strong auxiliary conjecture of zero nuisance covariance, this idealization is irksome and in some research situations cannot be well enough approximated to rely on robustness. This chapter derives a more general algorithm free of this idealizing conjecture, called *generalized* MAXCOV (no longer HITMAX, because the covariance-maximizing interval located is not necessarily that containing the hitmax cut).

GENERALIZED MAXCOV

The basic equation for deriving the MAXCOV algorithm (HITMAX or generalized) is a purely algebraic distribution-free decomposition identity—in fact, a set theoretical truism that holds even if the conjectured latent taxon has no real existence. In that situation, the search algorithm will reveal no clear maximum, and if a noise-determined pseudomaximum—a chancy or artifactual "highest local jog" in the covariance graph—were foolishly treated seriously, the several consistency tests we rely on will be violated, protecting against erroneous taxonic inference. (For a general theoretical and methodological discussion of the taxonicity conjecture and its testing, see Meehl, 1992.) This basic equation is, ignoring sampling error,

$$C_{yz}(x_i) = \quad pC_{yzt} + qC_{yzc} + p\,q\,(\bar{y}_t - \bar{y}_c)\,(\bar{z}_t - \bar{z}_c) \tag{1}$$

where

$C_{yz}(x_i) = \quad$ manifest (yz)-covariance of cases having a score x_i, hence, an empirical function of x;

$C_{yzt} \quad = \quad$ (yz)-covariance within the taxon, a constant;

$C_{yzc} \quad = \quad$ (yz)-covariance within the complement, a constant;

$\bar{y}_t,\ \bar{y}_c,\ \bar{z}_t,\ \bar{z}_c$ = means of the taxon and complement classes on indicators y and z, respectively;

$p,\ q \quad = \quad$ Proportions of the subset belonging to the taxon and complement classes, respectively.

   In the original MAXCOV-HITMAX procedure on the idealizing conjecture of no nuisance covariance ($C_{yzt} = C_{yzc} = 0$), the first two terms on the right vanish, so the left-hand manifest covariance equals the third term on the right. I call this the *validity mixture* term because its size depends on the two *crude validities* (mean taxon/complement differences, taken as constant absent sampling error or nontaxonic moderator effects) and the taxonic mixture $p{:}q$. If either the y or z indicator had zero taxonic validity, or if there were no taxon/complement mix (i.e., if $p = 0$ or $q = 0$), this validity mixture term would also vanish in any such population or sample. Since the validity mixture term is maximized when $p = q$, plotting the graph of the observable $C_{yz}(x_i)$ over x_i-intervals locates the hitmax interval by finding this graph's maximum. In that interval, $pq = \frac{1}{4}$, and knowing this allows us to solve for the mean difference product. Using that value, we can write quadratics in p_i for all other intervals, solve for p_i, and proceed as explained in Meehl (1973) to estimate all of the latent values.

If sizable nuisance covariance exists, the first two terms on the right do not vanish and the hitmax interval cannot be located by finding the empirical maximum of $C_{yz}(x)$ unless we know that the nuisance covariances are equal, whereby the sum $p_iC_{yzt} + q_iC_{yzc}$ is invariant over x-intervals. Even then, however, we cannot solve for the validity product because we cannot parse the right side into its nuisance covariance component and its validity mixture component. We can, however, proceed as follows: Choosing a cut at a sufficiently high value of x, we will have passed all or nearly all of the complement cases, so that cases lying above that cut will be nearly "pure taxon." Hence, in this region, the validity mixture term vanishes, as does the complement nuisance component, and only the component p_iC_{yzt} (where $p_i \approx 1$) remains, giving us an estimate of the taxon nuisance covariance. Similarly, we estimate the complement nuisance covariance from cases lying in the extreme low region of the x-distribution. Returning to Equation 1, designating the validity product as an unknown parameter θ

$$\theta = (\bar{y}_t - \bar{y}_c)\,(\bar{z}_t - \bar{z}_c), \text{ a constant} = K. \tag{2}$$

Simplifying subscripts as $\quad C_{yzt} = C_t,\ C_{yzc} = C_c$

and expanding Equation 1 in terms of $p_i (= 1 - q_i)$, we have (dropping the subscript i),

$$C_{yz}(x) = p(C_t - C_c) + (p - p^2)\,\theta + C_c \tag{3}$$

differentiating with respect to x and setting $= 0$ for a maximum,

$$\frac{dC(x)}{dx} = \frac{dp}{dx}(C_t - C_c) + \frac{dp}{dx}\theta - 2p\frac{dp}{dx} = 0 \tag{4}$$

dividing by $\dfrac{dp}{dx}$ $[\neq 0$ in region of interest$]$

$$(C_t - C_c) + \theta - 2p\theta = 0 \text{ at max} \tag{5}$$

so

$$p = \frac{\theta + (C_t - C_c)}{2\theta} \qquad \text{at max.} \tag{6}$$

At this maximum, $C_{yz}(x)$ has an observed numerical value, C_{max}. So at that value,

$$p(C_t - C_c) + p\theta - p^2\theta = C_{max} - C_c. \tag{7}$$

Plugging Equation 6 into Equation 7, we obtain

$$\left(\frac{\theta + (C_t - C_c)}{2\theta}(C_t - C_c)\right) + \left(\frac{\theta + (C_t - C_c)}{2\theta}\theta\right)$$
$$-\left(\left[\frac{\theta + (C_t - C_c)}{2\theta}\right]^2 \theta\right) + (C_c - C_{max}) = 0, \tag{8}$$

which, with some straightforward tedious algebra, yields

$$\theta^2 + (2C_t + 2C_c - 4C_{max})\,\theta + (C_t - C_c)^2 = 0 \tag{9}$$

a quadratic in θ. Its roots are

$$\theta = (2C_{max} - C_t - C_c) \pm 2\left[(C_t - C_{max})(C_c - C_{max})\right]^{1/2}. \tag{10}$$

This has the form

$$(a + b) \pm 2(ab)^{1/2} \tag{11}$$

since

$$a + b + 2(ab)^{1/2} = \left(a^{1/2} + b^{1/2}\right)^2 \tag{12}$$

and

$$a + b - 2(ab)^{1/2} = \left(a^{1/2} - b^{1/2}\right)^2 \tag{13}$$

the roots (Equation 11) are

$$\theta_1 = \left[(C_{max} - C_t)^{1/2} + (C_{max} - C_c)^{1/2}\right]^2 \tag{14}$$

$$\theta_2 = \left[(C_{max} - C_t)^{1/2} - (C_{max} - C_c)^{1/2}\right]^2. \tag{15}$$

Root θ_1 is selected by the physical situation that for the special case of zero nuisance covariance $C_t = C_c = 0$ it yields the correct value $\hat{K} = 4C_{max}$ in the hitmax interval, whereas θ_2 gives an impermissible $\hat{K} = 0$.

Having found θ, we proceed as in MAXCOV-HITMAX, using Equation 3 in each x-interval to get the interval's taxon rate p_i, the generalized quadratic algorithm for the taxon-proportion in an interval x_i being

$$p(x_i) = \frac{(K + C_t - C_c) \pm \sqrt{(K + C_t - C_c)^2 - 4K(C(x_i) - C_c)}}{2K}, \tag{16}$$

then $N_i p_i = N_{ti}$ the interval's taxon frequency, then $\Sigma N_{ti} = N_t$, and, finally, base rate $P = N_t/N$. The latent frequencies having been computed for each x-interval, we can obtain directly latent means, standard deviations, skewness, and kurtosis if desired. For any triad (x, y, z) of indicator variables, three MAXCOV procedures exist (using either x, y, or z as input indicator) and the three inferred latent distributions are thus obtained, as in MAXCOV-HITMAX.

ROBUSTNESS OF
THE ORIGINAL PROCEDURE

It is illuminating to ask why the original procedure is fairly robust under departures from the idealization of zero nuisance covariances within the categories (cf., even in my first technical report [Meehl, 1965, pp. 50–54], a reassuring numerical example for $r_t = .40$, $r_c = .20$; Meehl & Golden [1982, Table 5.2]; Meehl & Yonce [1995]). The General Covariance Mixture Formula for the observed (yz)-covariance in an x-interval includes the nuisance covariances

$$C_{yz}(x_i) = p_i C_t + q_i C_c + p_i q_i K$$

where K (treated as constant over intervals) is the product of the y and z separations, $K = (\bar{y}_t - \bar{y}_c)(\bar{z}_t - \bar{z}_c)$, and p_i, q_i are the taxon and complement proportions, respectively. Suppose the two nuisance covariances were equal, $C_t = C_c = C$, an auxiliary conjecture unlikely to be literally true in psychopathology but often an adequate approximation. Then the first two terms sum to $C(p_i + q_i) = C$, the neglected component being constant as we move through the intervals. The (erroneous, idealized) equation

$$C_{yz}(x_i) = K\, p_i q_i \tag{17}$$

employed instead of the correct relation

$$C_{yz}(x_i) = C + K\, p_i q_i \tag{18}$$

still locates the hitmax cut correctly by maximizing the variable term. However, solving for K via the hitmax interval relation $p_i = q_i = \frac{1}{2}$

$$C_{yz}(x_h) = \tfrac{1}{4} K \tag{19}$$

$$K = 4 C_{yz}(x_h) \tag{20}$$

yields an inflated estimate $\hat{K} > K$ [= true value of $\text{sep}_y \cdot \text{sep}_z$]. Relying on this erroneous $\hat{K}$ when we solve for the p_is in the other x-intervals, the quadratic algorithm (treating $C = 0$ again) is

$$p(x_i) = \tfrac{1}{2} \pm \left[\tfrac{1}{4} - \frac{C_{yz}}{\hat{K}} \right]^{1/2} \tag{21}$$

where the observed interval covariance is, in *latent* terms,

$$C_{yz}(x_i) = C + p_i q_i K \qquad \text{(true K)}. \tag{22}$$

Then our approximation for each p_i is

$$p_i = \tfrac{1}{2} \pm \left[\tfrac{1}{4} - \frac{C + p_i q_i \hat{K}}{C + \hat{K}} \right]^{1/2} \tag{23}$$

Rewriting the erroneous values in terms of two error multipliers $m(x_i)$ and M on K,

$$p_i = \tfrac{1}{2} \pm \left[\tfrac{1}{4} - \frac{p_i q_i \, m(x_i) \mathrm{K}}{\mathrm{MK}} \right]^{1/2} \tag{24}$$

where M is constant over x-intervals but $m(x_i)$ varies (since the fixed C added to the variable term $\mathrm{K} p_i q_i$ results in a varying *proportional* error), we have then for our taxon proportion estimate in each interval x_i

$$p(x_i) = \tfrac{1}{2} \pm \left[\tfrac{1}{4} - \frac{p_i q_i \, m(x_i)}{M} \right]^{1/2}. \tag{25}$$

The variable term is correct only at x_h, since in all other intervals $m(x_i)$ > M. We benefit from countervailing inflations in numerator and denominator, which partly explains the robustness, but $m(x_i)$ changes over intervals. In intervals other than the hitmax, the variable subtracted term is inflated; hence, the radicand is deflated. To the left of x_h, where one *adds* the radical to ½, one overestimates p_i. To the right of x_h, where the radical is *subtracted* from ½, p_i is underestimated. Hence, the values of $\hat{N}_{ti} = n_i p(x_i)$ are inflated in the region $x_i < x_h$ and deflated in the region $x_i > x_h$. For situations not too asymmetrical about hitmax (as when $P \doteq .50$), the sums of these opposite errors tend to cancel out in estimating $\hat{N}_t = \Sigma \hat{N}_{ti}$ from sums above and below x_h, and, hence, $\hat{P} = \hat{N}_t / N$ is not badly estimated. We note that when $P < .50$ (as is usual in psychopathology research), the asymmetrical countervailing errors lead to overestimation of the base rate P.

The somewhat surprising robustness of the original procedure under departure from the zero nuisance covariance idealization is illustrated in Table 1, based on error-free data (Gaussian table) for $\sigma_t = \sigma_c = 1$, separations $(\bar{y}_t - \bar{y}_c) = (\bar{z}_t - \bar{z}_c) = 2$, and five nuisance covariance configurations. As the preceding equations and text require, the peak covariance shifts toward the right whenever nuisance covariance is greater in the taxon than in the complement group, and more so for smaller base rates. That $C(yz)$ MAXCOV interval is, of course, not the hitmax interval unless the nuisance covariances are equal in taxon and complement. Even when the base rate is quite large (= .50), estimated $\hat{P}$ is unbiased when $C_t = C_c$. Large nuisance covariances and low base rate generates an upward bias in $\hat{P}$ that is unacceptably large ($\Delta\hat{P} = .07$), suggesting a need for the generalized procedure derived herein. The unavoidable tradeoff between bias (using the idealized procedure) and random sampling error (using the generalized procedure but often relying on somewhat unstable estimates of C_t and C_c) remains to be examined over the parametric configuration space. It is conceivable that a simple standard correction (downward) for situations where the MAXCOV graph strongly suggests a low P would do as well as the generalized, more elegant approach developed above.

Table 1 Error-Free MAXCOV Values With Various Combinations
of Nuisance Covariance

Configuration		Max(cov)			Maximum Interval			Estimated P		
Cov$_c$	Cov$_t$	$P=.50$	.25	.10	$P=.50$	.25	.10	$P=.50$	.25	.10
.00	.00	1.00	1.00	1.00	1.0	1.5	2.1	.49	.25	.10
.00	.25	1.13	1.13	1.13	1.1	1.6	2.2	.46	.23	.09
.25	.25	1.25	1.25	1.25	1.0	1.5	2.1	.49	.27	.14
.25	.50	1.38	1.38	1.38	1.1	1.6	2.2	.46	.26	.13
.50	.50	1.50	1.50	1.50	1.0	1.5	2.1	.49	.29	.17

Unfortunately, that question involves unsettled epistemological—not purely mathematical—issues in statistical inference theory (e.g., Bayesian rectangularity of priors).

ESTIMATING THE NUISANCE COVARIANCES

The use of Equation 3, as described above, requires that we have trustworthy estimates of the two nuisance covariances, as obtained from cases in the extreme (high and low) x-regions. Demarcating the "safe" x-regions is problematic, since we do not know how high a cut point must be to guarantee a negligible contamination of the taxon covariance estimate by the complement, and the same is true in the extreme low x-region. If we go out so far as to be very safe from taxon/complement mixture, the number of available cases in the demarcated region is dangerously small, except with very large initial samples. We have a tradeoff between random sampling error (demarcating a very extreme tail, and, hence, small N) and bias (systematic error due to appreciable complement class contribution to the manifest covariance). A rigorous analytic optimizing is presumably impossible without knowledge of the taxonic separation, and I have not tried to derive one since latent Gaussian distributions cannot be safely assumed in psychopathology and, in general, will be false.

With large samples, the obvious demarcation criterion would be the high (and low) x-regions where the observed (yz)-covariance has clearly become flat with changes in x. Because sampling error becomes important with a smaller number of cases, the covariances within successive x-intervals begin to fluctuate (apart from the systematic effect of decreasing taxon mixture) as we move out into relatively "pure" extreme regions far from the x-mean. Our problem is to decide when, in aiming to reduce random error by raising the N, we have located the upper cut so far down that undesired contribution by the complement class has become appreciable. I cannot currently offer a satisfactory answer to this. A crude nonparametric criterion would be the successive slopes of the interval covariance graph as we move downward. If the complement contribution is negligible in an x-region, increments and decrements of the (yz)-covariance will be random; hence, the slope *signs* (+) or (−) from interval to adjacent interval will be random. The probability of, say, three successive slopes being (− − −) is therefore $p = .125$, and, given a high prior that complement cases are being overtaken as we move down, this significance level might be a reasonable one at which to stop moving. Surely, we should stop at (− − − −), where $p < .07$. Or, looking at it the other way around, attempting a "positive" argument for minimal contamination (via a "positive" argument for flatness), one might set up a crude criterion of "near-zero" slope of adjacent line segments, say, $\Delta C_x = C(x_i) - C(x_{i+1}) \leq k$, then applying a sign test of "near-flatness" to the terminal segments. Another approach would be to define the x-intervals by blocks of equal frequency (deciles or, if N permits, vigintiles) and examine the Pearson rs in sets of adjacent blocks for homogeneity, testing their z_r-variance against the theoretical variance $\sigma^2 = (N - 3)^{-1}$. A third possibility asks, employing a suitable extrapolation algorithm, to what asymptote are the successive interval covariances converging as we move out? Perhaps a combination of procedures would be safest. Given thin data when far out, one must also hold down the effect of outliers (see, e.g., Cleveland, 1979, for an approach to this problem). It is reassuring that for sample size $N = 300$, $P = Q = \frac{1}{2}$, and a 2-*SD* taxon separation, the two top deciles will be about 98% uncontaminated by the complement class, providing 60 cases for estimating the nuisance covariance.

When $P \ll \frac{1}{2}$, as is the case in most psychopathology research, it is possible to demarcate a fairly large lower region of the x-distribution that will consist of nontaxon cases, with a subsample size permitting a trustworthy estimate of C_c. However, when the output covariance maximum (the taxonic "hump") is markedly displaced from center (due to small P), there may not be any flat x-region at the high side, and the graph may continue to fall or rise as we move farther out on x. In that situation, it may be appropriate to employ an extrapolation procedure, inferring the asymptote of $C_{yz}(x_i) = (p_i C_t + q_i C_c + p_i q_i K_{yz})$ as $p_i \to 1$, $q_i \to 0$, and $p_i q_i \to 0$. This asymptote estimates the desired nuisance covariance C_t for the taxon.

When the base rate is quite small (e.g., $P \leq .10$), the MAXCOV graph may not have a local maximum, since, unless the sample size is *very* great, there is not sufficient room far enough out to get past the hitmax interval (where $p_i \approx q_i$) so that the validity mixture term Kp_iq_i can begin to decline again. Error-free MAXCOV curves are shown in Figure 1. Nuisance covariance in the complement group is indicated

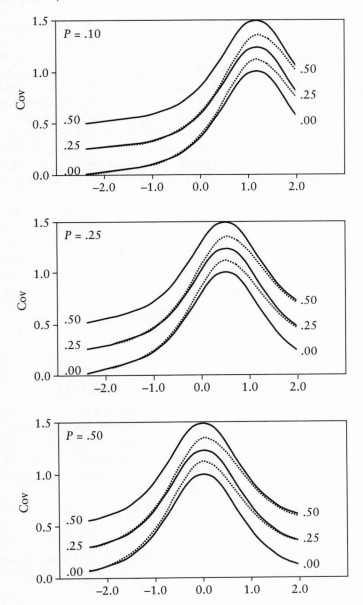

Figure 1   Error-free MAXCOV curves with different amounts
of nuisance covariance

at the left of the curves; taxon nuisance covariance is on the right. The MAXCOV peak shifts to the right with decreasing base rate (panels for $P = .50, .25, .10$) and also whenever there is greater nuisance covariance in the taxon group than in the complement (the latter situation is indicated by the dotted curves in each panel). Although a local maximum is clearly seen for the error-free curves in Figure 1, Monte Carlo runs on artificial data (incorporating random error) for $P = .10$ and a 2-SD separation may display either a (Tukey-smoothed) hump or a cusp (Meehl & Yonce, 1995). One cannot even be sure that $p_i \approx \frac{1}{2}$) in the "top" interval, since p_i may still be rising in the region; so $p_i q_i < \frac{1}{4}$, rather than $= \frac{1}{4}$ (as it is in a true hitmax interval where the taxon/complement mix is even).

My suggestion for this unfavorable case is an iterative bootstraps procedure, but I lack empirical evidence that it will work satisfactorily. The iterative sequence proceeds as follows. Writing the general covariance mixture equation for the observed x_i-interval covariance $C_{yz}(x_i)$ in latent terms,

$$C_{yz}(x_i) = p_i C_t + q_i C_c + p_i q_i K_{yz}, \tag{26}$$

we take as first approximation that the nuisance covariances C_t, C_c are equal $[= C_{yz}]$ and that the taxon proportion p_i in the C_{max} interval, whether a hump or a cusp, is $p_i = \frac{1}{2}$. Then

$$C_{yz(max)} = C_{yz} + \tfrac{1}{4} K. \tag{27}$$

To use this relation, we need to estimate the common covariance C_{yz}, which we achieve by calculating directly the observed covariance of the bottom half or third of the x-distribution, safely assumed almost wholly uncontaminated by taxon cases when the base rate is small and the maximum covariance is a hump or cusp located far to the right. Thus, if $N = 300$, there are 150 cases below the x-median, yielding a trustworthy "direct" estimate of $C_c (= C_{yz})$.

Putting this $\hat{C}$ in Equation 27 we solve for K,

$$\hat{K}_{yz} = 4(C_{max} - \hat{C}_{yz}). \tag{28}$$

Given these estimates $\hat{C}_{yz}$ and $\hat{K}$, writing the equation for each x-interval in the unknown p_i,

$$C_{yz}(x_i) = \hat{C}_{yz} + p_i q_i \hat{K}, \tag{29}$$

we solve for p_i, q_i per interval. In each interval, we compute the taxon *frequency* N_{ti}, given the interval's total frequency N (observed),

$$\hat{N}_{ti} = \hat{p}_i N_i \tag{30}$$

and $\hat{N}_{ci} = N_i - \hat{N}_{ti}.$ \hfill (31)

From these latent interval frequencies, we compute estimates of the latent means $\bar{x}_t$ and $\bar{x}_c$ and of the base rate $\hat{P}_x = \frac{1}{N}\overset{n}{\Sigma}\hat{N}_{ti}$ over all n-intervals.

Conducting this sequence with y as input and $C_{xz}(y_i)$ as output, we get another estimate $\hat{P}_y$, and of latent y-means $\bar{y}_t, \bar{y}_c$; similarly, we use z as input to get another estimate $\hat{P}_z$ and of the latent z-means $\bar{z}_t, \bar{z}_c$.

From the latent y- and z-means, we now *reconstitute* the $\hat{K}_{yz}$ (instead of inferring it from the observed (yz)-covariance with x as input) and, taking as a revised base rate estimate the average $\hat{P}_{yz} = \frac{1}{2}$ $(\hat{P}_y + \hat{P}_z)$, write a new grand covariance mixture equation for the *whole group* of cases,

$$C_{yz}(x) = \hat{P}_{yz}C_t + \hat{Q}_{yz}\hat{C}_c + \hat{P}_{yz}\hat{Q}_{yz}\hat{K}_{yz},\qquad(32)$$

now treating the taxon covariance as an unknown (hence, no carat on it in Equation 32) and solving for it (instead of assuming it $= C_t$).

Setting up equations analogous to Equation 32 with y and z as inputs, we obtain new approximations for C_{txz} and C_{txy} in the same manner. These values can then be employed in the generalized procedure described at the beginning of this chapter. If there is a MAXCOV "hump," that is clearly appropriate. If the graph is a cusp, we do not have an *observed* mathematical maximum, but relying on the error-free results, it may be safe to proceed as if the top interval is "like a maximum" for use of the generalized MAXCOV equation.

There is no vicious "circularity" here because we obtain the $\bar{y}_t, \bar{y}_c,$ $\bar{z}_t, \bar{z}_c$ components for reconstituting K_{yz} when we employ y and x as *input* indicators, but the $\hat{P}$ and $\hat{C}_t(yz)$ are inferred, employing the general equation with x as input variable. Since the formalism does not force convergence of these different epistemic paths to latent parameters, iterative agreement indicates the final estimates to be accurate and further corroborates the structural conjecture upon which the equations are predicated.

Estimating the two nuisance covariances is obviously a complicated, difficult matter that colleagues and I are currently exploring analytically and with Monte Carlo runs on artificial data. In this chapter, I have only sketched out what appear to be the main options. The availability and appropriateness of each undoubtedly depends on the parametric configuration, especially sample size, base rate, and taxonic separation—only the first of which is accurately known to the investigator. Assuming that the threshold question of taxonicity has been answered, one asks whether the MAXCOV graphs (three or more in number, e.g., 12 graphs given four indicators) display a flat region at the high end of the input variable. This inspectional impression must be corroborated by appropriate statistical tests (e.g., sign test on slopes of line segments, variance test on z_r-transformed (yz) correlations in the flat-looking x-intervals). If these tests indicate no change in the region, one concludes that the cases lying therein are almost "pure taxon," largely uncontaminated by complement class cases, so pooling these intervals one can compute C_t directly from the observations. In cases of low base rate, the iterative procedure may be an alternative. Monte Carlo investigation of estimating nuisance covariance with these procedures should provide more helpful guidelines for researchers.

I am grateful to Niels G. Waller and Leslie J. Yonce for helpful comments on this chapter, and to the latter for work on the chapter table and figure.

REFERENCES

Cleveland, W. S. (1979). Robust locally weighted regression and smoothing scatterplots. *Journal of the American Statistical Association, 74,* 829–836.

Gangestad, S., & Snyder, M. (1985). "To carve nature at its joints": On the existence of discrete classes in personality. *Psychological Review, 92,* 317–349.

Korfine, L., & Lenzenweger, M. F. (1995). The taxonicity of schizotypy: A replication. *Journal of Abnormal Psychology, 104,* 26–31.

Lenzenweger, M. F. (in press). Tracking the taxon: On the latent structure and base rate of schizotypy. In A. Raine, T. Lencz, & S. Mednick (Eds.), *Schizotypal personality.* New York: Cambridge University Press.

Lenzenweger, M. F., & Korfine, L. (1992). Confirming the latent structure and base rate of schizotypy: A taxometric analysis. *Journal of Abnormal Psychology, 101,* 567–571.

Meehl, P. E. (1965). *Detecting latent clinical taxa by fallible quantitative indicators lacking an accepted criterion* (Rep. No. PR–65–2). Minneapolis: University of Minnesota, Research Laboratories, Department of Psychiatry.

Meehl, P. E. (1973). MAXCOV-HITMAX: A taxonomic search procedure for loose genetic syndromes. In P. E. Meehl, *Psychodiagnosis: Selected papers* (pp. 200–224). Minneapolis: University of Minnesota Press.

Meehl, P. E. (1992). Factors and taxa, traits and types, differences of degree and differences in kind. *Journal of Personality, 60,* 117–174.

Meehl, P. E., & Golden, R. (1982). Taxometric methods. In P. Kendall & J. Butcher (Eds.), *Handbook of research methods in clinical psychology* (pp. 127–181). New York: Wiley.

Meehl, P. E., & Yonce, L. J. (1995). *Taxometric Analysis: II. Detecting taxonicity using covariance of two quantitative indicators in successive intervals of a third indicator (MAXCOV procedure).* Manuscript in preparation.

Nicholson, I. R., & Neufeld, R. W. J. (1994). *The problem of dissecting schizophrenia: Evidence for a dimension of disorder.* Manuscript submitted for publication.

Strube, M. J. (1989). Evidence for the *Type* in Type A behavior: A taxometric analysis. *Journal of Personality and Social Psychology, 56,* 972–987.

Waller, N. G., Putnam, F. W., & Carlson, E. B. (1994). *Types of dissociation and dissociative types: A taxometric analysis of dissociative experiences.* Manuscript submitted for publication.

Chapter 5

Peaked Indicators
A Source of Pseudotaxonicity
of a Latent Trait

Robert R. Golden and Mary J. Mayer
Albert Einstein College of Medicine

This chapter is based on the philosophical realists' view that an individual differences trait is a dispositional entity—often not directly observable and said to be "latent"—that causes a set of phenotypic indicators to be statistically intercorrelated across individuals (Meehl, 1986a; Tellegen, 1981). The researcher of individual differences traits in areas such as personality, behavior genetics, psychopathology, motivation, and the like often resorts to a statistical analysis of these associations to obtain a better understanding of the substantive nature of the trait. Although the set of conjectured indicators is often manipulated with regard to content, coverage, measurement, and so on, the primary interest is in the conjectured latent trait—usually regarded as the fundamental underlying causal factor. In this context, researchers such as Meehl and Golden have long been attempting to discover empirical criteria for distinguishing traits that are a matter of kind from those that are a matter of degree. This knowledge about a particular conjectured trait is critical to understanding its fundamental nature and also helps to settle issues regarding its measurement. In areas such as psychopathology and medicine, for example, clinicians and researchers alike wish to know if the fundamental causal factor underlying symptoms constituting an accepted behavioral syndrome such as autism in young children or clinical dementia in older adults is a matter of kind (produced by, for example, a gene, a virus, or a neurological or environmental threshold factor) or if it is a matter of degree (without a quasi-dichotomous effect on the indicators). Likewise, we often wish to test conjectures such as Meehl's (1962) that the trait

93

of schizotypy is partly a matter of kind because of the important role of a major gene in its etiology. Alzheimer's disease, believed to be one etiological cause of clinical dementia, has also been conjectured to have such a genetic taxonicity.

This problem of knowing if a trait is a matter of kind rather than a matter of degree is especially difficult at the beginning stages of research on a conjectured trait when there is no accepted criterion or standard that can be measured reliably and the only available indicators of the trait might be highly fallible.

In this chapter, we argue that for commonly used indicators in research on individual differences—those with ordered categories such as ratings and psychometric scales—it is sometimes difficult to distinguish a trait that is a matter of kind from one that is a matter of degree. When each indicator yields maximal discrimination with respect to the trait at approximately the same level of the trait, the set of indicators is said to be psychometrically *peaked*. In this situation, the precision of measurement as a function of trait level is not constant as is usually the case, but is a paraboliclike curve with a maximum at a middle value of the trait.

TWO KINDS OF LATENT TRAITS

In the framework of the realist, the question of whether a given latent trait underlying, say, the behavioral syndrome of clinical dementia is a matter of degree versus a matter of kind is not simply answered by fiat, but clearly it is an empirical one—about the real world. Specifically, it questions the existence of one or more natural categories of the trait that are often referred to as *natural subgroups* or *real types*. Following Meehl (1965), we prefer the use of the term *taxon* (and its plural *taxa*) over that of *subgroup* or *type*. By using the term taxon, we hope to convey the notion that we are referring to an entity, the latent trait, that is not arbitrarily defined—one that is quasi-dichotomous with respect to its effect on the indicators. Examples of such an entity include a gene, a germ, a basic lesion, or, as is more common (especially in traditional fields of individual differences), some sort of quasi-dichotomous threshold effect (environmental, learning, biological, and/or genetic) that results in a statistical clustering or association of the indicator scores. If a latent trait is such a quasi-dichotomous entity, we will call it dichotomously *taxonic*.

It is important to note that in the present framework it is the trait itself and not the set of indicators of the trait that has the property of taxonicity. More precisely, *taxonicity* refers to the nature of the causal effect of the trait on the indicators, that is, is it a smooth and continuous function (i.e., lacking a threshold) of the trait or is it discrete or discontinuous (i.e., with a threshold effect)? For example, the taxonicity of clinical dementia, which we will discuss further later in this chapter, has to do with the nature of a causal effect of a trait—neuronal loss or whatever may be the case—upon mental status, memory, and other similar indicators that are used for its diagnosis. However, even though such indicators have no role in the causal determination of the taxonicity of a trait, it is by analysis of the pattern of their statistical associations with each other that we hope to infer if the trait is taxonic or not.

QUASI-TAXONIC TRAITS
WITH THRESHOLD EFFECTS

In the field of medicine, there are many defects (neurological, physiological, structural, etc.) that are plausible candidates for taxonic threshold traits. As but one example, hypertension may be a taxonic trait—as it is closely associated with blood pressure—that has a threshold effect on such indicators as heart disease. In most traditional psychological domains of individual differences, we expect that a majority of taxonic traits will be of the threshold type.

Meehl has repeatedly made it clear that taxonicity itself is a matter of degree. In fact, there are relatively few conjectured latent traits that have a truly dichotomous effect on the indicators. We believe that most actual taxonic traits in traditional fields of individual differences, as well as in medicine and psychiatry, are probably quasi-dichotomous in that they are literally continuous but have ogival threshold effects that only approximate those of perfect step-function dichotomies, as illustrated in Figure 1. Although the causal effects of a perfectly dichotomous trait and those of a continuous trait with a perfect threshold are perfectly dichotomous, those for a quasi-taxonic threshold trait are ogival and can only approximate a step function.

PREVIOUSLY SUGGESTED CRITERIA
OF TAXONICITY

Statistical methods for the attempted detection of taxa usually analyze the statistical associations of the phenotypic indicators. If we are to use such a method to infer that a trait is either taxonic or dimensional, it is then necessary that the statistical associations of the indicators of a taxonic trait be generally distinguishable from those of a dimensional trait. An empirical criterion for taxonicity would involve specifying a set of such conditions regarding the associations of the indicator variables.

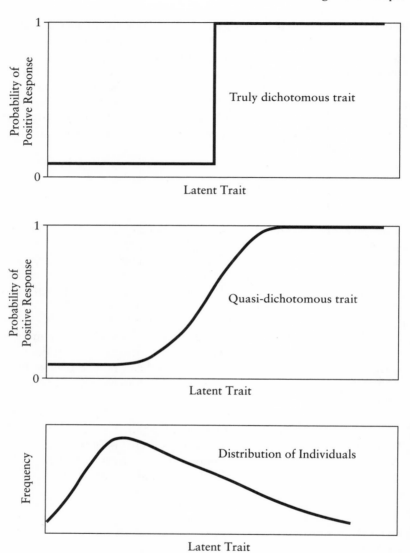

Figure 1   The indicator characteristic curve for a perfectly dichotomous
effect and for a quasi-dichotomous effect

A wide variety of taxometric methods has been developed by a number of researchers from various disciplines, usually for stated purposes
other than differentiating between taxonic and dimensional traits. These
include, to name but a few, the popular cluster analysis methods as
described by Fleiss and Zubin (1969), Blashfield (1976, 1984),

Blashfield and Aldenderfer (1978), Sneath and Sokal (1973), Mezzich and Solomon (1980), Hartigan (1975), Everitt (1980), and other prominent members of the Classification Society. These heuristic methods rest on plausible but arbitrary notions for characterizing taxa. Empirical trials of these methods suggest that they do not offer much promise for differentiating taxonic from dimensional traits (see Golden & Meehl, 1980). Attempts to explicate the notion of a taxon or type have been implicit in the development of more formal statistical models. The reasoning was intended to be simple: If the data for the indicator variables are closely fitted by such a theoretical model, then one can infer the existence of one or more taxa. The latent class models developed by Lazarsfeld and Henry (1968), Clogg (1977), Goodman (1975), Young, Tanner, and Meltzer (1982), Young (1983), Haberman (1979), Gibbons et al. (1984), and Rindskopf and Rindskopf (1986) posit that the indicators are uncorrelated within the taxon and the taxon complement. That is, if a mixed population for which the indicators are positively correlated can be divided into two subpopulations in such a way that indicators are uncorrelated within each, then it would seem likely that such a division could only result for a dichotomous taxonic trait. The so-called normal "mixture models" described in Titterington, Smith, and Makov (1985), and in Everitt and Hand (1981; also see Day, 1969; Hasselblad, 1968) posit that the indicators are normally distributed within the taxon and within the complement—a situation that would succeed if the indicators are sums of many components that are mutually independent within the taxon and its complement. A mathematically sophisticated treatment by Bartholomew (1987) shows that many of these models are formally related to each other and to the factor analytic model.

A major concern in this kind of research is that a finding of a taxonomic entity be one we can believe, that is, not likely to be spurious. We wish to know if the observed statistical clustering of the indicator scores reflects an actual taxonicity or if it is merely a *pseudotaxon* produced by, say, measurement properties of the indicators. Even though a pseudotaxon is artifactual, that is, is not caused by a taxonic trait, it can have face validity, the appearance of cohesiveness, and make good intuitive sense.

Meehl and Golden attempted to develop methods (Golden, 1982; Golden & Meehl, 1978, 1979, 1980, 1991, 1992; Meehl, 1965, 1973a, 1978a, 1978b, 1979, 1986a, 1986b; Meehl & Golden, 1982) that would overcome an obvious shortcoming of the cluster methods, normal mixture methods, and latent class methods—their propensity for pseudotaxa. They proposed the use of strong tests of the assumptions underlying the model through making intramodel numerical point estimations or other risk-taking predictions (as advocated by Popper, 1962). Use of these tests, called *consistency tests* by Meehl (1965), is an important way that the mathematics of these methods differs from previous cluster, normal-mixture, and latent class models. Some of these tests have been extensively studied by the Monte Carlo method (Meehl & Yonce, 1994).

However, the development and use of consistency tests does not preclude the possibility that pseudotaxonicity accounted for the result of a pilot study that used certain dichotomous *Minnesota Multiphasic Personality Inventory* (MMPI) items as indicators to detect a purported "schizoid taxon" in a sample of psychiatric patients who were nonpsychotic (Golden & Meehl, 1979). Attempts by Nichols et al. (1985) and Miller, Streiner, and Kahgee (1982) to replicate the construct validity of the resulting indicator scale met with failure—an indication that the taxometric method used may have led to a pseudotaxon.

In an application of the latent class method to the syndrome of tardive dyskinesia in autistic children (Golden, Campbell, & Perry, 1987), a phenotypic clustering that agreed very well with a diagnostic category was detected. Furthermore, application of the method to sets of indicators of neonatal brain dysfunction in a large sample of high-risk infants (Golden, Vaughan, Kurtzberg, & McCarton, 1988) and to sets of indicator scales for 24 disorders such as depression, general disability, fear of crime, and vision impairment in a large sample of older adults living in the community (Golden, Teresi, & Gurland, 1984) also resulted in detection of phenotypic clusterings that corresponded closely to diagnostic categories. When we consider each of these studies in terms of what we know now, we must ask whether the diagnostic category corresponds closely to the presence of a dichotomous entity or whether these are merely pseudotaxa caused by peaked indicators.

Finally, the Mendelian latent structure analysis model—developed by Matthysee, Holzman, and Lange (1986)—is an extension of the latent class model to include various genetic parameters but is based on the same fundamental assumption of independence of two dichotomous indicators (diagnosis of schizophrenia and disturbed eye tracking) within each of the two taxonomic classes. For it, the authors suggest that the taxonomic classes correspond to the presence and absence of a "latent trait which is genetically transmitted." The investigators are careful to state that they use their model only for hypothesis generation in an exploratory context. We are unable to determine if their model fits the data well, in part because of properties of the indicators.

CLINICAL DEMENTIA:
A TAXONIC TRAIT OR A PSEUDOTAXON?

Let us give a complete description of one illustrative example where we are unable to tell if the taxometric method has detected an actual taxonicity or has led us to a pseudotaxon. Several researchers have proposed a genetic theory of Alzheimer's disease. In this theory, it is hypothesized that only a certain class of people—those with a particular genetic constitution—have any predisposition for Alzheimer's disease. If the specific etiology of Alzheimer's disease includes a single dominant gene, and the only indicators available are highly fallible phenotypic ones, we again have the problem of estimating the probability that a person carries this gene without a generally acceptable criterion variable or a definitive diagnostic touchstone, sign, symptom, or trait that can be reliably measured. Memory impairment, viewed as the primary indicator of Alzheimer's disease, is not sufficient by itself for taxonomic purposes.

We attempted to test for taxonicity by using a taxometric model to analyze mental status indicator items. In this taxometric analysis, the mental status item scores were analyzed for a sample of 408 individuals who were 80 years and older and living in communities in New York City. All were nondemented at the start of the study, but 32 received a diagnosis of clinical dementia one year into the study. The mental status exam used was developed by Blessed, Tomlinson, and Roth (1968) and consists of simple questions testing knowledge of the year, month, day, and name of current and past presidents, and the name, age, address, and length of residence of the subject. With this method, the individual's responses are scored as either correct or incorrect, according to agreement with an accepted criterion source. The test has face validity for clinical dementia to the extent that failure to answer such questions correctly is evidently often due to impairment of memory, intellectual functioning, or orientation. Earlier studies provide some empirical evidence of the validity of this type of test for clinical dementia and Alzheimer's disease.

The latent class model used for this analysis requires the use of dichotomous indicators. All indicators are coded 1 for positive and 0 for otherwise. This method has been described in detail in Golden (1982). The model is based on the assumption that the latent within-taxonomic class covariances are each zero; under this assumption, we are able to derive estimates of the latent taxonomic class base rates and the latent valid and false positive rates for each of the indicators.

The validity of the latent class model is checked by the use of model-based consistency tests. These tests provide estimates of the errors of the parameter estimates due to inferred "assumption departure," compare the consistency of two or more estimates of the same parameter, and evaluate the estimated validity of the indicator. A series of these consistency tests is used in the method in an iterative fashion: When an indicator fails a test, it is removed and is not used in the remaining calculations. The tests are repeatedly applied to the indicators, and those failing the test are removed until none of the remaining indicators fails any of the tests. The consistency tests are calibrated so that for these real and artificial data trials, the failure of one more of the consistency tests succeeds if, and only if, the parameter estimates are not accurate enough for taxometric purposes.

The method has been tested by several empirical trials. First, was a study for a nephrotic renal kidney disease in children (Freeman, 1981; Golden & Freeman, 1983), the results of which were very encouraging in that the estimates of the base rate and the indicator valid and false positive rates were always within two standard errors of the actual values (Golden & Freeman, 1983). In another (unpublished) empirical trial, MMPI items that were known to discriminate between the sexes and were in the Masculinity-Femininity scale were used in a pseudoproblem in an attempt to detect a known underlying taxonomy of biological sex (for a similar study, see Golden & Meehl, 1980).

Also, extensive Monte Carlo runs combining various latent parametric situations and a wide range of sample sizes were conducted. An important part of that procedure was to study how well the consistency tests detect sample results as untrustworthy—as giving the "wrong" answer. These Monte Carlo trials have shown that accurate parameter estimation requires at least five indicators with validities (valid positive rate less the false positive rate) of .40 or more; that for such a set of indicators and a sample size of 500, a taxon base rate of .10 or even .05 is not too low; that indicator correlations within taxonomic classes need only be less than .20; and, generally, that the consistency tests accurately warn us if parameter estimates are not sufficiently accurate. Some illustrative Monte Carlo runs are described in Table 1.

Starting with 28 items, the application of the method resulted in the selection of nine "superitems"; model estimates of the valid and false positive rates for these items are given in Table 2. Those indicators that were highly correlated within the derived taxonomic classes were disjunctively combined to form superitems. As can be seen in the table, the items concerning the presidents' names, the names of months given backward, and the date of World War II have the highest construct validities. Those items concerned with the age and name of subject; location of the testing place; current month, year, and time of day; and date of World War I have somewhat less but clearly substantial validities.

Table 1   Results of Monte Carlo Trials of Latent Class Model

Trial	N	Valid Positive Rate	False Positive Rate	Within-Class Correlation	Actual Base Rate	Estimated Base Rate	Consistency Tests
1	100	.50	.05	0	.10	.10	Passed
2	200	.50	.05	0	.10	.16	Passed
3	500	.50	.05	0	.10	.11	Passed
4	800	.50	.05	0	.10	.09	Passed
5	500	.50	.05	0	.05	.08	Passed
6	500	.50	.05	0	.10	.12	Passed
7	500	.50	.05	0	.30	.29	Passed
8	500	.50	.05	0	.50	.50	Passed
9	500	.60	.05	0	.10	.09	Passed
10	500	.50	.05	0	.10	.13	Passed
11	500	.40	.05	0	.10	.13	Passed
12	500	.60	.05	0	.10	.12	Passed
13	500	.50	.10	0	.10	.13	Passed
14	500	.40	.10	0	.10	.12	Passed
15	500	.30	.10	0	.10	.19	Passed
16	500	.50	.10	0	.10	.08	Passed
17	500	.50	.05	.10	.10	.08	Passed
18	500	.50	.05	.30	.10	.07	Passed
19	500	.50	.05	.50	.10	.10	Passed
20	500	.50	.05	.70	.10	.11	Passed

Table 2   Estimates of Valid and False Positive Rates

	Valid	False
1. Age and date of birth	.555	.032
2. Present month and year	.536	.022
3. Day of week	.218	.008
4. Present and past presidents	.807	.146
5. Date of World War I	.335	.015
6. Date of World War II	.645	.109
7. Months backward	.819	.110
8. Name and address	.630	.014
9. Object recall test	.413	.085
Base rate	.110	.890

The estimate of the taxon base rate was .109, with an estimated error due to assumption departure of −.030; the corrected value is .079. The estimated errors due to assumption departure for the valid and false positive rates were each less than .05. These error estimates are of the same level of magnitude as would result from sampling error if we could sample directly from the taxon and the complement. Most important, each of these parameter estimates was within two standard errors of the corresponding directly observed value for diagnosed clinical dementia.

We used Bayes' theorem to obtain an estimate of the model-based probability of each individual being a member of the taxon. For most individuals, the probability of belonging to the taxon was either very close to zero (0 to .05) or very close to one (.96 to 1.00). Our previous Monte Carlo study suggested that such a U-shaped curve showing the frequency distribution of the probability that individuals would be taxon members is indicative of a nonspurious taxonomy.

A basic assumption of the method is that the indicators are uncorrelated in the taxon and in the complement. It follows that these correlations should also be close to zero for those classified in the taxon and for those classified in the complement. These correlations are given in Table 3 and indicate that for the two classification groups, this condition is approximately true. These results further confirmed the validity of the model.

The agreement between the classification "in" versus "out" of the dementia taxon and subsequent early clinical diagnosis of clinical dementia is given in Table 4. Of the 408 individuals, 32 were clinically diagnosed as having clinical dementia (most with Alzheimer's disease and a few with multiple infarct dementia or with other organic dementia). Diagnoses were made within a few months of the administration of the mental status and memory tests, which were administered at the end of the first year of the study. For the 32 concordant cases, there was clear agreement (no near misses) for these individuals: The total mental status score was always 8 or greater, and the taxometric probability of misclassification was nearly always less than .10 and usually less than .05. A cut score of 8 is the one agreed upon by clinicians for a diagnosis of clinical dementia.

Possibly of the most interest are the 14 individuals who were classified by the method as in the dementia taxon but who were not diagnosed as having clinical dementia. Of these 14 individuals, 8 had total mental status scores of 10 and above, with taxometric probabilities of misclassification less than .05. A review of the assessment records of the evaluation one year into the study revealed that 5 of these 8 individuals were most likely in the early stages of clinical dementia. The remaining 6 individuals had total mental status scores of 8 to 10 and

Table 3   Correlation Matrices for the Two Classification Subgroups

					Indicator				
	1	2	3	4	5	6	7	8	9
1		−03	−02	−03	01	−07	08	10	00
2	00		14	04	−04	00	−00	−02	−05
3	31	14		02	−03	03	03	−02	−04
4	11	23	−06		02	03	07	01	01
5	−05	08	−05	16		14	04	−04	−05
6	−10	17	−10	−02	08		11	02	01
7	13	20	−01	−06	−13	01		−05	06
8	−14	00	09	13	−02	06	−32		09
9	05	00	17	10	−18	−26	09	15	

Note. Decimals are omitted.
Lower triangle is classified in taxon; upper triangle is classified in complement.

Table 4   Diagnosis and the Taxometric Classification

Taxometric classification	Clinical Diagnostics of Clinical Dementia		
	Present	Absent	Total
Taxon	32	14[*]	46
Complement	0	362	362
Total	32	376	408

[*]5 were probable dementias at follow-up interviews and another 6 were not followed up because of death (3) or other reasons (3).

taxometric misclassification errors of .10 to .50 when classifications were made with the taxometric method.

In addition to the 5 individuals who probably did have clinical dementia within the following year, dementia status for 6 could not be reassessed (3 had died, 3 had dropped out of the study). Reassessment of the remaining 3 individuals two years into the study did not show any clear evidence of clinical dementia. We conclude that for the 402 individuals for whom data are available, the two methods of diagnosis are consistent for all but 3 to 8 individuals (depending on the true taxonomic status of the 5 individuals who eventually experienced what was probable clinical dementia); that is, most of the 14 discordant individuals probably had preclinical dementia and were initially classified correctly by the taxometric method. This small number of discordant cases can be easily explained by the unreliability in each of the two methods of classification.

Thus, we see that this analysis resulted in the accurate detection of a well-known manifest clinical syndrome in its full-blown or nearly full-blown state—that of clinical dementia. This was not what we had expected. We were specifically interested in attempting to detect a taxonicity due to a major gene for Alzheimer's disease—a specific cause of clinical dementia. Clinical dementia itself is a different entity. It is a syndrome for which there are many known etiological antecedents and probably many more that are not fully understood. Conjectured and/or known organic etiologies of clinical dementia in addition to Alzheimer's disease include hereditary neurogenerative diseases such as Huntington's chorea, intracranial tumors, meningitis, deficiency diseases, metabolic disorders, and brain damage due to trauma, cerebrovascular accidents, enzyme deficit, or toxic substances. General cognitive impairment can also be due to functional disorders such as schizophrenia and depression, other organic brain disorders, drug toxicity, nutritional deficiencies, and general cognitive traits such as low intelligence and poor memory, as well as environmental conditions resulting in lack of education, poor understanding of the language used for the testing, and so on.

We believe that while it would be grossly incorrect to infer that the present clustering and good fit of the taxometric model is due to effects of a single major gene, it may be that it is the result of a taxonic threshold trait. That is, it is possible, although not known, that the syndrome of clinical dementia is a unitary trait that is taxonic—possibly a parameter of the brain having to do with the quantity or proportion of nonfunctional brain cells that has a threshold effect on mental status indicators. Or the clustering may be due simply to measurement properties of the indicators; that is, the set of selected indicators is peaked and led us to a pseudotaxon. Could this be because the mental status items were selected first by Blessed et al. because they maximally discriminated the diagnostic class for clinical dementia (which approximately correspond to a certain level of mental status or cognitive dysfunction) and next by the iterative process of the taxometric method to maximize internal consistency?

THE DEMENTIA TAXON:
A MORE PROMISING ANALYSIS

We have indicated that we suspected the above analysis may very well be misleading with regard to the true nature of a dementia taxon.

Seven years after performing the above analysis, what do we know currently about such a taxon? First, we should note that there is much disagreement in the geriatrics literature as to the relationship between dementia and normal aging. Are the differences primarily a matter of degree or a matter of kind? Is dementia a behavioral syndrome with a fundamental common neuropathway or underlying factor such as neuronal loss? As but one example of those who believe differences are merely a matter of degree, Brayne and Calloway (1988) state that

> in the community, 'normal ageing,' benign senescent forgetfulness, and Senile Dementia of the Alzheimer Type (SDAT) do not fall into discrete categories but appear to lie on a continuum. Although these groupings are useful for planning treatment, the cut-off points are arbitrary. (p. 1266)

They further suggest that the model of a continuum does not contradict the concept that normal aging is *successful* (i.e., having few or no brain lesions of the SDAT type), *usual* (having an intermediate number of lesions), or *unusual* (having a large number of such lesions).

As but one example of those taking an opposite view, Terry and Katzman (1983) noted that "all of the morphologic abnormalities [of SADAT]...are found, although to a much lesser degree in the brain tissue of wholly normal aged people. It seems probable, therefore, that the disease represents a threshold phenomenon" (p. 54), which is described by them as a condition for which clinical symptoms are not manifested until after a certain number of tissue alterations have occurred. They further suggest the theory that individuals have unique thresholds that are dependent on their *reserve capacities*—reserve capacity is based on the amount of redundancy in a person's neural circuits, which, in turn, is relative to the number of "active synapses subserving each cerebral function" (p. 54).

We have argued earlier that the question of whether dementia is a matter of degree versus a matter of kind is not simply answered by fiat through the method of measurement, but clearly it is an empirical one about the real world. The second theoretical view is stronger, as it is more amenable to the risk of refutation, and we attempted to use a new taxometric method (a modification of that described in Golden, 1991, 1994)—one that requires quantitative indicators—to test the threshold as conjectured by Terry and Katzman.

Underlying the neuropsychologic indicators such as memory and cognitive tests are, of course, a large number of possible major causal factors that may range from those that are of a quasi-dichotomous nature to those that are of a quasi-continuous nature. In the development of this method, we suggested that if the causal effect of such a threshold on the indicators is sufficiently strong—relative to other underlying causal factors—then it will be amenable to statistical detection and corroboration.

It is only necessary that the neuropsychological indicators have adequate discriminant validity for the neuronal threshold. It is then possible, on the basis of analysis of internal statistical relationships among them, to end up with approximate estimates of their validities (for the neuronal threshold) and of the base rate of dementia.

With this new method, we analyze the statistical regression of each indicator on each of the other indicators for a mixed sample of individuals—some who, according to the Terry and Katzman conjecture, exceed their neuronal threshold and others who apparently do not. Although the validity of this method rests squarely on that of an auxiliary assumption—that when they occur within the subpopulation of individuals who exceed threshold and within the complementary subpopulation, such regressions are linear (or of another specified form) with homoscedasticity of the residual variance—model-based methods of indirectly testing this assumption can be developed. So far, this model has been sufficiently encouraging, both in theoretical development and in empirical application, to warrant its use for the present problem. For example, for the present sample of older individuals, we can accurately detect the biological sex taxa using height and weight as indicators.

When we used this method to analyze various pairs of intelligence and memory tests administered at baseline (i.e., when none of the individuals met criteria in the *Diagnostic and Statistical Manual of Mental Orders,* DSM-III, for diagnosis of dementia), we detected a taxon with an estimated base rate of .40 to .45, such that classification of individuals "in" versus "out" of the taxon had an 83% agreement with the later clinical diagnosis of "dementia" versus "normal." For a small subsample, this classification agreed better with pathologic diagnosis at autopsy than did clinical diagnosis at some point before death. Survival analysis of the time from baseline to diagnosis of dementia provided a probability estimate of .51 ($SE = .05$) for an individual being diagnosed demented when followed for the full 10 years of the study (i.e., they did not drop out of the study due to death or other reasons), which is very close to the estimated taxon base rate, just as it should be.

For our present discussion, then, because this later analysis evidently has accurately detected the dementia taxon, we have strong evidence that the former analysis produced a pseudotaxon that was, indeed, quite misleading. One might argue that the former analysis is also correct, but that it detected another taxon—one having to do with the full-blownness of the dementia. However, in that event, the taxon is not an interesting one to us, and the present method does not corroborate its existence.

A MODEL OF A DIMENSIONAL TRAIT

Because a clearly valid statistical criterion of taxonicity has been difficult to attain, it might be helpful at this time to consider a model of a dimensional trait and contemplate how one might be misled by a pseudotaxon. We will present such a theoretical model and we will use it to argue that where each indicator yields maximal discrimination with respect to the trait at approximately the same level of the trait, it is probably difficult to distinguish taxonic threshold traits from dimensional traits. Such a set of indicators is said to be peaked because the precision of measurement as a function of trait level is not constant (as is usual), but is instead a paraboliclike curve with a maximum at a certain point of the trait. That is, the apparent taxonicity is caused by a property of the set of indicators and is not a property of the trait itself. For dichotomous indicators, this ambiguity exists partly because for each of the two kinds of latent situations, the proportion that is positive can be approximately the same ogival-shaped function of the trait. The term *peaked* is used in educational measurement research to refer to a test that has a much higher precision of measurement at a certain point on the test or the underlying latent trait (Lord, 1980). Suppose that a latent dimensional trait F is normally distributed and that fallible indicators X_i $(i = 1, 2, 3...,n)$ of it are also continuous. Suppose further, that each X_i is simply a linear function of the trait F and a normally distributed factor U_i:

$$X_i = A_i F_i + b_i U_i ,$$

where U_i is uncorrelated with F (for $i = 1, 2, 3,...n$) and each of the U_is are uncorrelated with each other. Such a hypothetical ideal situation is dimensional simply because the latent trait is continuous. It follows that the X_is have a multivariate normal distribution. There is not a single characteristic of this multi-indicator distribution that somehow could lead to a pseudotaxonicity—the variance of an indicator X_i conditioned on the trait F is constant, the standard error in the estimation of F from the indicator scores is constant, and so on. Nevertheless, we believe that this can happen easily once we dichotomize the X_i scores. This is because the proportion of the scores for X_i that exceed any cut C_i is not a linear but an ogival function of F, as shown in Figure 2, which has a point of inflection where its rate of change with

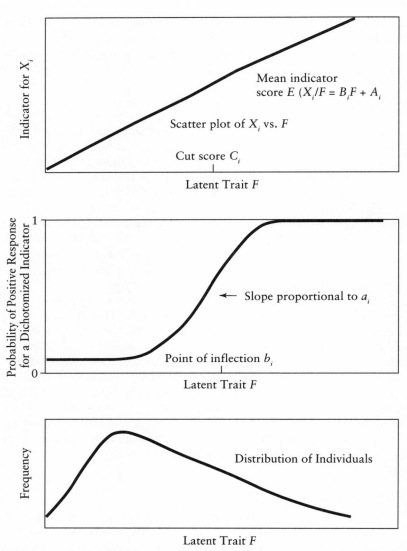

Figure 2   The continuous and dichotomous indicator characteristic curves for a dimensional trait F

respect to F is at a maximum. We see in Figure 2 that the curve for this ogival function has a very small positive slope for both low and high values of F, and that as F increases from low values to intermediate values, the slope increases at an increasing rate and reaches its maximum value at an inflection point $F = b_i$, where it begins to steadily decrease at a decreasing rate.

Such a model of dichotomous indicators is known as the *latent trait model*, and its use in item response theory has already been proposed for other purposes by Lord (1980), Lord and Novick (1968), Wright and Masters (1982), and Rasch (1960; see Hambleton & Cook, 1977, for a brief overview). In this model, the probability of a positive response or "indicator characteristic curve" is assumed to be a normal ogive function of the latent dimensional trait F,

$$(1/ \pi^{1/2}) \int_{-\infty}^{a_i (F - b_i)} \exp(- t^2 /2)dt.$$

The characteristic curve for an indicator i is a function of the two parameters denoted by a_i and b_i. The parameter a_i is proportional to the slope of the indicator characteristic curve at the point of inflection, which is the point where the ordinate (the probability of a positive response) is .50 and where the abscissa $F = b_i$. The latent variable F is defined, without loss of generality, to have a mean of 0 and a standard deviation of 1. The indicator b_i-value, which is usually between −3 and +3 units of F, is that point on the latent factor F at which the slope of the indicator characteristic curve is greatest, that is, where the indicator best discriminates higher from lower scores on F. The a_i-value—usually between 0 and 5—describes how discriminating the indicator is at the point of inflection, as it is proportional to the slope of the indicator characteristic curve at this point. The a_i-values and the b_i-values can be estimated by maximum likelihood methods, and, for each individual, the associated point on the factor F and its standard error can be estimated. Although for our purposes, the model consists of the assumptions of a single underlying factor and of monotonic indicator characteristic curves, it is often assumed for purposes of parameter estimation that at each point on the factor F, the positive responses to the indicators are pairwise independent.

Lord and Novick (1968) have shown mathematically that for a given set of continuous indicators, X_i, as described earlier, the set of cut scores can be determined such that when these indicators are so dichotomized, they have the same b_i-value (discriminate at the same point of the latent trait). They have also shown that each a_i-value is a monotonic function of the correlation of the continuous indicator X_i with the common factor or trait F. Thus, if the X_i indicators are highly correlated with the trait F, then the ogival shape will become close to that of a step function.

If the probability of a dichotomous indicator being positive is a linear function $c_i + d_i \text{pr}(X_i \geq C_i)$, then it approaches c_i for small values of F and approaches $c_i + d_i$ for large values of F. Thus, indicator characteristic curves that are not only ogival with respect to F but also have asymptotes of any magnitudes can easily be obtained by dichotomizing variables with a multivariate normal distribution.

PEAKED INDICATORS

If all of the indicators are rather sharply discriminating at about the same point on the latent dimensional trait, the set of indicators can be described as peaked. Within this model, it becomes obvious that if the indicators discriminate sharply enough at the same point on the latent dimensional trait, then the distribution for the total scale score (the sum of the dichotomous indicators) will be bimodal and will give the appearance of taxonicity. Grayson (1987) was one of the first to suggest the likelihood that this phenomenon makes it difficult, if not impossible, to distinguish categorical and dimensional views.

Further, from our theoretical model it can be seen that when indicators are sufficiently peaked, two latent subpopulations can exist that have relatively low indicator correlations within each. Both are defined by a cut at the abscissa of the common point of inflection. It is possible that such subpopulations generally satisfy taxonicity criteria that have been derived from taxometric models based on an assumption of independence of indicators within the taxon and within its complement. Such an assumption is made in most latent class and mixture models and in many of the early models developed by Golden and Meehl, but not in a method recently suggested by Golden (1994).

A proper selection of indicators may produce a scale that has uniform measurement error variance over a wide range of trait levels, whereas another selection of indicators can maximize the discrimination power of the scale over narrow range of level of the trait. If there are a large number of indicators, such as the items on a questionnaire or inventory, it is often possible to find one or more such subsets of items, each sufficiently peaked to produce a pseudotaxon. Eaves (1983) suggested that such properties of a scale can easily be engineered by the psychometrician. This means that for our purposes, any use of a peaked scale to detect a major gene must be considered suspect. Scales constructed for purposes of screening and/or diagnosis tend to be peaked (as they should be) and, therefore, when used to detect a taxon, will lead to ambiguous results.

In the typical situation, clinical psychologists have the job of assessing individual patients in order to decide which ones are at a sufficiently high level of the dysfunctional trait to receive a specific treatment. Because only fallible signs and symptoms of the trait are available to work with, it is impossible to avoid fallibility in the assignment of individual patients. After doing the best they can for a large number of patients, they may attempt to develop a scale that maximally discriminates between the two classes of patients. They may find that certain items work the best here—ones that make good sense to them—and they will focus attention on these symptoms in future patients. If they observe that patients tend either to have a fair number of these symptoms or not to have many at all, they may note the existence of an apparent clinical syndrome and begin to conjecture that there might be a dichotomous genetic or a biochemical dysfunction effect underlying the clinical syndrome. Finally, they turn to the statistician to analyze selected sets of symptoms for evidence of taxonicity, which is immediately forthcoming. The fact that the result could be a pseudotaxon is immediately evident.

As described earlier, peaked-indicator scales are often created by item selection, but they can also be the result of more subtle factors, such as when the symptoms selected are those that are, say, (a) perceived by the patient as serious enough to cause them to seek medical care or that interfere substantially with daily living, (b) used by the clinician as early signs of a dysfunction, or (c) perceived as manifest by the clinician or patient.

IMPLICATIONS FOR TAXOMETRIC RESEARCH

We have argued that for commonly used indicators with ordinal or nominal categories such as checklists, ratings, and questionnaire or test items and scales, it may be difficult to distinguish between the statistical associations of a dimensional trait and those of a taxonic trait. Although we have used an idealized model to illustrate the phenomenon of peaked indicators, we believe that indicators of actual traits are often peaked so as to behave in approximately the same manner.

In the earlier illustrative example of a taxometric analysis of indicators of clinical dementia, there remains a nagging suspicion that a pseudotaxon resulted from the indicators being peaked, even though the latent class model appeared to fit the data very well, the detected taxon was easily identified in terms of a plausible causal variable, and the values of the parameter estimates were in accord with those of a DSM-III diagnostic classification. We generated samples of artificial indicator scores according to the dimensional model so as to have values of the single and joint indicator population proportions that were the same as the actual sample proportions of the selected indicators. When these samples were analyzed by the latent class model, the results of the consistency tests and parameter estimations were indistinguishable from those of the actual data sample; that is, for a reasonable dimensional situation, the taxometric method produces a pseudotaxon.

In order to believe a detected taxon is the real thing, we must demonstrate that the indicators are not peaked. Evidently, the best way to solve this problem is to use continuous indicators that are obviously measured with the same precision at all levels, such as indicators that are measured in units such as weight, time, and distance, if at all possible.

SUMMARY

In this chapter, in order to simplify the discussion without losing generality, we restricted our discussion of dimensional traits to those that are said to be unidimensional and to taxonic traits that are quasi-dichotomous rather than polychotomous.

We emphasized that it is the trait that has the property of being taxonic or not. For example, the taxonicity of clinical dementia has to do with the nature of the brain and not with the nature of the mental status and memory test indicators used for its diagnosis. However, although the indicators, of course, have no role in the causal determination of the taxonicity of a trait, it is by analyzing the pattern of their statistical associations with each other that we hope to infer if the trait is taxonic or not.

We have suggested by means of a theoretical model that when each indicator yields maximal discrimination with respect to the trait at approximately the same level of the trait, taxonic threshold traits are currently difficult to distinguish from dimensional traits. In other words, a pseudotaxonicity can result when the measurement properties of the indicators of a dimensional trait are such that they are sufficiently peaked.

We suggest that by using indicators that are not peaked, we not only avoid the possibility of a pseudotaxon but also make it possible to demonstrate the impressive detection power of taxometric methodologies such as those developed and inspired by Meehl. For a specific taxometric method, the present conjectures regarding peakedness can easily be subjected to simulation tests.

REFERENCES

Bartholomew, D. J. (1987). *Latent variable models and factor analysis.* New York: Oxford.

Blashfield, R. K. (1976). Mixture model tests of cluster analysis: Accuracy of four agglomerative hierarchical methods. *Psychological Bulletin, 83,* 377–388.

Blashfield, R. K. (1984). *The classification of psychopathology: Neo-Kraepelinian and quantitative approaches.* New York: Plenum.

Blashfield, R. K., & Aldenderfer, M. S. (1978). The literature on cluster analysis. *Multivariate Behavioral Research, 13,* 271–295.

Blessed, G., Tomlinson, B. E., & Roth, M. (1968). The association between quantitative measures of dementia and of senile change in the cerebral grey matter of elderly subjects. *British Journal of Psychiatry, 114,* 797–811.

Brayne, C., & Calloway, P. (1988, June 4). Normal ageing, impaired cognitive function, and senile dementia of the Alzheimer's type: A continuum? *The Lancet,* 1265–1267.

Clogg, C. C. (1977). *Unrestricted and restricted maximum likelihood latent structure analysis: A manual for users.* [Working Paper 1977-04]. University Park, PA: Population Issues Research Office.

Day, N. E. (1969). Estimating the components of a mixture of normal distributions. *Biometrika, 56,* 463–474.

Eaves, L. J. (1983). Errors of inference in the detection of major gene effects in psychological test scores. *American Journal of Human Genetics, 35,* 1179–1189.

Everitt, B. S. (1980). *Cluster analysis* (2d ed.). New York: Halstead Press.

Everitt, B. S., & Hand, D. F. (1981). *Finite mixture distributions.* London: Chapman and Hall.

Fleiss, J. L., & Zubin, J. (1969). On the methods and theory of clustering. *Mutivariate Behavioral Research, 4,* 235–250.

Freeman, K. (1981). *Classification of patients with nephrotic syndrome.* Unpublished doctoral dissertation, Columbia University, New York.

Gibbons, R. D., Dorus, E., Ostrow, D. G., Pandey, G. N., Davis, J. M., & Levy, D. L. (1984). Mixture distributions in psychiatry research. *Biological Psychiatry, 19,* 939–961.

Golden, R. R. (1982). A taxometric model for detection of a conjectured latent taxon. *Multivariate Behavioral Research, 17,* 389–416.

Golden, R. R. (1991). Bootstrapsing taxometrics: On the development of a method for detection of a single major gene. In W. M. Grove & D. Cicchetti (Eds.), *Thinking clearly about psychology* (Vol. 2, pp. 259–294). Minneapolis: University of Minnesota Press.

Golden, R. R. (1994). *A regression-mixture model for detection of a quasidichotomous factor underlying a syndrome or disease.* Research Reports. New York: Biometrics Unit, Albert Einstein College of Medicine. Manuscript in preparation.

Golden, R. R. (1994). In pursuit of a gold-standard: Using fallible indicators to study the taxonicity of a behavioral syndrome. Manuscript in preparation.

Golden, R. R., Campbell, M., & Perry, R. (1987). A taxometric method for diagnosis of tardive dyskinesia. *Journal of Psychiatric Research, 21,* 101–109.

Golden, R. R., & Freeman, K. D. (1983). *Taxometric diagnosis of a latent disease without use of a criterion variable.* (Report No. B-34). New York: Columbia University, School of Public Health.

Golden, R. R., & Meehl, P. E. (1978). Testing a dominant gene theory without an accepted criterion variable. *Annals of Human Genetics, 41,* 507–514.

Golden, R. R., & Meehl, P. E. (1979). Detection of the schizoid taxon with MMPI indicators. *Journal of Abnormal Psychology, 88,* 217–233.

Golden, R. R., & Meehl, P. E. (1980). Detection of biological sex: An empirical test of six cluster methods. *Multivariate Behavioral Research, 15,* 475–494.

Golden, R. R., Teresi, J. A., & Gurland, B. J. (1984). Development of indicator scales for the Comprehensive Assessment and Referral Evaluation Interview Schedule. *Journal of Gerontology, 39,* No. 2, 138–146.

Golden, R. R., Vaughan, Jr., H. G., Kurtzberg, D., & McCarton, C. M. (1988). Detection of neonatal brain dysfunction without the use of a criterion variable: Analysis of the statistical problem with an illustrative example. In P. Vietze & H. G. Vaughan, Jr. (Eds.), *Early identification of infants at risk for mental retardation* (pp. 71–95). Orlando, FL: Grune and Stratton.

Goodman, L. A. (1975). A new model for scaling response patterns: An application of the quasi-independence concept. *Journal of the American Statistical Association, 70,* 755–768.

Grayson, D. A. (1987). Can categorical and dimensional views of psychiatric illness be distinguished? *British Journal of Psychiatry, 151,* 355–361.

Haberman, S. J. (1979). *Analysis of qualitative data, Vols. 1 and 2.* New York: Academic Press.

Hambleton, R. K., & Cook, L. L. (1977). Latent trait models and their use in the analysis of educational test data. *Journal of Educational Measurement, 12,* 75–96.

Hartigan, J. A. (1975). *Clustering algorithms.* New York: Wiley.

Hasselblad, V. (1968). Estimation of parameters for a mixture of normal distributions. *Technometrics, 8,* 431–444.

Lazarsfeld, P. F., & Henry, N. W. (1968). *Latent structure analysis.* Boston: Houghton Mifflin.

Lord, F. M. (1980). *Application of item response theory to practical testing problems.* Hillside, NJ: Erlbaum.

Lord, F. M., & Novick, M. R. (1968). *Statistical theories of mental test scores.* Reading, MA: Addison-Wesley.

Matthysse, S., Holzman, P., & Lange, K. (1986). The genetic transmission of schizophrenia: Application of mendelian latent structure analysis to eye tracking dysfunction in schizophrenia and affective disorder. *Journal of Psychiatric Research, 20,* 57–76.

Meehl, P. E. (1962). Schizotaxia, schizotypy, schizophrenia. *American Psychologist, 17,* 827–838.

Meehl, P. E. (1965). *Detecting latent clinical taxa by fallible quantitative indicators lacking an accepted criterion.* (Report No. PR-65-2). Minneapolis: University of Minnesota, Reports from the Research Laboratories of the Department of Psychiatry.

Meehl, P. E. (1973a). MAXCOV-HITMAX: A taxonomic search method for loose genetic syndromes. In P. E. Meehl (Ed.), *Psychodiagnosis: Selected papers.* Minneapolis: University of Minnesota Press.

Meehl, P. E. (1973b). *Psychodiagnosis: Selected papers.* Minneapolis: University of Minnesota Press.

Meehl, P. E. (1978a). Theoretical risks and tabular asterisks: Sir Karl, Sir Ronald, and the slow progress of soft psychology. *Journal of Consulting and Clinical Psychology, 46,* 806–834.

Meehl, P. E. (1978b). Specific etiology and other forms of strong influence: Some quantitative meanings. *Journal of Medicine and Philosophy, 2,* 33–53.

Meehl, P. E. (1979). A funny thing happened to us on the way to the latent entities. *Journal of Personality Assessment, 43,* 563–581.

Meehl, P. E. (1986a). Trait language and behaviorese. In T. Thompson & M. Zeller (Eds.), *Analysis and integration of behavioral units* (pp. 315–334). Hillside, NJ: Erlbaum.

Meehl, P. E. (1986b). Diagnostic taxa as open concepts: Metatheoretical and statistical questions about reliability and construct validity in the grand strategy of nosological revision. In T. T. Millon & G. L. Klerman (Eds.), *Contemporary directions in psychopathology* (pp. 215–231). New York: Guilford.

Meehl, P. E. (1991). Four queries about factor reality. *History and Philosophy of Psychology Bulletin, 3(20),* 16–18.

Meehl, P. E. (1992). Factors and taxa, traits and types, differences and degree and differences in kind. *Journal of Personality.*

Meehl, P. E., & Golden, R. R. (1982). Taxometric methods. In J. N. Butcher & D. C. Kendall (Eds.), *The handbook of research methods in clinical psychology* (pp. 127–181). New York: Wiley.

Meehl, P. E., & Yonce, L. J. (1994). Taxometric analysis I: Detecting taxonicity with two quantitative indicators using means above and below a sliding cut (MAMBAC procedure). *Psychological Reports, 74,* 1059–1274.

Mezzich, J. E., & Solomon, H. (1980). *Taxonomy and behavioral science.* New York: Academic Press.

Miller, H. R., Streiner, P. L., & Kahgee, S. L. (1982). Use of the Golden-Meehl indicators in the detection of schizoid-taxon membership. *Journal of Abnormal Psychology, 91,* 55–60.

Nichols, D. S., & Jones, R. E. (1985). Identifying schizoid-taxon membership with Golden-Meehl MMPI items. *Journal of Abnormal Psychology, 94,* 191–194.

Popper, K. R. (1962). *Conjectures and refutations.* New York: Basic Books.

Rasch, G. (1960). *Probabilistic models for some intelligence and attainment tests.* Copenhagen: Neilsen and Lydiche.

Rindskopf, D., & Rindskopf, W. (1986). The value of latent class analysis in medical analysis. *Statistics in Medicine, 5,* 21–27.

Sneath, P. H. A., & Sokal, R. R. (1973). *Numerical taxonomy.* San Francisco: Freeman.

Tellegen, A. (1981). Practicing the two disciplines for relaxation and enlightenment: Comment on the "Role of feedback signal in electromyographic biofeedback: The relevance of attention." *Journal of Experimental Psychology: General, 110,* 217–226.

Terry, R., & Katzman, R. (1983). Senile dementia of the Alzheimer type: Defining a disease. In R. Katzman & R. Terry (Eds.), *The neurology of aging.* Philadelphia: Davis.

Titterington, D. M., Smith, A. F. M., & Makov, U. E. (1985). *Statistical analysis of finite mixture distributions.* New York: Wiley.

Wright, B. D., & Masters, G. N. (1982). *Rating scale analysis.* Chicago: Mesa Press.

Young, M. A. (1983). Evaluating diagnostic criteria: A latent class paradigm. *Journal of Psychiatric Research, 17* (3), 285–296.

Young, M. A., Tanner, M. A., & Meltzer, H. Y. (1982). Operational definitions of schizophrenia: What do they identify? *The Journal of Nervous and Mental Disease, 170* (8), 443–447.

Part Three

New Findings on Traditional Individual Differences Variables

In the beginning, the field of individual differences was devoted to the following topics: measurement, group differences, for example, sex, age, race and nationality, social class, genius, and mental retardation; determinants of individual differences, for example, the mental-physical relationship, practice, and heredity vs. environment; and appraisal of the individual, for example, abilities, interests, and personality. The field is probably best known for its literature on group differences, which has periodically produced passionate controversy.

Part 3 of this volume samples topics that the field of individual differences has traditionally studied. In Chapter 6, Nancy Betz discusses gender-related differences in personality and, in particular, the once-unexamined and uncritically accepted construct of "masculinity"-"femininity." Betz traces the odyssey of this construct through such formulations as androgyny, instrumentality-expressiveness, nurturance-warmth versus dominance-poise, gender-schematics, and gender identity. She also reviews research on gender-related roles, behaviors, and attitudes. Betz's scholarly account provides a strong brief for good measurement as the necessary complement to good thinking in research.

In Chapter 7, David Campbell, who uses a variety of measurements to delineate a psychological characterization of an occupational group—U.S. army generals—offers another example of traditional individual differences research. Campbell finds a distinctive pattern of abilities, personality traits, vocational interests, and other psychological attributes that characterizes the generals. He discusses the implications of this personality syndrome for the selection and development of the leadership of our defense forces.

In Chapter 8, James Rounds searches for the structure of basic interests, following the trail from Guilford through Strong and Kuder to Jackson and today's investigators. He finds evidence for 19 to 28 basic interests that appear to "occupy" more space than is traversed by the popular Holland hexagon. Rounds shows how the new multivariate data-analytic methods—multidimensional scaling, in particular—can provide precise quantitative answers to questions previously addressed only qualitatively or subjectively.

To close out this section devoted to traditional individual differences, Niels Waller, David Lykken, and Auke Tellegen report on a study of occupational interests, leisure time interests, and personality in Chapter 9. They find the three to be separate domains by and large, but definitely related: Several noteworthy relationships among some variables across the three domains were found to exist. In an unexpected but welcome addition to this main study theme, Waller, Lykken, and Tellegen describe a new nonmetric multidimensional scaling method. They also provide persuasive evidence for the heritability and stability of the three sets of individual differences variables.

Chapter 6

Gender-Related Individual Differences Variables
New Concepts, Methods, and Measures

Nancy E. Betz
Ohio State University

INTRODUCTION

The empirical study of sex differences in psychological functioning has a long history in psychology, dating back to the early 1900s. Sex has, in fact, been one of the major variables brought to bear in attempts to understand and predict individual differences in behavior.

The original approach in these studies utilized sex as the independent variable and a wide range of cognitive and personality traits as the dependent variables. Thus, studies of sex differences in intelligence, abilities, and personality characteristics such as dominance and sociability proliferated. Reviews of this work, for example, the "vote counting" approach of Maccoby and Jacklin (1974), and meta-analytic reviews, for example, those by Eagly (1983), Feingold (1988), Hyde (1981, 1986), Linn and Petersen (1986), and Whitley, McHugh, and Frieze (1986) have largely suggested a lack of efficacy of sex per se as a predictor of individual differences in psychological traits.

In addition to a lack of either consistently found or practically (versus statistically) significant sex differences, researchers were frustrated by the apparent situational specificity of many observed differences. For example, Linn (1986), in a review of sex differences research reviews, concluded that variations in the characteristics of the experimental situation/task or other gender-related characteristics of the subjects were far more important to the nature and extent of observed differences than was sex per se. Similarly, researchers such as Deaux and Major (1987), Eagly (1987), Maccoby (1988, 1990), and Unger (1990), among others, have pointed out the large extent to which behaviors traditionally associated with sex vary according to social and interpersonal contexts. Finally, there has been considerable discussion of sex as a "stimulus variable," leading to the differential perceptions and assumptions that are based on the sex of the person being perceived (Deaux & Lewis, 1984; Matlin, 1987).

Although studies and discussions about sex differences will undoubtedly continue (e.g., the controversy over mathematical giftedness, as discussed by Benbow, 1988; Becker & Hedges, 1988; Humphreys, 1988), the focus of research has increasingly been on the conceptualization and measurement of what may be termed gender-related individual difference variables, that is, variables assumed to be related to, but not isomorphic with, sex. These gender-related individual differences variables have been studied as both independent and dependent variables, thus complicating what will be described as an already theoretically underdeveloped area of study. The following review will examine developments in the conceptualization and measurement of gender-related individual differences variables and will include in that examination gender-related personality traits (originally the concepts of masculinity and femininity), and gender-related roles, behaviors, and attitudes.

Most research attention has probably been focused on personality traits assumed to be gender-related by virtue of their association with social conceptions of "masculinity" and "femininity." Conceptualizations of these traits have included what Spence (1985) has called the single-factor and two-factor models and, currently, several proposed reconceptualizations of existing measures and concepts.

THE SINGLE-FACTOR MODEL

Until the mid-1970s, the dominant theoretical conception of masculinity and femininity represented what Spence (1985) has called the single-factor model, as extensively reviewed by Constantinople (1973). This model utilized empirical test construction procedures and was based on the following assumptions: (a) that there is a bipolar unidimensional construct definable such that extreme masculinity falls at one end and extreme femininity falls at the other, leading to the name "masculinity-femininity" to describe what is being measured; (b) that masculinity and femininity are mutually exclusive, that is, one can be masculine or feminine but not both; (c) that failure to be masculine if male or failure to be feminine if female is a sign of deviance, often in the form of homosexuality; and (d) that the concept can be measured by empirical item selection procedures using the two sexes or samples of heterosexuals versus homosexuals as criterion groups.

The first measure of masculinity-femininity was that of Terman and Miles (1936), who believed that "mental masculinity and femininity" was a central personality trait and that it acted as a core around which much of the rest of the personality was formed. Terman and Miles did not actually define the trait but selected for their masculinity-femininity test a group of items that yielded significant sex differences in item responses. Other measures of the trait were the MF scale of the *Strong Vocational Interest Blank* (SVIB), the MF scale of the *Minnesota Multiphasic Personality Inventory* (MMPI), Gough's (1952) Femininity (Fe) scale, later incorporated into the *California Psychological Inventory* (CPI), and Guilford's Masculinity (M) scale, later incorporated into the *Guilford-Zimmerman Temperament Survey*.

Although measures such as these were used extensively in clinical practice as well as research, both their conceptualization and measurement were seriously flawed. First, there was very little attempt to define the construct of interest, that is, masculinity-femininity, except in relationship to scale items on which the sexes were found to differ significantly. Thus, although *something* was being measured, that something was, in reality, "sex differences in item response," which, in itself, has little meaning or importance. As stated by Tellegen and Lubinski (1983):

> Sweeping genotypic labels, such as psychological femininity-masculinity, for mixed collections of gender-differentiating items are too pretentious. Even if a heterogeneous M-F scale represents a certain pool of important gender-differentiating attributes, the aggregate scale score does not necessarily measure anything as systematic as a personality trait. (pp. 448–449)

The lack of a logical definition of the trait was probably tolerated more so than might have been the case because of assumptions that one (meaning the researcher) knew intuitively what constituted masculinity and femininity—the idea that any adult could identify a masculine man or a feminine woman. Thus, such assumptions justified scale development, and then the existence of the scales encouraged test users to accept as self-evident the validity of the construct the scales purported to measure. The lack of a theoretical, as opposed to an empirical or intuitive, existence for masculinity-femininity led Constantinople (1973) to conclude that the concept was among the muddiest in all of psychology (p. 63).

Another serious problem with these scales was that research showed them to be neither bipolar nor unidimensional. Rather, they appeared to be multifaceted and to elicit response patterns countering the assumption of the mutual exclusivity of "masculine" versus "feminine" personality characteristics. Thus, new conceptions were needed, the first of which was represented by what Spence (1985) has called two-factor models.

TWO-FACTOR MODELS

Beginning in the 1970s, a number of writers (e.g., Bem, 1974; Constantinople, 1973; Spence, Helmreich, & Stapp, 1974) suggested that masculinity and femininity were appropriately conceptualized as separate, independent dimensions rather than as opposite ends of a single dimension. With this conceptualization, an individual of either sex could possess relatively high levels of both masculinity and femininity, relatively low levels of both, or a high level of one in combination with a low level of the other. In Bem's (1974) original formulation, a *balance* of masculine and feminine characteristics was postulated to be advantageous because balanced or androgynous individuals would have maximal behavioral flexibility and adaptability. Such individuals would be freer of artificial sex-role-related constraints on the extent of their behavioral and coping repertoires. For example, an androgynous individual would theoretically be able to display adaptive "masculine" behaviors (e.g., assertiveness, active problem solving) *and* adaptive "feminine" behaviors (e.g., giving emotional support to others) as would be appropriate to situational demands.

Measuring Androgyny

In 1974, Bem introduced the *Bem Sex-Role Inventory* (BSRI) as a measure of the two constructs of masculinity and femininity. Her substantive definitions were as follows: "In general, masculinity has been associated with an instrumental orientation, a cognitive focus on 'getting the job done,' and femininity has been associated with an expressive orientation, an affective concern for the welfare of others" (p. 156). Rather than select items assessing instrumental and expressive orientations, however, Bem (1974) compiled a list of 200 adjectives that seemed positive in value and either masculine or feminine in tone (p. 156). Items judged by undergraduate students to be significantly more desirable for males than for females were eligible for the masculinity scale, and vice versa for the femininity scale. The empirical method of item selection thus went considerably beyond the definitions given originally. For example, the Masculinity scale items "independent," "assertive," and "acts like a leader" seem related to an instrumental orientation, but the items "athletic" and "masculine" are less well related or, in the latter case, tautological. Similarly, the Femininity scale items of "affectionate," "compassionate," and "tender" seem appropriately "expressive," but "childlike," "shy," "gullible," and "feminine" do not appear to fit the original definition.

The *Personal Attributes Questionnaire* (PAQ; Spence et al., 1974) was constructed in a similar way, using items that had been rated as significantly more characteristic of one sex than the other. The original item pool, taken from the *Sex-Role Stereotype Questionnaire* of Rosenkrantz, Vogel, Bee, Broverman, and Broverman (1968), had been divided into "male-valued" items (those the pole rated more characteristic of males were also the more socially desirable pole), "female-valued" items (wherein the pole characteristic of females was more highly valued), and "sex specific" items (for which the socially desirable pole depended on the sex of the target). Spence et al. defined the male-valued items as reflecting instrumental behaviors and the female-valued items as descriptive of expressive behaviors. The next step was to define the "masculine" pole and, therefore, a masculinity score, as that rated more descriptive of males and, similarly, a "femininity" pole and score, as that rated more descriptive of females. Again, item content exceeded in scope the substantive definitions provided.

In addition to postulating and measuring concepts of masculinity and femininity, Bem (1974) postulated that, taken together, they represented a higher order, unidimensional concept of degree of "sex-typing." At one end of this continuum were highly sex-typed individuals (high masculine but low feminine or vice versa) and at the other end were "androgynous" individuals—those possessing a balance of masculinity and femininity. According to Bem (1977), the sex-typed individual is one who is highly attuned to cultural definitions of sex-appropriate behavior and who uses such definitions as the standard for guiding his or her behavior. Androgynous individuals, because they are theoretically less sensitive to cultural prescriptions, can behave more in concert with individual proclivities and situational demands.

Considerable controversy has surrounded attempts to specify the way in which—or whether—masculinity and femininity scores should be combined to indicate degree of sex typing. Bem (1974) originally proposed a simple balance score, where degree of sex typing versus androgyny was indicated by a *t*-ratio, derived from subtracting the masculinity score from the femininity score. Subjects would be classified as sex-typed if the androgyny *t*-ratio reached statistical significance and as androgynous if the absolute value of the *t*-ratio was less than or equal to one. This method of determining androgynous versus sex-typed orientation had at least one ultimately fatal flaw, however. Specifically, a score classified as androgynous could indicate a balance of high levels of both masculinity and femininity or low levels of both. Inasmuch as the items represent socially desirable characteristics, high versus low levels of both masculinity and femininity have different implications for behavior and functioning. In more recent conceptions, the low-low individuals (those possessing low levels of both attributes) have been referred to as "undifferentiated" rather than androgynous.

As an alternative to the *t*-ratio, both Bem (1977) and Spence et al. (1974) suggested a fourfold classification using a median split. Individuals above the median on both the Masculinity and Femininity scales were to be classified as androgynous, those above the median on one and below on the other were classified as "sex-typed" (if above the median on the own-sex scale) or "cross-sex-typed" (if above the median on the other-sex scale), and those below both medians were "undifferentiated."

Problems With Androgyny Models

A number of problems with the fourfold classification have been pointed out, and Spence and Helmreich no longer advocate its use. Tellegen and Lubinski (1983) note the loss of information when dimensional variables are replaced by categories. To begin with, any median split technique involves errors of classification. Even worse, however, the categories are often used in such a way that all dimensionality is lost. Specifically, Bem's rationale involved the concept of degree of sex typing, along which categories could theoretically be ordered, yet studies often convert BSRI or PAQ scores to four nonordered categories. Conversion to four nonordered categories, followed by one-way analysis of variance is incorrect—two-way ANOVA's retaining the underlying M and F dimensions would be more appropriate (or, better yet, regression analysis using the separate variables and their interactions).

In addition, Bem's (1974) original androgyny model implied an additive effect of masculinity and femininity on psychological well-being, that is, the androgynous individual is assumed to be the most healthy psychologically by virtue of possessing both instrumental and expressive characteristics. If, in fact, research would support the existence of the additive model, the concept of androgyny would, ironically, not be needed because any predictive and explanatory power could be attributed to the two scales contributing to it, that is, masculinity and femininity.

Unfortunately for those who are attached to the concept of androgyny, the additive model is in serious doubt. Lubinski, Tellegen, and Butcher (1981, 1983) and others have pointed out the strong relationship of masculinity, but not femininity, to indices of subjective well-being, countering assumptions of additivity. In addition to casting doubt on the validity of an additive model, these data call into question the need for the concept of androgyny and the use of a four-fold classification. Unless consistent relationships of a higher-order variable, however defined quantitatively, with other variables can be found, masculinity and femininity (or at least whatever is measured by the M and F scales) are sufficient concepts.

Lubinski et al. (1981, 1983) have suggested that, instead of an additive model, interactive models of the relationship of masculinity and femininity to other psychological variables should be developed and empirically examined. The substantive possibilities of this type of interaction are illustrated by Harrington and Andersen (1981), who describe a hypothetical example where "feminine" aesthetic sensitivity enhances the extent to which "masculine" engineering skills (and vice versa) lead to creativity in architects. More specifically, Tellegen and Lubinski (1983) urged researchers to utilize hierarchical regression analyses that include gender, measures of masculinity and femininity, and the interactions among all three. When data are appropriately analyzed, findings may be quite different from those reported using analyses less sensitive to either the underlying dimensionality or to potential interactions.

In addition to the fact that androgyny is not a useful concept unless it can be shown to be an interactive, versus simply additive, function of the dimensions of masculinity and femininity is the fact that two-factor models have done little to advance theoretical understanding of the concepts of masculinity and femininity (Spence, 1983, 1985; Tellegen & Lubinski, 1983). Specifically, no valid method has yet been devised to measure masculinity and femininity as global theoretical concepts, as the terms imply. The measures, whether derived from the single-factor or two-factor views, have validity only in an empirical sense, that is, in their elicitation of sex differences in item response patterns or in the perceptions of judges that males and females differ or should differ on the characteristic.

There is a critical distinction between empirical and theoretical uses of masculinity and femininity and other gender-related terms. In the former case, the terms are "nominal labels for observable qualities or events that are more closely associated with one gender than the other in a given culture. In the latter, they are used in a theoretical sense, referring to hypothetical properties of the individual" (Spence, 1985, p. 66).

Attempts to give substantive meaning to the concepts of masculinity and femininity began with Spence and Helmreich (1978) in their revision of the PAQ, restricting it to items reflective of their original definitions of masculinity and femininity, that is, as "instrumentality" and "expressiveness." They also recommended that these terms be used in reference to the scores yielded by the scales. Similarly, David Bakan's (1966) distinction between "agentic" (self-assertive, motivated to master) and "communal" (concerned with others, selfless) characteristics provides an alternative set of descriptive labels for what is measured by Masculinity and Femininity scales. Spence, Helmreich, and Holahan (1979) used the terms "unmitigated agency" and "unmitigated communion" to refer to two new scales, included in the *Extended Personal Attributes Questionnaire* (EPAQ). These scales were designed to tap the negative aspects of traditional masculinity and femininity, inasmuch as other measures used only positive trait descriptors.

Lubinski et al. (1981, 1983) argue that even "instrumentality" and "expressiveness," or "agency" and "communion," carry some surplus meaning. Lubinski et al. (1983) reported that the patterns of intercorrelations of the BSRI and EPAQ scales with other personality variables indicated that the F scales were related primarily to a cluster called "nurturance-warmth" and the M scales to a cluster labeled "dominance-poise." Because these terms are even closer to the manifest item content, they are descriptive of what is being measured without leading to excesses in interpretation.

Regardless of whether we call these dimensions instrumentality and expressiveness, or dominance-poise and nurturance-warmth, the fact is that the constructs of masculinity and femininity are no longer necessary if we are interested in the substantive meaning of these scales. Bem (1985) herself now questions whether masculinity and femininity are real, versus invented, entities. Some researchers continue to use the BSRI, PAQ, or other similar measures to assess sex typing (e.g., Dimitrovsky, Singer, & Simon, 1989; Frable, 1989; Ingram, Cruet, Johnson, & Wisnicki, 1988; Roos & Cohen, 1987), and Lenney (1991) provides an excellent review of such uses. Meanwhile, other researchers have turned their attention to attempts to reconceptualize this area of individual differences.

BEYOND TWO-FACTOR MODELS

Continuing activity in the study of gender-related traits can be described in terms of at least two different emphases. One involves a proliferation of new measures of masculinity and femininity. In Beere's (1990) handbook of tests and measures of gender-related concepts, there are 39 instruments in the section that includes the BSRI and

PAQ—scales such as the *Boyhood Gender Conformity Scale*, the *Effeminacy Rating Scale*, and the *Hyper-masculinity Scale* are illustrative. Another 18 measures, including the *Children's Androgyny Scale*, are contained in a Children and Gender section. Unfortunately, not all of these instruments were carefully developed and evaluated—many were probably used once and then forgotten (see Beere, 1990, and Lenney, 1991, for reviews). Proliferation of measures reflects vitality in a field, but it may be inversely related to both instrument quality and theoretical progress.

The second general direction, what Lenney (1991, p. 648) calls the "postandrogyny revolution," is based on concerns about the lack of theoretical substance of the masculinity, femininity, and androgyny concepts and on agreement that global concepts of masculinity and femininity—if they exist at all—cannot be either conceptualized or assessed using traditional trait concepts alone. Rather, there is general agreement that the domain is probably multidimensional (e.g., Edwards & Spence, 1987; Lenney, 1991; Spence & Helmreich, 1978; Spence & Sawin, 1984) and includes attitudes, behaviors, information processing, and social interaction. The extent to which newer approaches use the concepts of masculinity and femininity versus concepts such as gender identity (Spence, 1985), gender-related behavior (Deaux & Major, 1987), gender-schematic processing (Bem, 1985; see also Bem, 1993), sex-typing schemas (Martin & Halverson, 1983), gender-related individual differences (as used herein), or gender as a social category influencing social interactions (Maccoby, 1988, 1990) varies with the researcher.

One recent approach that continues to use the BSRI and related measures, although it abandons the constructs of masculinity and femininity, is Bem's (1981, 1985) "gender schema" theory. Bem (1985) concluded that because masculinity and femininity have not been shown to have an existence beyond a few gender-stereotypic personality traits, "human behaviors and personality attributes should no longer be linked with gender" (p. 222). Instead, Bem proposed that the BSRI and other measures of masculinity and femininity measure a trait that might be called "gender-schematization," describing the extent to which people use gender as an organizing principle of perception and cognition. Individuals fall on a continuum ranging from highly gender-schematic, relying heavily on gender in both the perception and interpretation of events or people, to gender-aschematic at the other end, placing little reliance on gender as an organizing principle. Those individuals who formerly would have been classified as sex-typed are viewed as gender-schematic, whereas individuals once described as androgynous are postulated to be gender-aschematic.

Also using the idea of gender schema are Markus and her colleagues (Crane & Markus, 1982; Markus, Crane, Bernstein, & Siladi, 1982), who propose two, rather than one, gender schema. Specifically, they propose that there is a schema that relies on masculinity as an organizing principle—theoretically, persons high in masculinity (BSRI-M) would be more responsive than those low in masculinity to male-related stimuli but would not differ vis-à-vis female-related stimuli. Conversely, high BSRI-F scores would enhance attentiveness to female stimuli.

Although gender schema theories have an intuitive appeal in some respects, for example, they allow study of the primacy of gender as an organizing construct versus other possible organizing constructs (Frable & Bem, 1985; Jacklin, 1989), consistent empirical support for the postulates of either the Bem or Markus versions is still wanting. For example, Frable and Bem (1985) cite the study of Taylor and Falcone (1982) as supportive of their gender schema theory, but the findings of neither Frable and Bem (1985), Edwards and Spence (1987), nor Payne, Connor, and Colletti (1987) were convincingly supportive of either one-factor or two-factor gender schema theories. Deaux, Kite, and Lewis (1985) and Edwards and Spence (1987) reported little evidence for gender-schematic processing at all, never mind relationships of schematicity to BSRI or PAQ sex typing.

Tellegen and Lubinski (1983) questioned the postulate of a direct relationship between degree of gender schematicization and sex typing versus androgyny of personality, as suggested originally by Bem. They reanalyzed data from Moran (cf. Bem, 1981) using appropriate hierarchical regression with interaction terms and reported that although same-sex-typed individuals were the most gender-schematic, the least schematic were not androgynous but cross-sex-typed individuals, that is, feminine-typed males and masculine-typed females. Tellegen and Lubinski (1983), therefore, suggest that gender is used as a central organizing construct only to the extent that one's own perceived characteristics fit the schema.

Another recent approach (Spence, 1985; Storms, 1979) retains the concepts of masculinity and femininity but uses them to refer to a global self-perception of oneself as masculine or feminine. Based on findings such as those of Pedhazur and Tetenbaum (1979) that responses to the BSRI items masculine and feminine are negatively correlated with each other and largely unrelated to other scale items, Spence (1985) concluded that the personal sense of being masculine or feminine is real and important, although it does not necessarily imply any other gender-related attributes. The theory is based on the empirically supported assumption that gender-linked differences vary across cultures, are multifactorial in structure, and are not necessarily correlated with one another. It implies that individuals differ widely in the gender-congruent versus gender-incongruent behaviors, attitudes, competencies, and personality characteristics displayed.

Spence proposes that the terms masculinity and femininity refer to *gender identity,* which is defined as a "basic phenomenological sense of one's maleness or femaleness that parallels awareness and acceptance of one's biological sex and is established early in life" (p. 91). Gender-related characteristics are important primarily as they help individuals maintain and protect their sense of gender identity, but as long as that identity remains secure (which Spence suggests it usually does), the extent to which one's behaviors, traits, or attitudes are gender congruent makes little difference to the individual.

Once established, gender identity plays little role in the acquisition of other traits and behaviors; rather, they develop from the unique constellation of genetic and environmental influences on the individual. There may be some critical developmental stages and/or tasks, such as adolescence, or events that threaten the sense of adequacy as a man or woman, such as divorce or the inability to bear or father a child, which elicit feelings of inadequacy and thus possibly compensatory gender-congruent behaviors. In general, however, gender identity is postulated as a stable condition in individuals with only idiosyncratic relationships to other gender-related attributes.

Implications of this theory for measurement and research include the necessity of conceptualizing and measuring separately the different domains of gender-related behavior and investigating what Spence (1985) calls the *internal calculus.* The internal calculus is the equation by which an individual incorporates self-knowledge of one's gender-related characteristics into a secure, versus less secure, sense of adequacy as a male or female. For example, under what conditions does lack of athletic ability threaten the self-concept of a male or lack of interest in having children threaten that of a female? What factors are related to the durability versus the vulnerability of one's sense of adequacy as appropriately masculine or feminine?

Storms (1979) developed a *Sex-Role Identity Scale,* designed to assess the global self-concept of one's masculinity and femininity. Storms (1979) and Edwards and Spence (1987) found that differences in endorsement of self-descriptive gender-related personality traits were related to differences in global perceptions of masculinity and femininity. A study by O'Heron and Orlofsky (1990) showed that lower gender identity and gender adequacy were related to lesser endorsement of BSRI-Masculine (Instrumental) traits in men, but both identity and adequacy were relatively independent of BSRI traits in women. Further, lower gender identity was related to indices of psychological maladjustment (e.g., higher anxiety and depression) in men, but, again, not in women. Thus, a global concept of gender identity does appear to have utility.

Finally, Edwards and Spence (1987) conducted a study designed to compare the utility of both gender schema and gender identity theories. Using the dependent variables of extent and nature of recall of gender-related words, no support for gender schema theories and limited support for gender identity theory was found. Clearly, further research of this type using a broader array of well-conceptualized and defined criterion variables is necessary before the theoretical utility (if any) of these theories and, it is hoped, others, will be demonstrated. The problem of poorly conceptualized and defined criterion variables is the subject of the next section.

OTHER GENDER-RELATED CHARACTERISTICS

One of the major problems with trait-based concepts of masculinity and femininity was the lack of consistent relationships of these measures to other gender-related variables. Furthermore, there has been a general lack of agreement about what the concepts of masculinity and femininity, assuming they reflect something real, should be related to. In terms of theory, lack of clear understanding of the construct is only the first problem. Lack of consensus (or even hypotheses) about what it should be related to leaves the construct isolated in a predictive sense.

Many researchers have assumed that masculinity and femininity should be related to other gender-related traits. For example, we might postulate that a "feminine" woman should be emotionally expressive and nurturant, that she would prefer the roles of homemaker and mother to that of career woman, that she would be competent at sewing and cooking but be unable to change a tire or repair a toilet, and that she would have relatively traditional attitudes toward the roles, rights, and responsibilities of women in our society. The research, however, does not support the existence of strong relationships among different domains. Thus, the assumption that any one of them, not to mention all of them, reflect the entities masculinity and femininity is inaccurate.

For example, factors analyses of several measures of masculinity-femininity should yield one or two factors, yet they yield evidence of multiple underlying factors (see Constantinople, 1973). Numerous other studies (e.g., Bem, 1974) support the lack of relationship between different domains of gender-related characteristics. In actuality, correlations between the BSRI and the PAQ and criterion behaviors are positive only when the criteria themselves require instrumental or expressive behaviors, thus reinforcing a more limited interpretation of what they measure. They do not appear to measure abstract concepts such as masculinity and femininity, sex-role orientation, or sex typing but, rather, constellations of personality traits best summarized as instrumentality and expressiveness, or "dominance-poise" and "nurturance-warmth." Thus, relationships with other gender-related variables are more likely the result of shared personality trait variance than shared masculinity or femininity.

It seems that multifactor conceptions of gender-related variables are needed in which the variables measured by current M and F scales are included (Spence, 1983). However, such theoretical advances depend on clear specification of the nature of the domain of gender-related characteristics, including both conceptual and operational definitions of characteristics postulated. In the next section, other gender-related variables, in addition to personality traits, will be briefly introduced.

GENDER-RELATED ROLES, BEHAVIORS, AND ATTITUDES

In this section, concepts and measures of gender-related roles, behaviors, and attitudes will be discussed together because they overlap considerably. The term *gender-related roles* will be used herein to refer to adult social role expectations for men and women, such as those of homemaker and childrearer for women and breadwinner and family decision maker for men. Within the domain of career pursuits, occupational sex segregation has, likewise, implicitly led to stereotypes of appropriate versus less appropriate occupations for men and women.

Beyond the realm of home and career involvement, however, are other classes of behavior typically associated with being male or female. These include competencies (e.g., the ability to repair a tire or prepare a meal), interests, and leisure time activities.

Finally, there are individual differences in attitudes about the *desirability* of sex-differentiated roles and behaviors. Originally studied as attitudes toward the roles of women, there also are now measures of attitudes toward the roles of men.

Gender-Related Roles

Early research in vocational psychology assumed that unless involuntarily unemployed, men would pursue careers or hold jobs. No individual variability in this choice among men was expected. Among women, however, research began to differentiate women according to a dimension of home versus career orientation and to study factors associated with that variable. Early studies, among the first of women's vocational behavior, compared the SVIB responses of homemakers to those of career-oriented women and found predictable differences in vocational interests, for example, high scores among the homemakers on the Housewife scale (Hoyt & Kennedy, 1958; Vetter & Lewis, 1964). Originally, groups were differentiated based on responses to an item about preferences for home versus career, and, later, the SVIB itself was used to differentiate orientations empirically (e.g., Rand, 1968).

Assumptions that women choose either home or career were gradually replaced by the realization that most women combine the roles in their lives. Thus, measures of career salience, that is, the importance of a career relative to other life roles, replaced the home versus career dichotomy. For example, Eyde's (1962) *Desire to Work Scale* requested respondents to rate their desire to work under various conditions of marital status, number and ages of children, and perceived adequacy of husband's income; level of career orientation was indicated by the range of conditions under which the woman continued to desire to work. A widely used measure of career salience is Greenhaus' (1971) 27-item *Career Salience Scale*. Other measures of career salience have been reviewed by Betz and Fitzgerald (1987).

Although measures of career salience were originally developed to study the vocational behavior of women, researchers have also begun to use them to study individual differences among men in the importance of work in their lives. For example, Nevill and Super's (1986) *Salience Inventory* was developed to assess the relative importance of six life roles, including both work and home roles among both men and women. Beere's (1990) handbook lists 26 scales assessing marital and parental roles (e.g., the *Motherhood Inventory* and the *Eversoll Father Role Opinionaire*), 24 assessing employee roles (*Attitudes Toward Male Nurses, Women in Science Scale*), and 30 assessing multiple roles (*Home-Career Conflict* measure, *Dual-Career Family Scales*). Thus, what began as the study of gender-traditional versus nontraditional role choices among women has now been expanded to assume that both men and women are likely to pursue a variety of life roles and that there are within-sex individual differences in the salience of these roles.

Gender-Related Behaviors

Orlovsky (1981; Orlofsky, Cohen, & Ramsden, 1985; Orlofsky & O'Heron, 1987a, 1987b; Orlofsky, Ramsden, & Cohen, 1982) has attempted to define and measure a domain of gender-related behaviors. The original 240-item *Sex-Role Behavior Scale* (SRBS; Orlofsky et al., 1982) assessed interests and behaviors in four areas: leisure activities, vocational interests, social/dating behaviors, and marital and primary relationship behaviors. Items reflecting each area were written and administered to large samples of college men and women for rating purposes. Behaviors that were rated as stereotypically masculine but were also viewed as appropriate for both sexes were called "male-valued" (after Spence & Helmreich, 1978), stereotypically feminine behaviors viewed as appropriate for both sexes were labeled "female-valued," and those behaviors both associated with and rated as appropriate for one sex only were labeled "sex-specific." For example, male-valued, female-valued, and female and male sex-specific items in the recreational activities domain include reading science fiction, gardening, knitting, and football, respectively. Note the implication of the sex-specific items, that is, that males who knit or females who play football risk social disapproval. Vocational interests items in the same categories included physician, social worker, and nurse or plumber. In social and dating behavior, deciding where to go on a date, taking special care with one's appearance, primping in front of the mirror, and helping opposite sex persons on with their coat are sample items. Finally, items in the realm of marital behavior included preparing income tax returns, buying the groceries, doing laundry, and doing the driving when out with one's spouse.

Orlofsky reported significant sex differences in all areas of behavior except for the male-valued occupations, which were equally preferred by women and men. Intercorrelations among male-valued scales ranged from .18 to .43, among female-valued scales from .37 to .50, and among sex-specific areas from .66 to .82 (but large sex differences on the sex-specific scales were suggested by Orlofsky to account for these correlations). Thus, the data suggested some degree of relationship between different domains of gender-related behavior, but, as with previous research, not enough to suggest that one underlying factor of masculinity versus femininity or sex-role orientation is being measured. More recently, Orlofsky and O'Heron (1987a) introduced a 96-item short form of the SRBS. Subjects rate each item on a five-point scale that measures how characteristic the behavior or activity is for them. Correlations of the M, F, and MF scales with the corresponding traits scales of the PAQ were in the .30s. Orlofsky's recent work has focused on the relationship of stereotypical and nonstereotypical trait and behavior orientations indices of psychological adjustment (Orlofsky & O'Heron, 1987b; O'Heron & Orlofsky, 1990).

Gender-Related Attitudes

Attitudes Toward Women's Roles   A gender-role–related attitudinal variable that has received considerable research attention is attitudes toward women's roles in society. Theorist researchers Spence and Helmreich (1972; Spence, Helmreich, & Stapp, 1973) operationalized the notion of "attitudes towards women's roles" and developed the *Attitudes Toward Women Scale* (AWS). The AWS's items are categorized into six groups representing the following themes: (a) vocational, educational, and intellectual roles (e.g., "Women with children should not work outside the home if they don't have to" and "Women should be given equal opportunity with men for apprenticeships in the skilled trades"), (b) freedom and independence (e.g., "The modern girl is entitled to the same freedom and regulation from control that is given to the modern boy" and "Most women need and want the kind of protection and support that men have traditionally given them"), (c) dating, courtship, and etiquette (e.g., "The initiative in dating should come from the man" and "A woman should be as free as a man to propose marriage"), (d) drinking, swearing, and dirty jokes (e.g., "Intoxication among women is worse than intoxication among men"), (e) sexual behavior (e.g., "If both husband and wife agree that sexual fidelity isn't important, then there's no reason why both shouldn't have extramarital affairs if they want to"), and (f) marital relationships and obligations (e.g., "It is insulting to women to have the 'obey' clause remain in the marriage service," "It is childish for a woman to assert herself by retaining her maiden name after marriage," and "In general, the father should have greater authority than the mother in the bringing up of the children").

Although the AWS and its various short-form adaptations (Spence et al., 1973) have been most commonly used in research in this area, another widely used measure of attitudes toward women's roles is Kalin and Tilby's (1978) *Sex-Role Ideology Scale* (SRIS). Developed to distinguish feminist from traditional sex-role ideologies, the SRIS consists of 39 seven-point bipolar items pertaining to work roles, parental responsibilities, personal relationships, special roles of women, abortion, and homosexuality. Beere, King, Beere, and King's (1984) *Sex-Role Egalitarianism Scale* assesses attitudes toward equality in marital roles, parental roles, employee roles, educational roles, and social-interpersonal-heterosexual roles. Dreyer, Woods, and James' (1981) 19-item *Index of Sex Role Orientation* measures the factors of home-career conflict, male-female division of household responsibilities, and attitudes toward women's work roles outside the home. Other measures include Lyson and Brown's (1982) nine-item measure that includes scales for role appropriateness (e.g., attitudes toward working after the birth of children) and social/marital equality between the sexes: Tetenbaum, Lighter, and Travis' (1984) 32-item scale assessing attitudes toward working mothers, and Knaub and Eversoll's (1983) scale assessing attitudes toward the timing of parenthood. Frable (1989) has assessed a construct she calls *gender ideology*, defined as the extent to which subjects accept rules designating gender-appropriate or -inappropriate behavior. Overall, Beere (1990) lists 56 measures of attitudes toward gender roles.

Although sex-role attitudes have been measured in a variety ways, research to date has yielded a fairly consistent pattern of findings. First, studies have shown that women's attitudes toward women's roles are more liberal than those of men (Hare-Mustin, Bennett, & Broderick, 1983; Mezydlo & Betz, 1980; Zuckerman, 1981) and that younger women are more liberal in their attitudes than older women (Slevin & Wingrove, 1983; Stafford, 1984). Recent research also indicates that women are becoming more liberal in their role expectations and values in comparison with women in previous studies (Lyson & Brown, 1982; Mezydlo & Betz, 1980; Stafford, 1984; Thornton & Freedman, 1979; Zuckerman, 1981).

In addition, attitudes toward women's roles have been found to be related to women's role choices, especially in terms of career involvement. Career-oriented women consistently express more liberal or feminist attitudes toward women's roles than do home-oriented women (e.g., Stafford, 1984; Tinsley & Faunce, 1980; see also Betz & Fitzgerald, 1987, for a comprehensive review of this literature). Liberal attitudes toward women's roles are also positively related to remaining single and to remaining childless if married (e.g., Dreyer et al., 1981). Thus, there are relationships of moderate magnitude between attitudes toward and actual selection of alternative role behaviors.

Attitudes Toward Men's Roles   A more recent development in the literature is a focus on the empirical and theoretical distinction of attitudes toward men's roles from attitudes toward women's roles. Although earlier measures of attitudes toward women's roles often alluded to men in comparison with women (e.g., with items such as "Intoxication among women is worse than intoxication among men" and "The father should have greater authority than the mother in the bringing up of the children" from the AWS), they did not actually measure attitudes toward men's roles. Just as global concepts of masculinity and femininity were erroneously assumed in personality research, a global concept of sex-role attitudes, which would vary from traditional to nontraditional and apply equally to men's and to women's roles, was assumed in attitude studies (Pleck, 1987). Pleck (1987) and others have pointed out the possibility that one may be relatively liberal with regard to the roles of one sex but relatively conservative with respect to those of the other. For example, a parent may be proud of a nontraditional daughter but disapprove of a nontraditional son, for example, one who stays home to care for children while his wife works.

Several scales designed to measure attitudes toward the male role as independently as possible from attitudes toward the female role have been developed recently. The *Brannon Masculinity Scale* (Brannon, 1985) assesses four components of traditional beliefs about male roles and behaviors, that is, that men should not be feminine, that men should be respected and admired for successful achievement, that men should never show weakness or uncertainty, and that men should seek adventure and risk and even engage in or tolerate violence if necessary.

In research using this scale in a sample of 233 male undergraduates from two New England colleges, Thompson and Pleck (1986) reported only weak relationships between attitudes toward the male role and attitudes toward the female role; thus, traditionalism versus liberality in attitudes is sex-specific. Thompson, Grisanti, and Pleck (1985), using the same data set, reported that attitudes toward the male role were moderately related to other aspects of male behavior norms, including the Type A behavior pattern, lower self-disclosure, and greater dominance over a partner in an intimate relationship.

Based on O'Neil's (1981) model of gender-role conflict and strain and related to Pleck's (1981) sex-strain paradigm, the *Gender Role Conflict Scales I and II* (GRCS-I, GRCS-II; O'Neil, Helms, Gable, David, & Wrightsman, 1986) assess attitudes toward and conflict with several potentially problematic aspects of the traditional male role. The aspects include restrictive emotionality; homophobia; need for power, control, and competition; restricted sexual and affectionate behavior; obsession with achievement and success; and health care problems. Factor analyses of the GRCS-I indicated four factors: success, power, and competition; restrictive emotionality; restrictive affectionate behavior between men; and conflicts between work and family relations. The GRCS-II yielded four factors of success, power, and competition, homophobia, lack of emotional response, and public embarrassment from gender-role deviance (e.g., "How uncomfortable would you feel carrying a woman's purse in front of people in a restaurant?").

Other measures of attitudes toward the male role included in Beere's (1990) 56 gender-role attitudes measures are the *Attitudes Toward the Male Role Scale* (Doyle & Moore, 1978) and *Attitudes Toward Males in Society.*

Synthesis

In general, the areas of gender-related roles, behaviors, and attitudes are characterized by a proliferation of largely unexamined measures, in combination with a dearth of construct explication or theory development. Probably the best research on gender-related roles has been done in vocational psychology, and Spence and Helmreich's work on attitude assessment has also been highly influential. In general, though, these concepts, their measures, and their relationships to other individual differences variables, gender-related and otherwise, represent an area at the beginning stages of exploration.

SUMMARY AND RECOMMENDATIONS

This chapter has provided an overview of the use of gender-related individual differences variables in psychology. Beginning with the study of sex differences in the early part of this century, concepts, measures, and research designs have become increasingly numerous and varied. Research on gender-related phenomena has grown as fast as any other area in psychology. Two fairly new journals, *The Psychology of Women Quarterly* and *Sex Roles,* were originated in order to publish research on sex and gender, and everincreasing numbers of studies of gender-related phenomena are found in traditional journals in psychology (e.g., the *Journal of Personality and Social Psychology*). The area has attracted continued interest and, for many, has been the object of sustained research productivity.

In spite of the flurry of activity, progress in understanding remains limited because the literature on gender-related phenomena is characterized by a bewildering, even intimidating, array of concepts and measures in combination with a relative lack of underlying or integrative theory. Concepts are, in most cases, poorly defined and operationalized. Substantive definitions may be insufficient or, worse, lacking altogether, and often the definition of the construct is assumed to be self-evident. Measures have proliferated—Beere's (1990) review lists 211 gender-role measures! Furthermore, attempts to place the construct in the context of a nomological network (Cronbach & Meehl, 1955) are thus far virtually nonexistent (with a few exceptions such as Deaux & Major, 1987).

Given the vagueness of definitions and the lack of a theoretical framework, attempts to measure the concepts may be doomed to failure. Because of limitations in length, this chapter did not generally focus on the psychometric quality of the measures described. This topic warrants a separate discussion. Some general statements may be made, however. First, some of the measures described herein have been extensively studied and have been revised to improve their psychometric quality, for example, the *Bem Sex-Role Inventory* and the *Personal Attributes Questionnaire*. Even with these measures, however, issues of construct validity are not entirely settled. Most other measures have been used in only one or a few studies, and their psychometric qualities have not been investigated adequately.

Based on the work reviewed herein, it is recommended that much more attention be devoted to construct definition, theory construction, and measurement. The first step in this process is acknowledgment that the postulation of global, inclusive, comprehensively explanatory theoretical concepts such as sex role, or masculinity-femininity has, to date, remained unsupported by empirical data. As stated by Spence, Deaux, and Helmrich (1985),

> the various components of gender-related phenomena are infuriatingly free to vary among themselves, defying those theorists who would seek a simple and sovereign concept. (p. 172)

Thus, we need to attend to the conceptualization and measurement of more limited and homogeneous domains of behavior. Homogeneous, measurable domains of behavior can then be placed in a theoretical structure postulating their interrelationships and relationships to criterion measures. A good theory can serve the same purpose as an all-inclusive concept, namely, comprehensiveness and explanatory power.

What is needed, in short, is a moratorium on instrument development without a priori attention to the careful definition of constructs of interest and the postulation of a nomological network within which they are embedded. Integrative theories, rather than more constructs and measures, are in especially short supply.

In conclusion, it is clear that the importance of gender as an individual differences variable has not diminished but has, rather, increased markedly over the years. Unfortunately, enthusiasm for the topic has outstripped the care with which it has been approached. Researchers interested in sex and gender as individual differences variables may wish to slow down and devote considerably more attention to issues of definition, measurement, and theory construction if the potential of these variables to contribute to the understanding of human behavior is to be realized.

I would like to thank Martin Heesacker of the University of Florida for his comments on an earlier draft of this manuscript.

REFERENCES

Bakan, D. (1966). *The duality of human existence.* Chicago: Rand McNally.
Becker, B. J., & Hedges, L. V. (1988). The effects of selection and variability in studies of gender differences. *Behavioral and Brain Sciences, 11,* 183–185.
Beere, C. (1990). *Gender roles: A handbook of tests and measures.* New York: Greenwood Press.

Beere, C. A., King, D. W., Beere, D. B., & King, L. K. (1984). The sex role egalitarianism scale: A measure of attitudes toward equality between the sexes. *Sex Roles, 10,* 563–576.

Bem, S. L. (1974). The measurement of psychological androgyny. *Journal of Consulting and Clinical Psychology, 42,* 155–162.

Bem, S. L. (1977). On the utility of alternative procedures for assessing psychological androgyny. *Journal of Consulting and Clinical Psychology, 45,* 196–205.

Bem, S. L. (1981). Gender schema theory: A cognitive account of sex typing. *Psychological Review, 88,* 354–364.

Bem, S. L. (1985). Androgyny and gender schema theory: A conceptual and empirical integration. In T. B. Sonderegger (Ed.), *Nebraska Symposium on motivation: Psychology and gender.* Lincoln: University of Nebraska Press.

Ben, S. J. (1993). *The lenses of gender.* New Haven, CT: Yale University Press.

Benbow, C. P. (1988). Sex differences in mathematical reasoning ability in intellectually talented preadolescents: Their nature, effects, and possible causes. *Behavioral and Brain Sciences, 11,* 169–183.

Betz, N. E., & Fitzgerald, L. F. (1987). *The career psychology of women.* New York: Academic Press.

Brannon, R. (1985). A scale for measuring attitudes about masculinity. In A. Sargent (Ed.), *Beyond sex roles* (pp. 110–116). St. Paul, MN: West and Co.

Constantinople, A. (1973). Masculinity-femininity: An exception to the famous dictum? *Psychological Bulletin, 80,* 389–407.

Crane, M., & Markus, H. (1982). Gender identity: The benefits of a self-schema approach. *Journal of Personality and Social Psychology, 43,* 1195–1197.

Cronbach, L. J., & Meehl, P. E. (1955). Construct validity in psychological tests. *Psychological Bulletin, 52,* 281–302.

Deaux, K. (1984). From individual differences to social categories: Analysis of a decade's research on gender. *American Psychologist, 39,* 105–116.

Deaux, K. (1985). Sex and gender. *Annual Review of Psychology, 36,* 49–81.

Deaux, K., Kite, M. E., & Lewis, L. (1985). Clustering and gender scheme: An uncertain link. *Personality and Social Psychology Bulletin, 11,* 387–397.

Deaux, K., & Lewis, L. L. (1984). Structure of gender stereotypes: Interrelationships among components and gender label. *Journal of Personality and Social Psychology, 46,* 991–1004.

Deaux, K., & Major, B. (1987). Putting gender into context: An interactive model of gender-related behavior. *Psychological Review, 94,* 369–389.

Dimitrovsky, L., Singer, J., & Simon, S. (1989). Masculine and feminine traits: Their relation to suitedness for and success in training for traditionally masculine and feminine army functions. *Journal of Personality and Social Psychology, 57,* 839–847.

Doyle, J. J., & Moore, R. J. (1978). Attitudes toward the male role scale (AMR): An objective instrument to measure attitudes toward the male's sex role in contemporary society. *JSAS Catalog of Selected Documents in Psychology, 8,* 35.

Dreyer, N. A., Woods, N. F., & James, S. A. (1981). ISRO: A scale to measure sex role orientation. *Sex Roles, 7,* 173–182.

Eagly, A. H. (1983). Gender and social influence: A social psychological analysis. *American Psychologist, 38,* 971–981.

Eagly, A. H. (1987). *Sex difference in social behavior: A social-role interpretation*. Hillsdale, NJ: Erlbaum.

Edwards, V. J., & Spence, J. T. (1987). Gender-related traits, stereotypes, and schemata. *Journal of Personality and Social Psychology, 53,* 146–154.

Eyde, L. D. (1962). *Work values and background factors as predictors of women's desire to work*. Columbus, OH: Bureau of Business Research.

Feingold, A. (1988). Cognitive gender differences are disappearing. *American Psychologist, 43,* 95–103.

Frable, D. E. S. (1989). Sex typing and gender ideology. *Journal of Personality and Social Psychology, 56,* 95–108.

Frable, D. E. S., & Bem, S. L. (1985). If you are gender schematic, all members of the opposite sex look alike. *Journal of Personality and Social Psychology, 49,* 459–468.

Gough, H. (1952). Identifying psychological femininity. *Educational and Psychological Measurement, 12,* 427–439.

Greenhaus, J. H. (1971). An investigation of the role of career salience in vocational behavior. *Journal of Vocational Behavior, 1,* 209–216.

Hare-Mustin, R. T., Bennett, S. K., & Broderick, P. C. (1983). Attitudes toward motherhood, gender, generational, and religion comparisons. *Sex Roles, 9,* 643–660.

Hare-Mustin, R. T., & Marecek, J. (1990). *Making a difference: Psychology and the construction of gender*. New Haven, CT: Yale University Press.

Harrington, D. M., & Andersen, S. M. (1981). Creativity, masculinity, femininity, and three models of psychological androgyny. *Journal of Personality and Social Psychology, 41,* 744–757.

Hoyt, D. P., & Kennedy, C. E. (1958). Interest and personality correlates of career-motivated and homemaking-motivated college women. *Journal of Counseling Psychology, 5,* 44–49.

Humphreys, L. G. (1988). Sex differences in variability may be more important than sex differences in means. *Behavioral and Brain Sciences, 11,* 195–196.

Hyde, J. S. (1981). How large are cognitive gender differences? A meta-analysis using $w2$ and d. *American Psychologist, 36,* 892–901.

Hyde, J. S. (1986). Gender differences in aggression. In J. S. Hyde & M. C. Linn (Eds.), *The psychology of gender* (pp. 51–66). Baltimore: Johns Hopkins University Press.

Ingram, R. E., Cruet, D., Johnson, B. R., & Wisnicki, K. S. (1988). Self-focused attention, gender role, and vulnerability to negative affect. *Journal of Personality and Social Psychology, 55,* 967–978.

Jacklin, C. N. (1989). Female and male: Issues of gender. *American Psychologist, 44,* 127–133.

Kalin, R., & Tilby, P. (1978). Development and validation of a sex role ideology scale. *Psychological Reports, 42,* 731–738.

Knaub, P. K., & Eversoll, D. B. (1983). Is parenthood a desirable adult role?: An assessment of attitudes held by contemporary adult women. *Sex Roles, 9,* 355–362.

Lenney, E. (1991). Sex roles: The measurement of masculinity, femininity, and androgyny. In J. P. Robinson, P. R. Shaver, & L. S. Wrightsman (Eds.), *Measures of personality and social psychological attitudes*. San Diego: Academic Press.

Linn, M. C. (1986). Meta-analysis of studies of gender differences: Implications and future directions. In J. S. Hyde & M. C. Linn (Eds.), *The psychology of gender* (pp. 210–232). Baltimore: Johns Hopkins University Press.

Linn, M. C., & Petersen, A. C. (1986). A meta-analysis of gender differences in spatial ability: Implications for mathematics and science achievement. In J. S. Hyde & M. C. Linn (Eds.), *The psychology of gender* (pp. 67–101). Baltimore: Johns Hopkins University Press.

Lott, B. (1990). Dual natures or learned behavior: The challenge to feminist psychology. In R. Hare-Mustin & J. Maracek (Eds.), *Making a difference* (pp. 65–101). New Haven, CT: Yale University Press.

Lubinski, D., Tellegen, A., & Butcher, J. N. (1981). The relationship between androgyny and subjective indicators of emotional well-being. *Journal of Personality and Social Psychology, 40,* 722–730.

Lubinski, D., Tellegen, A., & Butcher, J. N. (1983). Masculinity, femininity, and androgyny viewed and assessed as distinct concepts. *Journal of Personality and Social Psychology, 44,* 428–439.

Lyson, T. A., & Brown, S. S. (1982). Sex role attitudes, curriculum choice, and career ambition. *Journal of Vocational Behavior, 20,* 366–375.

Maccoby, E. E. (1988). Gender as a social category. *Developmental Psychology, 26,* 755–765.

Maccoby, E. E. (1990). Gender and relationships: A developmental account. *American Psychologist, 45,* 513–520.

Maccoby, E. E., & Jacklin, C. N. (1974). *The psychology of sex differences.* Stanford, CA: Stanford University Press.

Markus, H., Crane, M., Bernstein, S., & Siladi, M. (1982). Self schemas and gender. *Journal of Personality and Social Psychology, 42,* 38–50.

Martin, C. L., & Halverson, C. F. (1983). The effects of sex-typing schemes on young children's memories. *Child Development, 54,* 563–574.

Matlin, M. (1987). *The psychology of women.* New York: Holt, Rinehart and Winston.

Mezydlo, L., & Betz, N. E. (1980). Perceptions of ideal sex roles as a function of sex and feminist orientation. *Journal of Counseling Psychology, 27,* 282–285.

Nevill, D. E., & Super, D. E. (1986). *Manual for the Salience Inventory: Theory, research, and application.* Palo Alto, CA: Consulting Psychologists Press.

O'Heron, C. A., & Orlofsky, J. L. (1990). Stereotypic and non-stereotypic sex role trait and behavior orientations, gender identity, and psychological adjustment. *Journal of Personality and Social Psychology, 58,* 134–143.

O'Neil, J. M., Helms, B. J., Gable, R. K., David, L., & Wrightsman, L. S. (1986). Gender Role Conflict Scale: College men's fear of femininity. *Sex Roles, 14,* 335–350.

O'Neil, J. S. (1981). Patterns of gender role conflict and strain: Fear of femininity in men's lives. *Personnel and Guidance Journal, 60,* 203–210.

Orlofsky, J. L. (1981). Relationship between sex role attitudes and personality traits and the Sex Role Behavior Scale-1: A new measure of masculine and feminine role behaviors and interests. *Journal of Personality and Social Psychology, 40,* 927–940.

Orlofsky, J. L., Cohen, R. S., & Ramsden, M. W. (1985). Relationship between sex role attitudes and personality traits and the Revised Sex Role Behavior Scale. *Sex Roles, 12,* 377–391.

Orlofsky, J. L., & O'Heron, C. A. (1987a). Development of a short form Sex Role Behavior Scale. *Journal of Personality Assessment, 51,* 267–277.

Orlofsky, J. L., & O'Heron, C. A. (1987b). Stereotypic and nonstereotypic sex role trait and behavior orientation. Implications for personal adjustment. *Journal of Personality and Social Psychology, 52,* 1034–1042.

Orlofsky, J. L., Ramsden, M. W., & Cohen, R. S. (1982). Development of the Revised Sex Role Behavior Scale. *Journal of Personality Assessment, 46,* 632–638.

Payne, T. J., Connor, J. M., & Colletti, G. (1987). Gender-based schematic processing: An empirical investigation and reevaluation. *Journal of Personality and Social Psychology, 52,* 937–945.

Pedhazur, E., & Tetenbaum, T. (1979). Bem Sex Role Inventory: A theoretical and methodological critique. *Journal of Personality and Social Psychology, 37,* 996–1016.

Pleck, J. H. (1981). *The myth of masculinity.* Cambridge, MA: MIT Press.

Pleck, J. H. (1987). The contemporary man. In M. Scher, M. Stevens, G. Good, & G. Eichenfield (Eds.), *Handbook of counseling and psychotherapy with men.* Newbury Park, CA: Sage.

Rand, L. (1968). Masculinity or femininity: Differentiating career-oriented and home-oriented college freshmen women. *Journal of Counseling Psychology, 15,* 444–449.

Roos, P. E., & Cohen, L. H. (1987). Sex roles and social support as moderators of life stress adjustment. *Journal of Personality and Social Psychology, 52,* 576–585.

Rosenkrantz, P. S., Vogel, S. R., Bee, H., Broverman, I. K., & Broverman, D. M. (1968). Sex role stereotypes and self-concepts in college students. *Journal of Consulting and Clinical Psychology, 32,* 287–295.

Slevin, K. F., & Wingrove, C. R. (1983). Similarities and differences among three generations of women in attitudes toward the female role in contemporary society. *Sex Roles, 9,* 609–624.

Spence, J. T. (1983). Comment on Lubinski, Tellegen, and Butcher's "Masculinity, femininity, and androgyny viewed and assessed as distinct concepts." *Journal of Personality and Social Psychology, 44,* 440–446.

Spence, J. T. (1985). Gender identity and its implications for the concepts of masculinity and femininity. In T. B. Sonderegger (Ed.), *Nebraska symposium on motivation: Psychology and gender* (pp. 59–98). Lincoln: University of Nebraska Press.

Spence, J. T., Deaux, K., & Helmreich, R. L. (1985). Sex roles in contemporary American society. In G. Lindzey & E. Aronson (Eds.), *The handbook of social psychology* (3d ed., pp. 149–178). New York: Random House.

Spence, J. T., & Helmreich, R. L. (1972). The attitudes towards women scale: An objective instrument to measure attitudes toward the rights and roles of women in contemporary society. *JSAS Catalog of Selected Documents in Psychology, 2,* 66–67.

Spence, J. T., & Helmreich, R. L (1978). *Masculinity and femininity: Their psychological dimensions, correlates, and antecedents.* Austin: University of Texas Press.

Spence, J. T., Helmreich, R. L., & Holahan, C. K. (1979). Negative and positive components of psychological masculinity and femininity and their relationships to neurotic and acting out behaviors. *Journal of Personality and Social Psychology, 37*, 1673–1682.

Spence, J. T., Helmreich, R. L., & Stapp, J. (1973). A short version of the Attitudes Toward Women Scale. *Bulletin of the Psychonomic Society, 2*, 21–22.

Spence, J. T., Helmreich, R. L., & Stapp, J. (1974). The Personal Attributes Questionnaire: A measure of sex role stereotypes and masculinity-femininity. *JSAS Catalog of Selected Documents in Psychology, 4*, 43.

Spence, J. T., & Sawin, L. L. (1984). Images of masculinity and femininity: A reconceptualization. In V. O'Leary, R. Unger, & B. Wallston (Eds.), *Sex, gender, and social psychology*. Hillsdale, NJ: Erlbaum.

Stafford, I. P. (1984). Relation of attitudes towards women's roles and occupational behavior to women's self-esteem. *Journal of Counseling Psychology, 31*, 332–338.

Storms, M. D. (1979). Sex role identity and its relationship to sex role attributes and sex role stereotypes. *Journal of Personality and Social Psychology, 37*, 1779–1789.

Taylor, S. E., & Falcone, H. T. (1982). Cognitive bases of stereotyping: The relationship between categorization and prejudice. *Personality and Social Psychology Bulletin, 8*, 426, 432.

Tellegen, A., & Lubinski, D. (1983). Some methodological comments on labels, traits, interaction, and types in the study of "femininity" and "masculinity": Reply to Spence. *Journal of Personality and Social Psychology, 44*, 447–455.

Terman, L. L., & Miles, C. C. (1936). *Sex and personality*. New York: McGraw-Hill.

Tetenbaum, T. J., Lighter, J., & Travis, A. (1984). The construct validation of attitude towards working mothers scale. *Psychology of Women Quarterly, 8*, 69–78.

Thompson, E. H., Jr., Grisanti, C., & Pleck, J. H. (1985). Attitudes toward the male role and their correlates. *Sex Roles, 13*, 413–427.

Thompson, E. H., Jr., & Pleck, J. H. (1986). The structure of male role norms. *American Behavioral Scientist, 29*, 531–544.

Thornton, A., & Freedman, D. (1979). Changes in the sex role attitudes of women: 1962–1977. *American Sociological Review, 44*, 831–842.

Tinsley, D. J., & Faunce, P. S. (1980). Enabling, facilitating, and precipitating factors associated with women's career orientation. *Journal of Vocational Behavior, 17*, 183–194.

Unger, R. (1990). Imperfect reflections of reality. Psychology constructs gender. In R. Hare-Mustin & J. Maracek (Eds.), *Making a difference* (102–149). New Haven, CT: Yale University Press.

Vetter, L., & Lewis, E. C. (1964). Some correlates of homemaking versus career preference among college home economics students. *Personnel and Guidance Journal, 42*, 593–598.

Whitley, B. E., Jr., McHugh, M. C., & Freize, I. H. (1986). Assessing theoretical models for sex differences in causal attributions. In J. S. Hyde & M. C. Linn (Eds.), *The psychology of gender*. Baltimore: Johns Hopkins University Press.

Zuckerman, D. M. (1981). Family background, sex role attitudes, and the goals of technical college and university students. *Sex Roles, 7*, 1109–1126.

Chapter 7

The Psychological Test Profiles of Brigadier Generals
Warmongers or Decisive Warriors?[*]

David P. Campbell
Center for Creative Leadership
Colorado Springs, Colorado

The world has always been at war, and wars are run by generals. Generals plan for war, prepare for war, execute wars, and, in the aftermath, often have great influence on the postwar world.

Because of their central role in times of great conflict, military leaders have probably had more influence on history than any other occupational group, with the possible exception of politicians. Witness the impact, for example, of Alexander the Great, Julius Caesar, and Napoleon.

The impact on our own country of military leaders such as George Washington, Robert E. Lee, Ulysses S. Grant, and Dwight D. Eisenhower has been enormous, especially as many of them subsequently began political careers and thus further influenced events. George Washington, our first military commander in chief and, later, our first president, is perhaps the most dramatic example. Other more recent cases include George Marshall, who, as chairman of the Joint Chiefs of Staff, oversaw our military policy during World War II, and then, as secretary of state, initiated the Marshall Plan, which rebuilt and stabilized Western Europe; and Douglas MacArthur, who, as commander of the Pacific Theater, prosecuted the war against Japan,

---

[*]A version of this chapter was presented as an invited address to the division of industrial and organizational psychology on 20 August, 1987, at the meetings of the American Psychological Association in New York City.

and then, as commander of occupied Japan, was the chief architect of the current Japanese democratic system, which has proven to be so effective.

What kind of people are top military commanders? In psychological terms: How bright are they? What kind of personalities do they have? What are their vocational interests? What values do they hold?

In the last nine years, through our programs at the Center for Creative Leadership (CCL), we have had the rare opportunity to study some of these questions through the medium of standardized psychological assessment techniques. Roughly 160 Army general officers have participated in our one-week Leadership Development Program (LDP) course. At any one time, the army has about 400 generals, so we have tapped a reasonably large percentage of the total group. Because testing general officers is no simple matter, a few comments about how we need to collect the following test data might be relevant.

The LDP course is quite psychological in tone, as opposed to either exhortative or technical. The course components include standardized psychological tests, assessment center exercises in which each individual is observed and rated on several performance dimensions, peer and subordinate evaluations, and small group exercises that are videotaped and then played back to the participants.

All data collected from and about these individuals are given back to them in ways that are specifically designed to help them make personal use of the information. None of the individual's data are given to the sponsoring organization, which specifically means that the army does not have access to the test information for each individual officer, although they do receive overall summaries for the entire group.

This emphasis on the individual's privacy is worth some elaboration. One reason that our leadership course has become so popular is that the participants, which include a wide range of powerful people, find the course to be a psychologically safe environment in which to consider some important personal issues: What kind of a leader am I? How do others see me? Which of my characteristics have been strengths and which ones weaknesses? In which situations am I most effective? What kind of subordinates do I have difficulty with, and why? Where do I want to lead my organization to next? and What kind of personal challenges do I want to take on, and what is the best approach to ensure success?

A sizable portion of the course focuses on the individual's career aspirations. Even general officers are still trying to decide what they want to be when they grow up, and the topic of personal future planning is seen as one of the most important segments of the course.

Although it sounds trite to say it, we do focus on the whole person. We encourage people to think about the entire context of their lives, not just their career, but also about their close relationships (or, in our population, more often the lack of them), their families, their communities, their health, their finances, and anything else that is important to them.

For some years now, the Army General Officer Management Office has recommended that each newly appointed brigadier general attend the course. We do not know how the recommendation to attend the course is transmitted to each individual officer. Although most participants come to the class with at least mild acceptance of the assignment—and many with enthusiasm—a few have made it clear that they have little time for this "psychological stuff," that they came because they were ordered to, and that they do not expect to learn anything new or useful.

With a few inevitable exceptions, their final course evaluations indicate they have all completed the course with a positive feeling. Indeed, we are now told that the general officer grapevine gives our center high marks as a worthwhile activity. For example, the following letter was received a few years ago from a former participant, Brigadier General James Dozier. General Dozier had attended the LDP course in August 1981. Later that fall, he was kidnapped by the Italian Red Brigade and was held for about six weeks until he was rescued by the Italian police. A few weeks after his release, I received this letter:

Dear Dave:

Just a quick note to let you know that the week that I spent with you and your staff in Greensboro this past summer stood me in good stead during the six weeks that I spent as an unwelcome guest of the Red Brigades here in Italy....

Sincerely,
James L. Dozier
BG, USA

THE SAMPLES

For comparison purposes, data from three samples are presented in this chapter:

1. Army Brigadier Generals ($N = 163$). These data probably generalize to general officers in the other services, but the military does not agree. In fact, it is remarkable to listen to army, air force, navy, and marine officers talk about the differences between the leadership styles of the military services—they believe they live in different worlds!

2. High-Level Corporate Executives (N ranges from 74 to 139). These are civilian executives with job titles of CEO, president, or vice president, who have also attended the program.

3. CCL Norm Sample (N = approximately 1,000). Our usual participant group, which includes a variety of managers and technical workers from corporate, governmental, educational, and public service organizations. Both of the first two samples are embedded in this one. The numbers vary for any one measure, both because of the usual problems of missing data and because data have been drawn from a variety of reports.

BASIC DEMOGRAPHIC DATA

Table 1 includes basic demographic data for the three samples on age, sex, and race. As the table illustrates, course participants are typically white males in their forties. The generals were in this basic age range, although a few years older.

All three samples were predominantly male. Although we make an effort to include women in every course, the percentage of female participants is small. It is even smaller in the corporate and military samples. Males continue to be the major benefactors of leadership training in our society.

The samples were predominantly white, but the army is making greater strides than either CCL or the civilian world in working with African-American leaders. Roughly 10% of the officers in the army (approximately 10,000 out of a total 90,000 officers) are African-American, so the number of African-American generals attending our course is representative of the overall army population.

Table 2 shows the educational level for the three samples, and here the most dramatic difference between the groups appears. Even though both the CCL Norm Sample and the High-Level Corporate Executive Sample are well educated—about 90% of each have college degrees and roughly one-third have graduate degrees—the general officers have even more formal education. All individuals in the sample have a college degree, 88% have a master's degree, and 9% have a doctoral-level degree. The higher echelon of the United States Army is uncommonly well educated.

THE COGNITIVE ABILITY TEST

Table 3 presents the mean scores on the *Shipley Institute of Living Scale* (SILS), a short, 20-minute, 40-item IQ test. It is a quick, relatively effective screening device that provides a reasonable index of

Table 1   Age, Sex, and Race Statistics for Three Samples

	Brigadier Generals (N = 163)	High-Level Corporate Executives (N = 139)	CCL Norm Sample (N = 1,002)
Age			
Mean	47	44	41
S.D.	2.4	7.2	8.0
Sex			
Male	98%	97%	86%
Female	2%	3%	14%
Race			
Native American	0%	0%	1%
African-American	10%	1%	3%
Asian	1%	1%	1%
Hispanic	1%	1%	2%
White	86%	96%	92%
Other	2%	1%	1%

Table 2   Educational Level in Percentages for Three Samples

Highest Level Attained	Brigadier Generals (N = 163)	High-Level Corporate Executives (N = 139)	CCL Norm Sample (N = 1,002)
High school graduate	0	2	3
Some college	0	10	11
College graduate	3	55	43
Master's degree	88	19	29
Doctorate	9	11	11
Other	0	3	3

Table 3   Cognitive Ability (IQ) Using the *Shipley Institute of Living Scale*

	Brigadier Generals (N = 162)	High-Level Corporate Executives (N = 137)	CCL Norm Sample (N = 1,477)
Mean	124	121	118
S.D.	6.5	6.8	7.1

general mental ability. Longer, more precise measures of the mental abilities would have been preferred, but logistical difficulties preclude that possibility.

As the data indicate, the brigadier generals tested were bright people, with an average score of 124, which is a full standard deviation above our other two samples and at the 95th percentile of the general population. Because the SILS has a low ceiling—the maximum possible score is only 140—these average scores are almost certainly underestimates.

Summary statistics conceal individual variation, so the distributions of scores are also shown. Figure 1 shows the frequency distribution of the brigadier generals on this IQ measure; again, the data look impressive, especially noting the large grouping at the top of the distribution.

The demographic and cognitive test scores indicate that the brigadier generals were slightly older, better educated, and more intelligent than either the High-Level Corporate Executive Sample or the CCL Norm Sample, which is all the more impressive because these latter groups are quite impressive in their own right. This combination of personal attributes showed up as a high level of experience and self-confidence during their participation in the leadership course, a theme that will be repeated in the remaining data, especially in the next block of information, which is based on their performance in the small group problem-solving exercises.

THE BEHAVIOR ASSESSMENT RATINGS

Early in the Leadership Development Program, each person participates in two small group exercises called "Leaderless Group Discussions." In these exercises, six people are seated around a table, given a problem to solve, and then the group is left alone to work out the solution. One of the exercises is "competitive," where the resources are such that only one person can win; the other is "cooperative," where the group must pool their resources together to achieve a solution. This difference in the exercises is not pointed out to the participants until after the exercises are completed.

During the exercises, each participant is observed by staff members and rated on the following factors:

- Activity Level

- Led the Discussion

- Influenced Others

- Problem Analysis

- Task Orientation

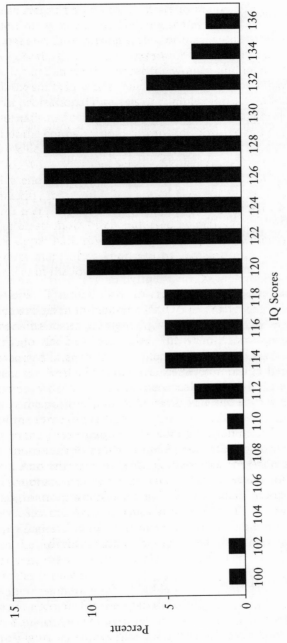

Figure 1   Distribution of IQ scores of brigadier generals (*N* = 162) using the *Shipley Institute of Living Scale*

- Motivated Others
- Interpersonal Skills
- Verbal Effectiveness

Although the results are reported to each participant on all eight rating factors, we know from the intercorrelations that there are basically two dimensions being tapped by the ratings: task orientation and relationship orientation.

In addition, after the exercise each person is rank ordered on overall effectiveness by (a) themselves, (b) the other people in the group (their peers), and (c) our staff members. This rank order is reported as a number from 1 to 6, with 1 being the highest.

The assessment ratings and the rank orderings for the three samples are shown in Figure 2 for the competitive exercise and in Figure 3 for the cooperative exercise. (In both figures, the scale for the rankings is reversed from that of the ratings, with low scores being high, i.e., more desirable.)

What is immediately apparent from Figures 2 and 3 is that the Brigadier General Sample was consistently higher in performance than the other two samples, with the High-Level Corporate Executive Sample being rated higher than the CCL Norm Sample. The differences were usually in the two-point range, which is roughly one-third of a standard deviation—not a huge difference, but definitely notable. In this standardized exercise, with standardized ratings, the general officers demonstrated a clear and consistent, though modest-sized edge, when compared with the other two samples.

The data for the individual rating scales show that there was a noticeable tendency for the brigadier generals to be rated relatively higher on those scales tapping the Task Orientation factor, compared with the scales tapping the Relationship Orientation factor. Furthermore, the relative differences were larger for the competitive exercise than they were for the cooperative exercise. The same pattern appears in the Self-Peers-Staff rank orderings. These patterns of ratings and rankings suggest that when competitiveness and forcefulness are required, the brigadier generals stand out. When cooperativeness and harmony are required, their relative standing is lower.

THE PSYCHOLOGICAL INVENTORIES

We use several psychological inventories in the program, including the *California Psychological Inventory* (CPI), the *Myers-Briggs Type Indicator* (MBTI), the FIRO-B, and the *Strong-Campbell Interest Inventory* (*Strong-Campbell*). Each serves a specific and different purpose.

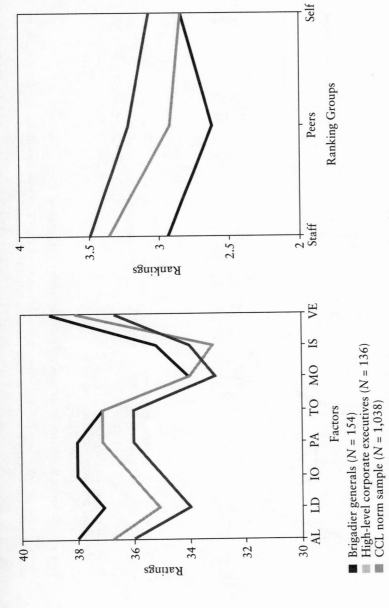

Figure 2 Behavioral assessment competitive exercise ratings and rankings

Note. AL = Activity Level, LD = Led the Discussion, IO = Influenced Others, PA = Problem Analysis, TO = Task Orientation, MO = Motivated Others, IS = Interpersonal Skills, and VE = Verbal Effectiveness.

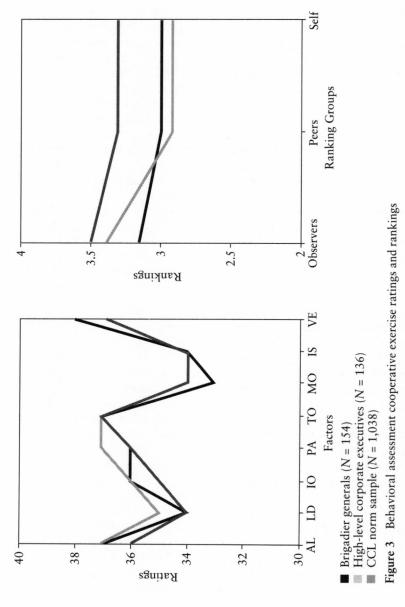

Figure 3 Behavioral assessment cooperative exercise ratings and rankings

Note. AL = Activity Level, LD = Led the Discussion, IO = Influenced Others, PA = Problem Analysis, TO = Task Orientation, MO = Motivated Others, IS = Interpersonal Skills, and VE = Verbal Effectiveness.

California Psychological Inventory

The *California Psychological Inventory* (CPI) is a 462-item questionnaire designed to measure certain *folk concepts,* that is, factors frequently invoked when people are describing other individuals. The CPI is oriented toward positive descriptions, which means that scores above the population mean are associated with healthy psychological functioning. An exception might be in the extremely high ranges, where obsessions can sometimes be noted.

The CPI averages for the three samples are presented in Figure 4. The population average for each of these scales is 50, with a standard deviation of 10.

Figure 4 is a rich collection of data, but space constraints prohibit a full discussion. Instead, only four main points will be made here. First, the general elevation of the entire profile for all three samples indicates that these samples contain individuals who are, on the average, psychologically healthy. Although low-scoring deviants can always be buried in the averages, that generally is not the case here. The more likely source of pathology, especially among the generals, is the obsession that may come from high scores. This brings up the second point: The three highest scores for the general officers were on the Dominance, Self-acceptance, and Achievement via Conformance scales.

The Dominance scale reflects self-perceived leadership ability, persistence, and social initiative. Very high scores, such as those in Figure 4, can also indicate an aggressive, demanding, and possibly self-centered personality. The Self-acceptance scale assesses a sense of personal worth and the capacity for taking action. The Achievement via Conformance scale reflects a desire for structure and clearly prescribed criteria for performance assessment. However, it should be noted that the generals, like the other two samples, also scored high on the Achievement via Independence scale, which indicates a desire for autonomy and intrinsically motivating rewards. The scores suggest that all three samples are achievement-oriented in a broad sense.

The third noteworthy point is that the generals scored significantly higher than the other two samples on the Responsibility and Socialization scales, which taken together reflect planfulness, dependability, social maturity, personal integrity, and an alertness to ethical and moral issues. This is where their sense of duty becomes clearly apparent.

Fourth, the general officers' scores were relatively lowest on the Flexibility scale, which says something about their willingness, or lack thereof, to consider new, innovative solutions to problems. This score indicates that they tend toward the conventional in their stance toward new ideas. However, their score is not low—it is actually right on the population average—but it appears low because most of their other scores are high.

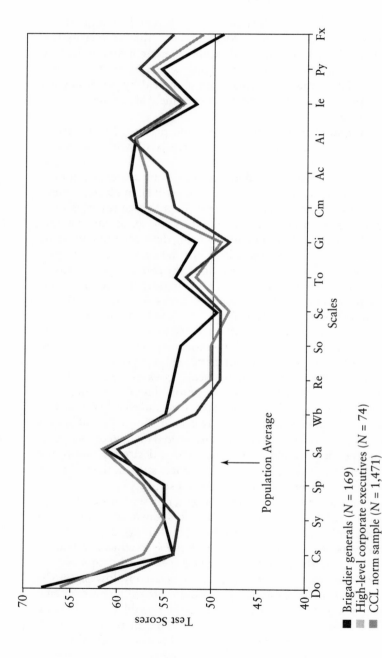

Figure 4 *California Psychological Inventory* scores for three samples

Note. Do = Dominance, Cs = Capacity for Status, Sy = Sociability, Sp = Social Presence, Sa = Self-acceptance, Wb = Well-being, Re = Responsibility, So = Socialization, Sc = Self-control, To = Tolerance, Gi = Good Impression, Cm = Communality, Ac = Achievement via Conformance, Ai = Achievement via Independence, Ie = Intellectual Efficiency, Py = Physical-mindedness, and Fx = Flexibility.

Again, to draw attention to the dispersion of individual cases, Figure 5 shows the distribution of the individual scores for the generals on the CPI Dominance scale. Clearly, we are not dealing with shrinking violets here.

The Myers-Briggs Type Indicator

The *Myers-Briggs Type Indicator* (MBTI) has achieved a sizeable following in many circles, and that is certainly true in the U.S. military. It is used in the military academies and in the advanced military educational institutions, such as the Army War College in Carlisle Barracks, Pennsylvania, and the National Defense University in Washington. In general, its use has probably been beneficial, not so much because of its psychometric qualities but because it vividly illustrates the concept of individual differences in ways that the layperson finds quite meaningful.

The MBTI has the following four scales: Extraversion-Introversion, Sensing-Intuition, Thinking-Feeling, and Judging-Perceiving. After completing the inventory, each individual receives a score on each scale that assigns him or her to one end of the dimension or the other, that is, Extraversion or Introversion, Thinking or Feeling, and so on:

- Extraversion (E) versus Introversion (I)—a preference for the outer world of people and things versus the inner world of ideas and concepts

- Sensing (S) versus Intuition (N)—a preference for immediate, real, and practical facts versus intuitive hunches and imagined possibilities

- Thinking (T) versus Feeling (F)—a preference for rational analysis emphasizing fairness versus an emotional analysis emphasizing feelings

- Judging (J) versus Perceiving (P)—a preference for decisive action achieving closure versus open-ended spontaneity

The 16 possible combinations of these four bipolar dimensions are arranged into what is known as the MBTI Type Table, and the percentages of each type for the three samples are shown in Table 4.

Two conclusions are immediately apparent from Table 4. First, in none of the three samples are the percentages evenly distributed across the 16 types. Second, only a few composite types account for a majority of each sample: four types account for 59% of the CCL Norm Sample, three types account for 61% of the High-Level Corporate Executive Sample, and only two types—ISTJ and ESTJ—account for 56% of the Brigadier Generals Sample. (This lack of individual differentiation is one of the features that is absent from the MBTI.)

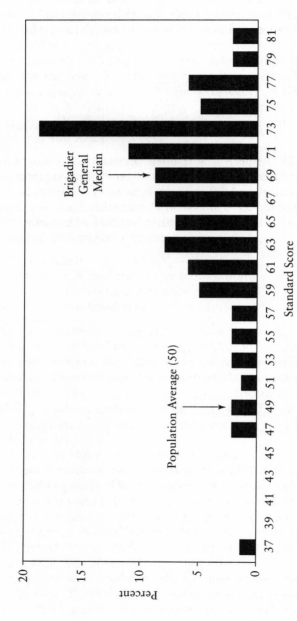

Figure 5   CPI Dominance scale scores for brigadier generals (*N* = 159)

Table 4   Percentage of the 16 MBTI Types in Three Samples

ISTJ	ISFJ	INFJ	INTJ
——— 28%	——— 3%	——— 1%	——— 9%
- - - 26%	- - - 0%	- - - 1%	- - - 8%
——— 21%	——— 2%	——— 2%	——— 11%

ISTP	ISFP	INFP	INTP
——— 5%	——— 2%	——— 1%	——— 3%
- - - 5%	- - - 1%	- - - 3%	- - - 4%
——— 4%	——— 0%	——— 3%	——— 7%

ESTP	ESFP	ENFP	ENTP
——— 4%	——— 1%	——— 2%	——— 3%
- - - 4%	- - - 4%	- - - 0%	- - - 6%
——— 4%	——— 1%	——— 4%	——— 6%

ESTJ	ESFJ	ENFJ	ENTJ
——— 28%	——— 3%	——— 1%	——— 7%
- - - 20%	- - - 3%	- - - 1%	- - - 15%
——— 18%	——— 3%	——— 2%	——— 13%

——— Brigadier generals (N = 161)
- - - High-level corporate executives (N = 111)
——— CCL norm sample (N = 1,262)

The two dominant types, ISTJ and ESTJ, are described in the booklet *Introduction to Type* (Myers, 1993) as follows (paraphrased here):

- ISTJ. Serious, quiet, earn success by concentration and thoroughness. Practical, orderly, matter-of-fact, logical, realistic, and dependable. Take responsibility. Make up their own minds as to what should be accomplished and work toward it steadily, regardless of protest and distractions.

- ESTJ. Practical realists with a natural gift for business or engineering. Not interested in subjects they see no use for, but can apply themselves when necessary. Like to organize and run activities. Tend to run things well, though they may sometimes forget to consider other people's feelings and points of view.

The description of these two types is quite consistent with the earlier pattern of scores produced by the CPI for the sample, and the fact that 56% of the top army leadership falls into this STJ category tells something about the psychological feel of the military environment.

FIRO-B

The FIRO-B is a short questionnaire that asks people to report how they behave in three different categories:

- Inclusion—"How often do you include others in your social activities?"

- Control—"How often do you try to control others?"

- Affection—"How often do you express warmth and affection toward others?"

The answers to these questions are reported as Expressed Behaviors. The same questions are asked about what the person wants from other people:

- Inclusion—"How often do you want others to include you in their social activities?"

- Control—"How often do you allow others to control your activities?"

- Affection—"How often do you want other people to express warmth and affection toward you?"

The answers to these questions are reported as Wanted Behaviors.

Scores are then given on six scales, as is shown in Table 5, which also includes a brief description of how high scores on each of them should be interpreted.

The FIRO-B means for each of the three samples are presented in Figure 6.

In looking at Figure 6, two notable patterns are immediately evident. The first is the high level of Expressed versus Wanted Control reported by all three samples, but, in particular, by the generals. What they are saying here is, "I want to be in charge of most of the people, most of the time, and I don't often want others to be in charge of me."

The second notable pattern is the high level of Wanted versus Expressed Affection. What this pattern is saying is, "I don't want to act warm and affectionate toward many people, but I want them to act warm and affectionate toward me." We see this pattern often within the managerial world. It is lonely out there, and people often make themselves even lonelier by the way they act. They want interpersonal warmth, but they often will not allow themselves to show it.

Once again, to make the point about individual variability, FIRO-B score distributions for the brigadier generals are presented in Figure 7. Averages conceal the individual richness and the enormous range of individual differences in these patterns.

Table 5   High FIRO-B Score Explanations

	Inclusion	Control	Affection
Expressed	Shows high social energy; initiates a lot of social interactions	Wants to be in charge of everything and everyone, at all times, and in all places	Expresses personal warmth easily and often toward others
Wanted	Wants to be included in the social plans of others	Willing to let others make decisions	Wants others to express warmth and affection toward them often

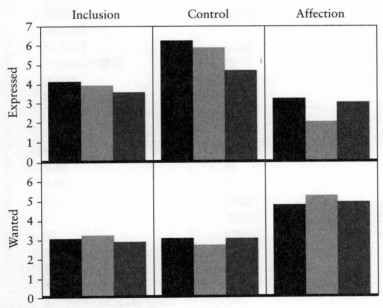

Brigadier generals ($N = 162$)
High-level corporate executives ($N = 137$)
CCL norm sample ($N = 1,485$)

Figure 6   FIRO-B mean scores for three samples

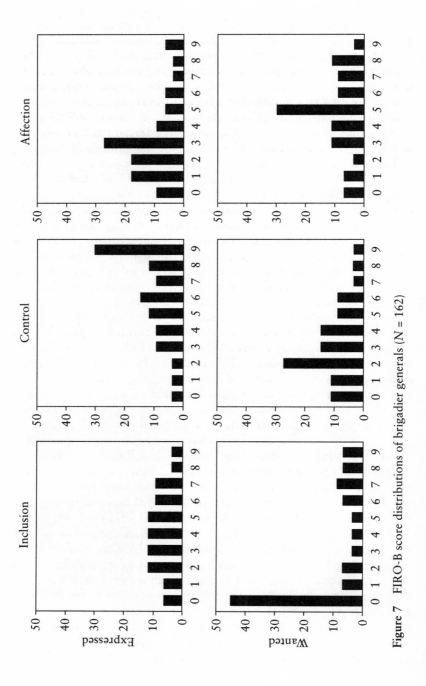

Figure 7 FIRO-B score distributions of brigadier generals (*N* = 162)

To illustrate, patterns of two officers in this sample suggest two very different social approaches. Table 6 shows the FIRO-B result patterns of 30 brigadier generals. One pattern (2/0, 0/1, 0/3) indicates a very cautious person; the 2/0 on Inclusion suggests that he does not want to give much socially to others and wants even less in return. An astonishing 44% of the Brigadier General Sample scored zero on Wanted Inclusion. This score is also often seen in our corporate groups, and clinical experience suggests that the explanation is that these people already lead impossibly busy social lives. Consequently, when confronted with a question such as, How often do you want other people to invite you to their social activities?, they most often answer "Rarely or Never." The Control score of 0/1 is also startling in a brigadier general because it indicates that "I don't want to be in charge of anyone, anywhere, anytime," nor do "I want anyone in charge of me." The Affection score (0/3) indicates an individual who is very guarded outwardly, but who inwardly is seeking interpersonal warmth.

In marked contrast, the second pattern (9/9, 9/8, 8/9) suggests a completely different dynamic. This "socially manic" pattern would be interpreted for the Inclusion scales (9/9) as a person reporting a strong drive to initiate social activities and an equally strong wish to be included by others; this person does not wish to miss a single coffee break conversation, football pool, or TGIF party. His control scores (9/8) indicate an obsessive need to take charge, but an equally strong willingness to follow others. His Affection scores (8/9) show that he is eager to be warm and affectionate to everyone and has an almost desperate desire to be loved indiscriminately in return. This pattern is a warning sign for Type A behavior, and this officer has in fact had some severe heart attacks. These score reports are used in the individually tailored feedback sessions given to each person, and a pattern like this would get a lot of attention.

The Strong-Campbell Interest Inventory

Figure 8 shows the average scores of the three samples on the Basic Interest Scales of the *Strong-Campbell Interest Inventory* (*Strong-Campbell*). These scales are normed on a mean of 50, with a standard deviation of 10.

The dramatic spike on the brigadier generals' profile is on the Military Activities scale; their mean score was 73, almost 2½ standard deviations above the population mean. Other noteworthy high scores for the generals are 58 on the Adventure scale and 59 on the Business Management scale. Not surprisingly, these people like action, and, once again, the evidence is clear that they like to be in charge. They also scored fairly high on the Athletics, Public Speaking, and Law/Politics scales.

Table 6 FIRO-B Results for 30 Brigadier Generals

Inclusion	Control	Affection	Inclusion	Control	Affection	Inclusion	Control	Affection
6/0	9/3	2/4	6/6	9/4	3/8	7/6	5/5	3/4
3/0	5/0	3/3	3/5	9/4	4/3	3/0	7/1	1/2
6/1	2/1	3/3	5/8	7/2	3/9	1/0	3/5	2/3
5/0	5/0	3/5	3/6	5/2	1/6	7/2	9/3	3/5
7/8	2/2	2/8	8/9	3/6	8/9	5/4	8/0	3/4
1/0	7/2	2/5	5/0	0/4	5/5	3/3	6/3	3/6
4/0	8/2	3/6	5/2	7/0	4/4	5/4	5/3	2/8
2/0	4/4	2/4	5/7	9/3	3/7	6/6	1/4	3/6
4/0	6/1	3/6	3/4	7/2	0/1	4/0	6/6	0/0
0/0	3/0	1/5	2/9	9/8	2/9	2/0	0/1	0/3

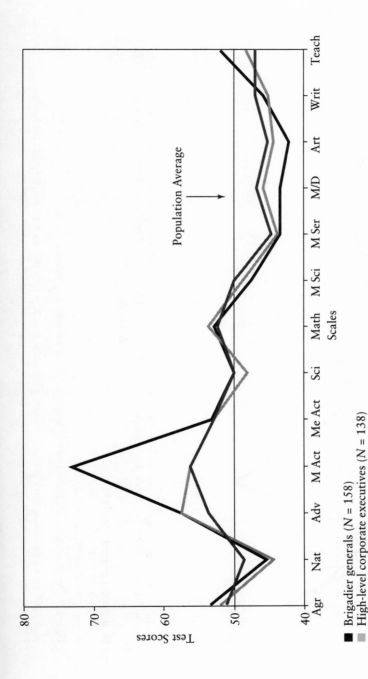

Figure 8 *Strong-Campbell* Basic Interest Scales for three samples

Note. Agr = Agriculture, Nat = Nature, Adv = Adventure, M Act = Military Activities, Me Act = Mechanical Activities, Sci = Science, Math = Mathematics, M Sci = Medical Science, M Ser = Medical Service, M/D = Music/Drama, Writ = Writing, and Teach = Teaching.

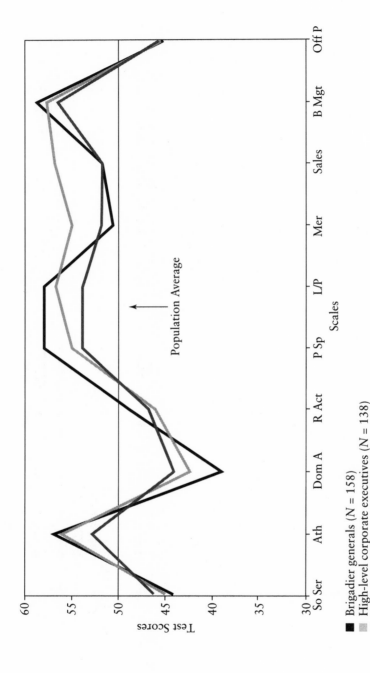

Figure 8 *Strong-Campbell* Basic Interest Scales for three samples (continued)

Brigadier generals (*N* = 158)
High-level corporate executives (*N* = 138)
CCL norm sample (*N* = 1,235)

Note. So Ser = Social Service, Ath = Athletics, Dom A = Domestic Arts, R Act = Religious Activities, P Sp = Public Speaking, L/P = Law/Politics, Mer = Merchandising, B Mgt = Business Management, and Off P = Office Practices.

Their low Basic Interest scores were on the Art, Music/Dramatics, and the Domestic Arts scales. These individuals are not particularly attracted by the finer activities of life.

Again, two distributions of individual scores are presented here to demonstrate the variability of the sample. Figure 9 shows the remarkable distribution of scores on the Military Activities scale for the brigadier generals. Figure 10 shows the distribution for the Music/Dramatics scale scores for the brigadier generals, illustrating that this is not a strong area of interest for most of these officers.

DECISIVE WARRIORS OR WARMONGERS?

Working from the test and demographic data presented above, as well as other anecdotal evidence and personal experience, we seem to have identified a notable personality syndrome—the aggressive adventurer—which has the following characteristics: dominant, competitive, action-oriented, patriotic men who are naturally drawn to physically adventuresome, militaristic activities and who are repulsed by artistic, literary, musical, and nurturing activities.

Further, this pattern, when accompanied by a high sense of social responsibility and personality integrity, as indicated by high scores on the CPI Responsibility and Socialization scales, can be described as a "decisive warrior." In the absence of the high scores just mentioned, this pattern may well be labeled "warmonger."

Given this conclusion, we can speculate about some selection and development issues; specifically, are we selecting the right people for leadership at the highest military levels? Are we finding and promoting the decisive warriors and eliminating other less desirable types, including the warmongers?

INDIVIDUAL SELECTION VERSUS DEVELOPMENT OF SYSTEMS

In my early days as a psychologist, I was strongly influenced in my thinking about such topics by my training and subsequent faculty activities at the University of Minnesota, which is perhaps the premier university in the world in terms of its focus on traditional psychological testing. The Minnesota thinking focused heavily on the individual, as opposed to either groups or larger systems, and the Minnesota point of view recommended solutions emphasizing selection and promotional decisions. This approach, based on individual differences, still has great appeal for me; it is hard to escape one's early training.

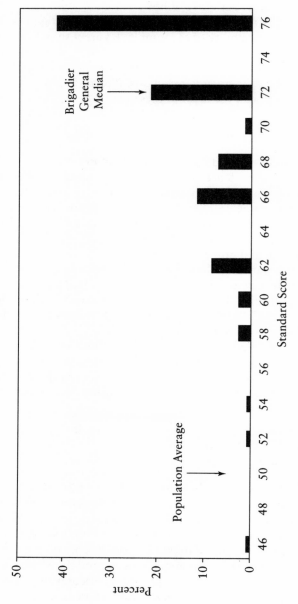

Figure 9 *Strong-Campbell* Military Activities Basic Interest Scale scores for brigadier generals ($N = 156$)

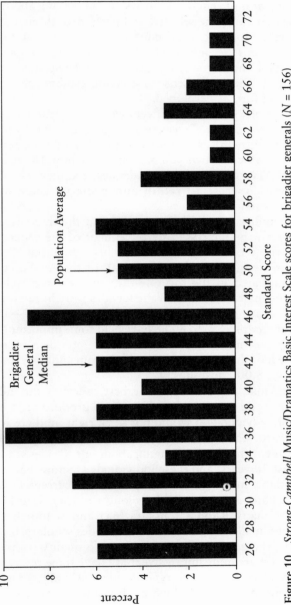

Figure 10 *Strong-Campbell Music/Dramatics Basic Interest Scale scores for brigadier generals (N = 156)*

However, more recently, I have found an expanded truth in the form of APA Division 14, with its focus on organizational psychology, which puts far more emphasis on systems. Thinking about individuals and how they might be selected and promoted, though important, is not enough. More attention must be given to the culture in which these individuals are embedded. Although decisions about individuals are important, the surrounding sociopolitical environment may be even more crucial. There is no sense in selecting good people if they are not retained and further developed.

For example, all general officers were once lieutenants—there are hardly any exceptions. Consequently, to influence the kind of people who become generals, one must first understand how people become lieutenants, which throws you back studying how 18-year-olds decide to enter ROTC or the military academies, and then try to understand what forces operate to retain and promote them during their formative years.

If one studies the admissions process at the three academies, one can't help but be impressed by the caliber of the cadets. I am most familiar with the Air Force Academy's procedure, but West Point and Annapolis are quite similar. Almost all of the Air Force Academy's cadets graduated in the top one-fifth of their high school classes; 10% of the males and 20% of the females were in the top 1%. Their average College Board scores are high—around 1250—and a sizable majority, perhaps 75% to 80%, have held some important high school leadership positions, such as student body president or athletic team captain. All of them appear to be able to run endlessly and to be able to do about 8,000 push-ups.

In particular, the quality of the best cadets at the military academies, the group that one would hope will produce the most generals, is astonishingly good—I would put them right up there with the best that Harvard, Yale, Princeton, and Iowa State can produce. The Air Force Academy has been averaging about one Rhodes scholar per year for the last 30 years, and these individuals are now making their way into the higher military ranks. One of them is currently Commandant of the Air Force Academy. With its longer history, West Point has had twice that many Rhodes scholars (61) and is fourth among U.S. universities in all-time production of Rhodes scholars.

Clearly, the academies are selecting top quality people, and their best products are quite impressive, but I have some reservations about what they are doing for their typical cadet. Each fall, the military academies admit roughly 1,300 high-quality students each—students who have already demonstrated the capacity and motivation for outstanding achievement. Then, for four years the academies treat their cadets as if they were untrustworthy adolescents. For all practical purposes, the cadets are deprived of the necessity or opportunity for making any significant personal decisions. They are told where to live and how to live, right down to exactly how their washcloths are to be folded. They are told what to eat, where to eat, and when to eat. They are told what to study, where to study, and when to study. They are told, in excruciating detail, what to wear. Their finances are monitored; their car ownership is controlled; their social life, such as it is, is highly structured. They are taught enormous respect for rank, so much so that to the civilian observer, it appears that rank usually over-powers all other personal characteristics. They are taught that any deviation from the norm is suspect, that all problems have answers, and that personal and organizational discipline is the solution to all dilemmas.

All of this is done under the guise of leadership training, which appears to me to be a dubious strategy. Holding a bright, young ca-pable person in such a cocoon for four years may not be the best way to prepare him or her to shoulder the responsibilities of leadership.

I do recognize that the military academies are constantly changing and evolving and that many changes that I consider improvements have come about in the last two or three decades; for example, the admission of women and minorities and the gradual liberalization of the curriculum. And I do recognize the political power of tradition and, thus, the difficulty of moving rapidly. As one of the senior offic-ers at the Air Force Academy told me, "Changing the curriculum here is the political equivalent of moving a cemetery."

MILITARY RETENTION OF "WISE" LEADERS

The central issue is whether or not the U.S. military, having attracted and trained excellent young people, can retain enough of the best of them to fill the diplomatic, political, and leadership roles at the top of the military establishment. Although there are many attractive fea-tures of a military career that should work to retain good people, such as the possibilities for excellent postgraduate education and opportu-nities for responsible commands at early ages, there are repelling forces also. The military, like all other large bureaucracies, including corpo-rations and universities, is capable of imposing seemingly senseless policies and practices on itself in a way that can drive good people right up the wall and out the door. The military's peculiar obsession with short hair is only one of the milder examples.

Give me a week on any military base anywhere with access to the troops, and I will come up with a half dozen illustrations of how the military bureaucracy tends to drive out the rational. One quick example: On U.S. military bases there is usually a policy requiring the posting of evacuation plans in all buildings so that people will know how to escape quickly in the event of a fire. You know the kind; they show the building floor plan with a large red "X" showing "You Are Here" and a red arrow showing the escape route. On some army posts, there are Quonset-hut-type shelters with both ends knocked out so that tanks and trucks can drive in one end for shelter while pulling maintenance, and then drive on out the other end. On at least one army base, soldiers were expected to post evacuation plans in their shelters, which were already basically open to the world. If you were a young, capable soldier, how would you feel about the quality of leaders who required such things?

When I have raised such questions in military settings, I usually have received some version of the following reaction:

> Charlie Brown (to Snoopy, dressed in his World War I flyer's outfit): The vet said we're going to have to start watching your diet.
>
> Snoopy: That's easy for him to say. He doesn't have to eat in the mess hall with the troops.
>
> Charlie Brown: I also had a little trouble explaining why you were wearing a helmet and goggles.
>
> Snoopy: Civilians don't understand anything!

Which brings me back to my point—that it is not sufficient just to select good people. You have to put them in an environment where quality is appreciated and nurtured.

THE AGGRESSIVE ADVENTURER

The world is a dangerous place; there are evil people out there who wish to do us great harm. Although terrorist acts provide the most visible, immediate evidence of danger, the build up of massive military forces, along with the clear intention of oppressing other nations, is the more frightening threat.

Given the necessity of protecting ourselves from such threats with military might, the general officers that we have now are outstanding—they are bright, well educated, experienced, responsible, and well indoctrinated in democratic ways. Furthermore, in the few ways we have had of evaluating them in comparison with civilian leaders, the generals come across as more impressive. In that regard, we are a fortunate society.

But a larger question is: Why do we need them? Why is the world a dangerous place? Where do the risks come from? Why is military might essential?

One reason that the world is a dangerous place may be that other countries also have their share of men with this personality syndrome—the aggressive adventurer is a universal phenomenon. To the extent that this is true, military conflict may arise simply because there are people in the world who are psychologically disposed to seeking it, especially because in many other countries, unlike the United States, such people have not been exposed to the ameliorating influences of higher education and a culture dominated by the democratic process. In societies where the individual's "life, liberty, and pursuit of happiness" is not recognized as a governmental goal, the instigation of conflict, that is, warfare, may come much more naturally and might, we even say, instinctively, to people with these personality characteristics.

If data could be gathered, I believe they would show that the themes making up this personality syndrome would be replicated in most of the world's military leaders, though not necessarily accompanied by the high scores on the Responsibility and Socialization scales that we have found in our sample of U.S. generals. Other cultures have not always had the tradition of substantial formal education for their fighters, and, of course, few other societies have had the benefits of 200 years of democracy.

When I present this theory, that is, that the presence of aggressive adventurers leads to international conflict, my military friends challenge me on this conclusion. They say that there is not one shred of evidence that what I am proposing is true, that there is no data to support this conclusion. That is a sobering challenge, one that I cannot answer empirically. Consequently, I must be very clear that what I am expressing are simply my opinions, and that many more intelligent, experienced people disagree with me.

Although I believe that the presence of the aggressive adventurer syndrome in other countries that do not have highly educated military leaders and which do not have an entrenched system of democratic checks and balances is likely to lead to armed conflict, I cannot prove that. One of the main reasons that the world is a dangerous place may be that such men in other countries—men equally energetic, equally eloquent, equally fueled by the self-righteousness of their own causes—are not always bound by our democratic constraints. All they need to wage war is political power and weapons. Unlike our military leaders, they are not operating under the constraints of personal morality and legislative principles.

What I am saying is that the personality pattern identified above can be considered, in the absence of any softening patina of education and democracy, to be the warmonger profile. I believe that men with such patterns will scheme to collect funds to secure lethal weapons, that they will strive to recruit young people into military units where they will be taught to kill, that they will argue mindlessly that their particular beliefs are the only truth, and that people who think differently are evil and wicked and therefore should be dispatched from this earth. And because they are forceful, motivated, and persistent, they may well be quite successful in imposing their will upon others.

Even though I am impressed with the characteristics of our general officers as effective commanders of a combat army, I am less sanguine about the prospects of them instinctively understanding the concept of achieving world peace without bloodshed. I wish I saw more evidence of military leaders who have a healthy skepticism toward the use of military action to resolve international disputes, of creative leaders who value the world of innovation, of thoughtful but practical philosophers who respect the value of unproductive beauty and who have some sense of the interlocking nature of human aspirations.

Yet even here, I may be wrong. Based on the following news item, I may be underestimating our current generals:

> After an afternoon in the Pentagon's super-secret chamber, "the tank," General Alfred M. Grey complained about "too many intellectuals" at the top of the armed services. He said what is needed is not intellectuals but "old-fashioned gunslingers" who like a good fight and don't spend all their time with politicians. (*Colorado Springs Gazette Telegraph*, April 17, 1987)

If the Marines are worried about too many intellectuals in the higher military ranks, then perhaps it is not a bad thing.

My own prediction of our military future is that there are going to be relatively few occasions where our classic hard-charging military types will be turned loose to fight against others like them from the other side. Instead, I think we have moved into an era where diplomatic ingenuity, interpersonal sensitivity, and creative vision are going to be the essential weapons for the preservation of peace. Can anyone believe, for example, that *any* war of *any* nature will bring lasting peace to the Middle East? The eventual solution will surely have to be a long, gentle evolution of ideas in which the use of violence will eventually be renounced as completely ineffectual in producing a world that will be safe for our children.

However, as we wait for and hopefully encourage that evolution to occur, we need to depend on our own decisive warriors for our own national security. Consequently, we need a strong military establishment, one especially that has funds for selecting, training, educating, and expanding the horizons of the leaders who are going to take over the top military positions.

A CLOSING NOTE

Despite my few misgivings, I have been impressed by most of the officers that I have been working with, and I want to close on a positive note. Most of these general officers, including the one woman general that I have met, have been personally delightful as well as extremely competent. The other civilians in our courses who have worked with these officers for a week have been almost uniformly impressed by their intelligence, capabilities, and dedication to this country. I doubt that any other major military power in history has had a more intelligent, well-educated, effective, experienced, honest, loyal group of career military officers, hundreds deep, as the U.S. Army has now. As a group, these officers are not only maintaining a world-class defense organization, they are also running a remarkably effective social institution, one that is handling racial relations better than the rest of society, an institution that is grappling more successfully with the new role of women than are most civilian institutions, an organization that is making the volunteer army work, and, most importantly, a military organization that for 200 years has never strayed from under proper civilian control, even when it felt it was being irrationally restrained.

The world *is* a dangerous place, and we *do* need our decisive warriors, many of whom have made searing personal sacrifices so that people like myself can exercise the freedom to engage in this sort of psychological research and candidly discuss their characteristics. I am grateful to them for such opportunities.

I would like to acknowledge the assistance of Martha Hughes, Ellen Van Velsor, and Lieutenant Colonel William Derrick in analyzing the data reported here.

REFERENCES

Colorado Springs Gazette Telegraph, 17 April 1987.
Myers, I. B. (1993). *Introduction to type.* Palo Alto, CA: Consulting Psychologists Press.

Chapter 8

Vocational Interests
Evaluating Structural Hypotheses

James Rounds
University of Illinois at Urbana-Champaign

Have hexagon, will travel.—John Holland

...A definitive structure of interests has not been established.
—Frederic Kuder (1977, p. 170)

The focus of this chapter is on recent attempts to identify and classify basic interest dimensions, the structural hypotheses proposed to represent how these interests are interrelated, and the implications that this research effort has for current conceptions of the structure of interests. It will be my contention that recent factor analytic research has expanded the number and types of interests and that the two-dimensional models of Roe and Holland do not adequately represent the complexity of the interest space when viewed from the perspective of basic interest dimensions.

SEARCHING FOR THE STRUCTURE OF INTERESTS

John Holland's proposal that there are six types of interests and that the organization of these interest types represents a hexagon has indeed traveled far. Kuder's disclaimer notwithstanding, Holland's personality types of Realistic (R), Investigative (I), Artistic (A), Social (S), Enterprising (E), and Conventional (C), referred to collectively as RIASEC, have dominated vocational interest assessment and research. Holland's work has been influential because it provides a classification and methodology that links scores on interest inventories to

177

occupations. The success of Holland's RIASEC interest and occupational classification has led to extensive revision of widely used interest measures, the accepted use of interest scales constructed with inductive and deductive rather than the contrast-group strategies pioneered by Strong and Kuder, and a renewed emphasis on an important forerunner of Holland's work, Roe's interest classification.

It is important to remember in the face of enthusiasm for these models, that the project that laid the groundwork for Holland's and Roe's structure of interest models was the search for basic interest dimensions. Some of the first applications of factor analysis (Guilford, Christensen, Bond, & Sutton, 1954; Strong, 1943; Thurstone, 1931) to interest data identified dimensions that were the forerunners of Roe's and Holland's interest classifications. In fact, because vocational interest theory has been underdeveloped (Dawis, 1980), factor analysis has primarily been used to develop theoretical constructs to advance vocational interest theory. And although the inappropriate use of factor analysis has been routinely criticized and there is not necessarily any basis for expecting that the "basic dimensions" of interests will be "discovered" in the structure of correlation matrices (Burisch, 1986), it is no exaggeration to say that our current understanding of the interest domain, our approach to describing vocational interests, and the emergence of theoretical models have been largely the result of factor analytic research.

Kuder's (1977) factor analytic research, for example, is one major instance of a continued focus on the search for basic dimensions of vocational interest. Presenting the research in which he reviewed six factor analyses of the *Kuder Occupational Interest Survey's* (KOIS) 600 response proportions (involving 217 occupational groups totaling 48,189 subjects) and compared these factor analytic results with Guilford's factors, Kuder concluded that there seems to be a limited number of "basic generalized dimensions" related to a heterogeneous group of occupations, superimposed on numerous specific factors. Because of the extensive literature on interest factors, Kuder did not attempt an integrative review to identify basic and specific interest factors or the relationship among these factors, although his research suggests a hierarchical arrangement of interests.

Guilford's Structural Analysis

The fact that factor analytic work can be perceived to possess a respectable genealogy in vocational interest literature is evident in its persistent return to certain insights. Roe's (1956) and Holland's (1958, 1985a) interest categories can be traced directly to Guilford, Christensen, Bond, and Sutton's (1954) study of structural properties of interest scales (for convenience, future references to this study will use only Guilford's name). Guilford factored 95 scales (10 items per scale) rationally constructed to represent 33 primary hypotheses regarding the nature of interests. Of the 28 interpretable factors from the two analyses, seven factors were defined as vocational interest factors. By 1954, as noted by Guilford, six of these factors were well established, having been identified in a number of prior studies. These six are as follows:

1. *Mechanical Interest*—contains items of mechanical manipulation, construction, and design, and items pertaining to working with equipment or tools. Secondary loadings reflected interest in manual activities, outdoor activities, and precision (exact or detail work).

2. *Scientific Interest*—contains items of science theory and investigation, with secondary loadings on thinking activities (mathematical and logical), precision (exactness and detail), and aesthetic appreciation (literature, music, and visual arts).

3. *Aesthetic Expression*—contains primarily items reflecting interest in performance in the fields of musical, literary, dramatic, and visual arts, with secondary loadings on items referring to the appreciation of these arts.

4. *Social Welfare*—involves interest in helping people (Altruism—Welfare of Others, Personal Services, and Health and Healing scales) and controlling others (Control of Others—Coercion, Dominance, and Persuasion scales). There are also strong loadings on verbal expression (explanation, clarification, and persuasion), with secondary loadings on business contact and clerical work.

5. *Business Interest*—contains items representing business variables of administration, selling, and contact. Verbal expression, pertaining to persuasive writing, also defined this factor.

6. *Clerical Interest*—contains items representing interest in bookkeeping and routine calculation tasks, with secondary loadings on scales of business contact and administration, and mathematical thinking and precision.

In addition to this list of well-known factors, Guilford proposed adding a seventh factor from a list of 28 interpretable factors: Outdoor-Work Interest, involving a liking for manual, outdoor work such as agriculture, forestry, and construction.

Rereading Guilford

When we look at these factors and compare them with the interest categories presented by Roe and Holland, we can indeed see a remarkably direct correspondence between their interest categories and Guilford's factors. In addition, with few exceptions (see Kuder's, 1977, discussion of the Cultural Interest factor), reviews of Guilford's study (e.g., Hansen, 1984; Holland, 1976; Roe, 1956; Rounds & Dawis, 1979; Super & Crites, 1962) and test construction efforts (e.g., Holland, 1985b; Knapp & Knapp, 1984; Lunneborg, 1981) have cited and focused exclusively on the seven factors just listed. (One review, Brookings & Bolton, 1986, unaccountably finds an "artistic thinking" factor in Guilford's study.) But it is worth returning to the Guilford study to note that additional vocational factors can be identified in the findings. These are listed below, with Guilford's descriptions:

1. *Adventure versus Security*—a liking for exploration and risk-taking activities at one pole and an interest in comfort and sedentary activity and the avoidance of risk taking at the opposite pole.

2. *Thinking*—an interest in understanding and working with mathematical and philosophical concepts and principles. (The thinking factor could justifiably be labeled "Mathematics" because the highest loading was on the Mathematics Concept scale. Other scales defining this factor, consonant with a "Mathematics" label, were Thinking–Problem Solving and Office Activity–Number Manipulation.)

3. *Precision*—an interest in doing detailed or exacting operations with precision instruments.

4. *Cultural Interest*—a fairly broad interest in cultural areas. The scales with the highest loadings were Civics, Verbal Expression–Elucidation, and Verbal Expression–Development, reflecting an interest in politics and speaking to explain, clarify, and persuade. Secondary loadings reflect interest in aesthetic appreciation in the areas of drama, music, and visual arts, and aesthetic expression in literature.

5. *Physical Fitness Interest*—with its highest loading on the Physical Activity–Athletics scale. (Discussing the remaining scales defining this factor, Guilford [p. 22] noted that "Watch athletic teams practice," "Be a leader so as to get more recognition for your work," and "Put a group through its regular setting-up exercises" have obvious common elements, although these items are from Amusement, Recognition, and Dominance [scales], respectively.")

Because factor analytic interest research seems, at this point in its history, to be phylogenetically tied to the Guilford study, we may well take a hint from Kuder's (1977) observation:

> It can be noted in passing that the possibilities of the GCBS [Guilford, Christensen, Bond, & Sutton, 1954] study have yet to be exploited fully regarding those factors that may appear on the surface to have no vocational significance, but that may be found to have such significance if only given the chance. (p. 201)

A rereading of the Guilford monograph and a reexamination of the 28 factors shows, interestingly, that five factors the authors considered nonvocational would now be considered vocational interest factors. A review of current vocational interest inventories shows the relevance of these factors, and recent factor analytic studies have identified similar factors as well, as will be discussed below.

CATALOG OF INTEREST FACTORS

At this point, it would seem that a catalog of interest factors identified since the pioneering Guilford study would be extremely useful. We might take as an example the ETS (French, Ekstrom, & Price, 1963) catalog of reference tests for aptitude and ability factors. The ETS kit has proved useful not only as a standard set of tests for defining factors but also, and more significantly, as a basis for the development of cognitive ability requirement classificatory systems (Fleishman & Quaintance, 1984). A catalog of vocational interests could serve similar functions for vocational researchers. It would enable researchers to exploit fully the significant work of precursors, as well as obviate much needless repetition. Furthermore, such a catalog would be an important tool for further scrutiny of the underlying assumptions as well as of the factors identified in past and ongoing research. Such a catalog could also facilitate interpretation and comparison across the many factorial studies of vocational interests.

Study Selection

Care must be exercised in the selection of studies to be included in a catalog of vocational interest factors inasmuch as selection of variables and, to a lesser extent, subject sampling must be used to determine what factors can appear and at what level they will appear. The catalog that follows is based on the studies identified in Table 1, which also provides details about their methodology. These studies are among the few factor analytic studies of interests reported since Guilford's study that have adequately sampled the interest domain and used sufficiently large subject samples (see also Waller, Lykken, & Tellegen, this volume).

Table 1   **Description of Factor Analytic Studies**

Study	Variable	N	Sample Description
Guilford et al. (1954)	95 scales	600	Airmen
		720	Male air force officers, cadets, and OCS candidates, no older than 27 years
Jackson (1977)	2,400 items	1,600	Females and males
	34 JVIS scales	1,292	Female high school students
		1,163	Male high school students
Kuder (1977)	217 occupational groups	48,189	600 KOIS response proportions for each group were correlated
Rounds & Dawis (1979)[a]	347 SVIB items	1,000	Women-in-General norm group
		2,500	Women randomly sampled from 25 occupations, stratified according to HOC, M age = 42 yrs, M tenure = 12 yrs
	357 SVIB items	1,000	Men-in-General norm group
		3,600	Men randomly sampled from 25 occupations, stratified according to HOC, M age = 42 yrs, M tenure = 16 yrs
Droege & Hawk (1977)	307 items	590	Women from nine states, 50% high school and college students; 50% USES applicants, trainees, employed workers
		525	Men (same description as above)

Note. HOC = Holland Occupational Classification, JVIS = *Jackson Vocational Interest Survey*, KOIS = *Kuder Occupational Interest Survey*, and SVIB = *Strong Vocational Interest Blank*.

[a] Five samples were studied; excluded from the present discussion are factor analytic results based on a sample of 1,874 male rehabilitation clients.

The purposes of these analyses varied. The Jackson (1977) study and the Droege and Hawk (1977; see also U.S. Department of Labor, 1979) study focused on scale development and only secondarily were concerned with theoretical questions about the appropriate number and type of distinctions to be made within the interest domain. Guilford et al.'s (1954), Kuder's (1977), and Rounds and Dawis' (1979) purpose was to search for the best theoretical framework to represent the interest domain. Jackson's research, like Guilford's and Droege's (for convenience, I will reference only the first author's name), was based on an a priori idea of the types of interest factors to be identified. Items were written or scales were constructed according to definitions of the vocational interest disposition to be appraised. The Basic Interest Scales of the *Strong Interest Inventory* (*Strong;* then called the *Strong Vocational Interest Blank*, SVIB; Campbell, 1971) influenced the selection and definition of dimensions for Jackson. Previous factor analyses and studies were the primary sources for Guilford's hypotheses. In the case of Droege's report on the *U.S. Employment Service Interest Inventory* (USES), items were written to correspond to Cottle's (1950) five bipolar factors. Kuder and Rounds, however, began with the assumption that the KOIS and SVIB items adequately represented the vocational interest domain because these item sets have been shown consistently to differentiate a wide variety of occupational groups and to be related to occupational choice. Their analyses, compared with Guilford's and Jackson's, were more exploratory than confirmatory, although prior research certainly informed their decisions about what factors to retain and interpret.

The subject samples studied also varied across the analyses. With the exception of Guilford's airmen and officers, the studies sampled both men and women. The Kuder, Rounds, and Droege studies relied on heterogeneous samples varying in age and geographic location, drawn from a variety of occupations. Jackson used high school and college students. The majority of subjects in all studies were probably drawn from the middle and upper middle class. The size of the samples varied from 590 females and 525 males in the Droege study to 48,189 respondents from 217 male and female occupations and college major groups in the Kuder study. In summary, the purposes, units of analysis, item type, analytical techniques, and subject samples varied among these five studies, lending confidence to possible findings of replicated factors from cross-study comparisons.

Although Guilford's study has been uniformly cited as the benchmark for comparing factor analytic results, Jackson's recent factor analytic studies have made good use of advances in factor analytic methodology and scale development—many of these advances contributed by Jackson himself—and they must now be considered pre-eminent. Jackson's sample of the vocational interest domain is considerably more extensive than Guilford's, and his analyses were replicated on female and male samples. Table 2 organizes the list of interest factors according to the 26 primary and 8 second-order work role factors reported by Jackson (1977, pp. 43–44). Kuder's (1977, pp. 183–201) 16 factors were drawn from his most extensive analysis (factor analysis VI); 7 factors identified in this analysis but not reported in Table 2 are Typical Response, Femininity-Masculinity, Adult Women, Adult Men, Young Women, Young Men, and Occupational Dissatisfaction. Guilford's 12 factors were discussed above. Rounds' factors are reported separately by sex inasmuch as men and women responded to different item sets. Included are the 14 male factors and 13 female factors that met the requirements of the same-sex sample congruency tests. Droege's 11 factors do not include Physical Performing, a scale later added to the USES, but not identified in their analyses.

The factors displayed in Table 2 were matched across the six studies, taking into consideration the scale and item factor loadings, the descriptions and definitions given by the investigators, and, in the case of Kuder's study, his discussion of the similarity of KOIS factors and Guilford's factors. (For the USES factors, viz. the Droege study, primary source material was unavailable.)

THREE CONCEPTUAL LEVELS
OF GENERALITY: GENERAL INTEREST,
BASIC INTEREST, AND OCCUPATION INTEREST

The factors shown in Table 2 represent three conceptual levels of generality: general interest, basic interest, and occupation interest. These conceptual levels have a counterpart in the writings on trait definitions and distinctions (Lubinski & Thompson, 1986; Meehl, 1986; Tellegen, 1991). I will make use of Meehl's (1986) reconstruction of Cattell's (1950) trait notions to further explain and refine the general interest, basic interest, and occupation interest definitions and distinctions I am proposing. Broadly speaking, interest items and scales involve preferences for *behaviors* (response and activity families), *situations* (the context in which the preferred behaviors occur, usually occupations or physical settings), and *reinforcer systems* (outcomes or reinforcers associated with the behavior and situation). On the response side, vocational interests are usually characterized by a shared property of the activities (Selling, Technical Writing, Teaching) and are often implied in the objects of interest (Mathematics, Physical Science, Religion) or inferred as a latent entity (Enterprising, Inquiring,

Table 2 General Interest and Basic Interest Factors From Five Studies

Jackson (1977)	Kuder (1977)	Guilford et al. (1954)	Rounds & Dawis (1979)		Droege & Hawk (1977)
			Male samples	Female samples	
Logical	*Science-Mathematics*	*Science Interest*	*Scientific Activity*		*Scientific*
Mathematics		Thinking	Mathematics	Mathematics	Mechanical
Physical Science	Engineering				Industrial
Engineering					Plants and Animals
					Protective
Practical	Skilled Trades	Mechanical Interest	Mechanical Activity	Mechanical Activity	Accommodating
Skilled Trades		Precision			
Nature-		Outdoor-Work Interest	Nature		
Agriculture					
Adventure		Adventure vs. Security	Military Activity		
Personal Service			Security vs. Adventure		
Family Activity				Domestic Arts	
	Physical Education	Physical Fitness Interest	Athletics	Athletics-Adventure	
	and Therapy				
Inquiring					
Life Science	Food-Nutrition				
Medical Service	Medical Professions		Medical Science	Medical Science	
Social Science	Behavioral Sciences				

Table 2 General Interest and Basic Interest Factors From Five Studies (continued)

Jackson (1977)	Kuder (1977)	Guilford et al. (1954)	Rounds & Dawis (1979) — Male samples	Rounds & Dawis (1979) — Female samples	Droege & Hawk (1977)
Expressive Creative Arts Performing Arts	*Artistic*	*Aesthetic Expression*	*Aesthetic*	*Aesthetic* Aesthetic Appreciation Fashionable Appearance	*Artistic*
Helping Social Service Elementary Education Teaching	Social Welfare	Social Welfare	*Social Service*	Teaching	Humanitarian
Communication Author- Journalism Technical Writing	Literary Journalism Library Science	*Cultural Interest*			

Table 2 General Interest and Basic Interest Factors From Five Studies (continued)

Jackson (1977)	Kuder (1977)	Guilford et al. (1954)	Rounds & Dawis (1979) Male samples	Rounds & Dawis (1979) Female samples	Droege & Hawk (1977)
Enterprising	*Influencing People-Social Approval*		*Meeting and Directing People*	*Meeting and Directing People*	*Leading-Influencing*
Human Relations					
Management					
Professional Advising					
Law	Agriculture-Law-Political Science				
	Religious Activity		Public Service Religion	Religion	
		Clerical Interest		Clerical Activity	Business Detail
		Business Interest	Business Contact	Business Contact	Selling
Conventional					
Finance					
Office Work					
Business					
Sales	Sales				
Supervision					

Note. General interest factors appear in italics.

Leading-Influencing). On the stimulus side, a shared property of the context (Outdoor-Work, Office Work, Industrial) is invoked to explain interest covariation. Vocational interests are rarely characterized by their association with reinforcers, and when they are, it usually occurs in the context of expressed interests (Rounds, Dawis, & Lofquist, 1979) or Holland's environment formulations (Rounds, Shubsachs, Dawis, & Lofquist, 1978).

General interest factors, sometimes called *occupational themes* or *second-order factors,* are what Kuder and Guilford referred to as "basic generalized dimensions" related to a heterogeneous group of occupations. These general interests are close to what Meehl means by *source traits*: The elements of the activity family (or occupational family) are dissimilar and an internal entity is postulated to explain their covariation. Jackson's Logical, Guilford's Science Interest, and Rounds' Science Activity are examples of similar general interest factors. Holland's interest types (which are dimensional traits, not taxa), Roe's interest categories, and Prediger's theory-based dimensions are also examples of general interests.

At the lowest level of generality are occupation interest factors that comprise a circumscribed set of work activities that are dissimilar in character and which usually reference a specific occupation. Meehl's rubric of surface quasi traits or environmental mould traits is an apt description. As shown in Table 2, occupation interest factors are inconsequential to these analyses. Jackson's Elementary Education and Kuder's Library Science are examples of occupation interest factors.

The majority of replicated factors in Table 2 are specific interest factors, typically called *basic interest* dimensions. These basic interest factors comprise work activities that transcend particular situations (occupations) and occupy a level of generality between general interest factors and occupation interest factors. Meehl's definition of surface traits comes to mind: The elements of the activity family have similar content. Basic interest factors can be considered subdomains, and when they covary, they are reference dimensions (general interest factors). Most people describe their vocational interests using the language of basic interests. Examples of similar basic interest factors are Jackson's Skilled Trades, Kuder's Skilled Trades, Guilford's Mechanical Interest, and Rounds' Mechanical Activity.

Making distinctions between basic interest factors and occupation interest factors in Table 2 is relatively easy, compared with distinguishing basic interest factors and general interest factors. Comparisons within studies show that factors at different conceptual levels—basic interest and general interest—occasionally appear in the same analysis. The exception is Jackson's analyses. The clarity of his results is due to two methodological features. First, he used high-density sampling of items to define the basic factors. In contrast, the Kuder and Rounds studies, because of the nature of the data, had little control over variable sampling. Without such controls, variation in the level for the same factor can occur. Second, Jackson extracted first-order and second-order factors, allowing the direct mapping of basic interest factors onto general interest factors. Kuder used the Wherry-Wherry hierarchical rotation method but stopped the analysis before a clear solution at the general interest level was established. The remaining analyses relied on orthogonal rotations and did not search for higher-order factors. Because of these methodological differences among studies, which can lead to confusion about the theoretical level or order of the factors that appear in Table 2, Jackson's study, which avoids such confusion, is the best guide to the structure of interests.

Given the above, Jackson's results can be considered an initial upper-bound estimate of the number and types of distinctions to be made within the vocational interest domain. Table 2 shows that 16 of 25 basic interest factors (excluding Elementary Education) and 5 of 8 general interest factors from Jackson's study were identified in at least one other study. Jackson's nine basic interest factors that did not replicate, possibly because of limited variable samples, can usually be mapped onto general interest factors in other studies. For example, basic interest items for Creative Arts (visual arts), Performing Arts, and Author-Journalism (literary arts) were found to collapse into an Artistic general interest factor in the Rounds and Droege studies.

Table 2 also shows that Jackson's list does not include three replicated basic interest factors: Athletics, Protection, and Religious Activity. Adding these basic interest factors to Jackson's factors, it can now be said that 19 to 28 basic interest factors have been identified and that these numbers are the best estimate of the lower and upper bounds of the types of distinctions that can be made within the interest domain. Waller, Lykken, and Tellegen (this volume) identify 4 of the 9 nonreplicated Jackson factors (Physical Science, Creative Arts, Performing Arts, Law) and also the three replicated basic interest factors that were added to Jackson's list, lending support to the conclusion about the number and kinds of distinctions that can be made at the basic interest level. One caveat is especially necessary about this conclusion: Nonprofessional interests may not be well represented in this basic interest catalog. The items and scales that enter into these factor analyses involve interests that are more related to differences among professional and managerial occupations than they are to differences among skilled, semiskilled, and unskilled occupations.

The basic interest catalog has the practical advantage of guiding scale development, but its primary purpose was to demonstrate that the number and types of distinctions in the interest domain are much larger than hitherto stated and that, when these distinctions are taken into consideration, our knowledge of general interest factors will be significantly affected. The remainder of this chapter will evaluate structural hypotheses associated with general interest and basic interest dimensions. In the next section, I will examine how well the general interest categories and dimensions of Roe, Holland, and Prediger fit the hypothesized circular structure of interest. I will then go on to contend that the circular structure of interests is a poor representation of the complexity of the interest space when viewed from the perspective of basic interest dimensions.

STRUCTURE OF GENERAL INTERESTS

Roe's and Holland's general interest themes have received by far the greatest attention because of their purported centrality to vocational choice and satisfaction and their usefulness in the development of occupational classifications. A representation of Roe's (1956) and Holland's (1973, 1985a) circular model of interest fields and types is shown in Figure 1. Although Roe (1956; Roe & Klos, 1969) hypothesized a circular ordering, the internal relationships among the interest fields were never specified. Holland, on the other hand, proposed a structural hypothesis, formally called the *calculus assumption,* that defines the internal relationships among the interest types such that the distances between the types are "inversely proportional to the theoretical relationships between them" (Holland, 1973, 1985a, p. 5), that is, adjacent types on the hexagon are most related, whereas opposite types are least related, with alternating types having an intermediate level of relationship. The calculus assumption serves the purpose of defining two key concepts in Holland's theory: consistency and congruence.

Holland's Structural Hypotheses

Holland's order hypothesis has received considerable attention following Holland, Whitney, Cole, and Richards' (1969) demonstration that a circular arrangement best describes the interrelationships among *Vocational Preference Inventory* (VPI) RIASEC scales. This initial paper stimulated a series of related investigations involving a variety of measures, samples, and data analytic methods. By far, the most comprehensive assessment of the RIASEC arrangement has been Prediger's (1982) study. He used Cooley and Lohnes' (1971) FACTOR program, a principal component technique for the extraction of arbitrary factors, to examine the extent to which two theory-based dimensions— Data/Ideas and Things/People—fit each of 24 sets of Holland scale

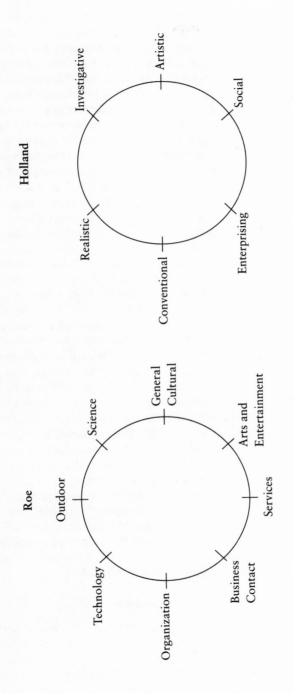

Figure 1   Representations of Roe's (1956) and Holland's (1973, 1985a) circular interest models

intercorrelations. Prediger reported finding the RIASEC scale arrangement for 23 of the 24 spatial representations. (Prediger's paper also raises an important issue about response set variance and interest measurement and techniques used to recover structure, which space considerations do not allow us to discuss here; see also Davison, 1985, and Waller, Lykken, and Tellegen in this volume.) Although these and other results (see Rounds & Zevon, 1983, for a review of multidimensional scaling studies; see also Fouad, Cudeck, & Hansen, 1984, for an application of confirmatory factor analysis) clearly support a polygonal RIASEC arrangement of interest types, these approaches cannot be considered precise tests of Holland's structural hypothesis. Because of their methodology—visual inspection of spatial representations—these studies address the simple circular order expectation of RIASEC, but not the expectations about the internal relations among the six types, that is, Holland's calculus assumption.

When more precise tests have been conducted to evaluate the calculus assumption, Wakefield and Doughtie's (1973) hypothesis-testing strategy has usually been applied (e.g., Gati, 1982; Lunneborg & Lunneborg, 1975; Rounds, Davison, & Dawis, 1979). The Wakefield and Doughtie procedure uses a binomial test to assess the magnitude of the number of violations of the calculus assumption: The distance between the six adjacent types (RI, IA, AS, SE, EC, CR) should be less than the distance between the six alternating types (RA, IS, AE, SC, ER, CI), and the distances between alternating types should be less than those for the opposite types (RS, IE, AC). Applications of this inference procedure have been frequently cited to support the calculus assumption (e.g., Holland, 1985a, 1985c). Hubert and Arabie (1987), however, have recently criticized Wakefield and Doughtie's procedure, showing that their simple binomial test is based on the inappropriate assumption that the order relations are independent, when, in fact, "violation or nonviolation of some order relations necessarily implies the violation or nonviolation of others" (Hubert & Arabie, 1987, p. 175). Their demonstration that the Wakefield and Doughtie (1973) approach is incorrect indicates, at the very least, that prior research using this procedure must be reevaluated and reopens the question about the viability of Holland's calculus assumption.

Evaluation of Holland's Structural Hypothesis

Evaluation of Holland's structural hypothesis has become a rather overwhelming task. The number of published intercorrelation matrices since the 1970s has increased substantially, due to the commercial development of interest inventories to assess Holland types. Any attempt to evaluate each matrix for Holland's order hypothesis and to integrate these findings across measures and samples is becoming a formidable task. Given these problems of integrating literature on structural relations, a secondary analysis of these matrices using three-way (individual differences scaling) multidimensional scaling would be a fairly parsimonious approach to the spatial representation of numerous matrices from heterogeneous sources. Although my present purpose is to produce a summary configuration or group solution using RIASEC correlation matrices, three-way scaling can also be used to examine individual differences among the sources (measures and samples).

Method   In a test of Holland's structural hypothesis, three-way scaling as implemented in ALSCAL (Young, Takane, & Lewyckyj, 1978) and SINDSCAL (Pruzansky, 1975) was applied to intercorrelation matrices for Holland's six types. (Both ALSCAL and SINDSCAL were applied because they optimize the fit of the INDSCAL model in different ways and can result in different solutions [Arabie, Carroll, & DeSarbo, 1987]). The primary sources for the data were test manuals, journals, and American College Testing Program technical reports. These sources were searched for the years 1965 to 1986. Test manuals for all major instruments assessing Holland's six types were reviewed: *Vocational Preference Inventory, Self-Directed Search, Strong-Campbell Interest Inventory, American College Testing Program Interest Inventory, Career Assessment Inventory,* and *Career Decision-Making System.* The journals included, but were not limited to, the *Journal of Vocational Behavior, Journal of Applied Psychology, Journal of Counseling Psychology, Journal of Occupational Psychology,* and *Measurement and Evaluation in Counseling and Development.*

Table 3 shows that 60 correlation matrices were located. (The unconstrained and constrained RSQ values shown in Table 3 will be discussed below.) The majority of the matrices came from scale correlations of Holland's measures with 20 data sets for the VPI and 12 data sets for the *Self-Directed Search* (SDS). The data sets are about equally divided between female and male samples. Few of the studies in Table 3 are satisfactory on sampling grounds. Most of the matrices were generated from nonprobability samples—convenience samples, one possible reason for prior divergent findings. Exceptions are the data collected by American College Testing Program (e.g., Hanson, Prediger, & Schussel, 1977; Holland, Whitney, Cole, & Richards, 1969; Lamb & Prediger, 1981) and the *Strong-Campbell Interest Inventory* general reference sample (Hansen & Campbell, 1985). Although these samples were not generated from strict probability sampling plans, there were efforts to guarantee that enough cases were obtained from relevant strata.

Table 3   Data Source Description and Unconstrained and Constrained RSQ Values by Measure

Data Source	N	Sex	RSQ		Sample Description
			UC[a]	C[b]	
Vocational Preference Inventory					
1. Holland (1965)	362	M	.92	.85	Grade 12, National Merit finalists
2. Holland (1965)	277	F	.84	.72	Grade 12, National Merit finalists
3. Holland (1965)	103	M	.74	.76	Employed adults
4. American College Testing Program (1968)	2,433	F	.89	.69	College students
5. Holland, Whitney, Cole, & Richards (1969)	1,234	M	.97	.76	10% sample, 2-year college students
6. Wakefield & Doughtie (1973)	373	M/F	.82	.82	Intro. psychology students
7. Crabtree & Hales (1974)	759	M	.71	.56	Grades 12, 17 rural school districts
8. Crabtree & Hales (1974)	672	F	.76	.59	Grades 12, 17 rural school districts
9. Holland (1975) [from Folsom (1971)]	191	M	.71	.58	Grades 9–12
10. Holland (1975) [from Folsom (1971)]	175	F	.63	.52	Grades 9–12
11. Holland (1975)	200	M	.80	.77	Employed adults
12. Lunneborg & Lunneborg (1975)	235	M/F	.92	1.00	Intro. psychology students
13. Gottfredson, Holland, & Holland (1978)	378	F	.93	.83	Employed adults and college students, M age = 27
14. Gottfredson, Holland, & Holland (1978)	354	M	.94	.91	Employed adults and college students, M age = 31
15. Holland (1979)	347	F	.54	.60	College freshmen
16. Holland (1979)	344	M	.90	.65	College freshmen
17. Athanasou, O'Gorman, & Meyer (1981)	101	M	.78	.50	Grades 9–12, Australian students
18. Athanasou, O'Gorman, & Meyer (1981)	99	M/F	.66	.58	Grades 9–12, Australian students
19. Athanasou (1982)	129	M	.78	.55	Age 15–45, Australian guidance clients
20. Athanasou (1982)	116	F	.79	.73	Age 15–45, Australian guidance clients

Table 3 Data Source Description and Unconstrained and Constrained RSQ Values by Measure (continued)

Data Source	N	Sex	RSQ UC[a]	RSQ C[b]	Sample Description
Self-Directed Search					
21. Holland (1972); also Holland (1979, 1985c)	344	M	1.00	.90	College freshmen
22. Holland (1972); also Holland (1979, 1985c)	347	F	.99	.90	College freshmen
23. Holland (1979, 1985 [from Power et al., 1979])	313	F	.86	.68	Grade 9 and 10
24. Holland (1979, 1985c [from Power et al., 1979])	200	M	.62	.49	Grade 11
25. Tuck & Keeling (1980)	247	M	.84	.76	Grades 11 and 12, New Zealand
26. Tuck & Keeling (1980)	252	F	.72	.34	Grades 11 and 12, New Zealand
27. Holland (1985c)	173	F	.57	.47	Age 14–18, miscellaneous sample
28. Holland (1985c)	172	F	.55	.54	Age 19–25, miscellaneous sample
29. Holland (1985c)	176	F	.73	.65	Age 26–74, miscellaneous sample
30. Holland (1985c)	114	M	.62	.61	Age 14–18, miscellaneous sample
31. Holland (1985c)	84	M	.56	.72	Age 19–25, miscellaneous sample
32. Holland (1985c)	99	M	.90	.76	Age 26–74, miscellaneous sample
Strong Vocational Interest Blank					
33. Campbell & Holland (1972)	150	M/F	.95	.84	Miscellaneous sample, Set II scales (Form TM399)
34. Hansen & Johannson (1972)	150	M/F	.92	.88	Same sample as data set No. 33, Set II scales (Form TW398)
35. Bull (1975)	147	M/F	.66	.62	New Zealand college students majoring in psychology

Table 3 Data Source Description and Unconstrained and Constrained RSQ Values by Measure (continued)

Data Source	N	Sex	RSQ		Sample Description
			UC[a]	C[b]	
Strong-Campbell Interest Inventory					
36. Campbell (1977)	201	F	.86	.66	Miscellaneous sample
37. Campbell (1977)	200	M	.84	.82	Miscellaneous sample
38. Prediger & Johnson (1979)	2,178	M/F	.77	.69	University freshmen
39. Rounds (1981)	420	M	.83	.67	Adult vocational assessment clients
40. Rounds (1981)	421	F	.91	.98	Adult vocational assessment clients
41. Campbell & Hansen (1981)	300	M	.84	.78	Miscellaneous sample, M age = 33
42. Campbell & Hansen (1981)	300	F	.96	.90	Miscellaneous sample, M age = 35
43. Wigington (1983)	1,140	F	.82	.78	University vocational counseling clients
44. Wigington (1983)	993	M	.88	.91	University vocational counseling clients
45. Hansen & Campbell (1985)	300	M	.81	.62	Sample stratified by occupation and level, M age = 38
46. Hansen & Campbell (1985)	300	F	.78	.73	Sample stratified by occupation and level, M age = 38
ACT Vocational Interest Profile					
47. Rose & Elton (1982)	327	F	.73	.64	Vocationally unstable college student clients
48. Rose & Elton (1982)	280	F	.58	.49	Vocationally stable college student clients

Table 3   Data Source Description and Unconstrained and Constrained RSQ Values by Measure (continued)

			RSQ		
Data Source	N	Sex	UC[a]	C[b]	Sample Description
ACT Interest Inventory—Unisex Edition					
49. Hanson, Prediger, & Schussel (1977)	914	M	.66	.57	Grade 11, Career Planning Program national norming sample
50. Hanson, Prediger, & Schussel (1977)	937	F	.74	.66	Grade 11, Career Planning Program national norming sample
51. Lamb & Prediger (1981)	1,247	M	.87	.91	Grade 12, UNIACT AAP norms sample
52. Lamb & Prediger (1981)	1,693	F	.84	.85	Grade 12, UNIACT AAP norms sample
Career Assessment Inventory—Vocational Edition					
53. Johansson (1976)	363	M	.76	.49	Miscellaneous adult sample
54. Johansson (1976)	298	F	.78	.59	Miscellaneous adult sample
Career Assessment Inventory—Enhanced Edition					
55. Johansson (1986)	703	F	.73	.58	Miscellaneous sample
56. Johansson (1986)	488	M	.59	.59	Miscellaneous sample
Career Decision-Making Inventory—English Edition					
57. Harrington & O'Shea (1982)	815	NR	.53	.54	High school and college students

Table 3   Data Source Description and Unconstrained and Constrained RSQ Values by Measure (continued)

Data Source	N	Sex	RSQ		Sample Description
			UC[a]	C[b]	
Career Decision-Making Inventory—Spanish Edition					
58. Harrington & O'Shea (1982)	148	NR	.57	.56	High school and college students, Mexican-American sample
59. Harrington & O'Shea (1982)	64	NR	.53	.41	High school and college students, Puerto Rican sample
60. Harrington & O'Shea (1982)	267	NR	.66	.55	High school and junior students, Spanish language sample

Note. RSQ values from ALSCAL analysis.
NR = not reported.
[a]UC = unconstrained RSQ
[b]C = constrained RSQ

Table 4   RIASEC Stimulus Coordinates for the Two-Dimensional ALSCAL
           and SINDSCAL Solutions and Prediger's Theory-Based Dimensions

	ALSCAL		SINDSCAL		Prediger (1982)	
Category	1	2	1	2	D/I	T/P
Realistic	.00	1.47	−.07	.58	.00	2.00
Investigative	1.01	1.03	.33	.49	1.73	1.00
Artistic	1.41	−.71	.62	−.22	1.73	−1.00
Social	−.04	−1.29	.08	−.47	.00	−2.00
Enterprising	−.91	−.75	−.33	−.39	−1.73	−1.00
Conventional	−1.48	.25	−.63	.01	−1.73	1.00

Note. ALSCAL and SINDSCAL solutions are based on 60 matrices referenced in Table 3.
D/I = Data-Ideas dimension; T/P = Things-People dimension.

Results   Table 4 shows the RIASEC stimulus coordinates from the
ALSCAL and SINDSCAL two-dimensional solutions for the 60 correlation matrices. These stimulus coordinates are plotted in Figure 2.
The fit of the data to the two-dimensional models seems satisfactory:
ALSCAL solution accounted for 77% of the variance and SINDSCAL
solution accounted for 80%. (The three-dimensional solutions showed,
as expected, a slightly better fit, with the ALSCAL solution accounting for 87% of the variance and the SINDSCAL accounting for 86%.
Because the increment in variance for three dimensions is small and
because the focus here is on Holland's circular model, the two-dimensional solution was retained.)
    The ALSCAL and the SINDSCAL configurations are very similar
(scale values from SINDSCAL shown in Table 4 have been multiplied
by a factor of 2.3 for display purposes). These solutions, however,
show a minor difference in the orientation of the coordinate axes. The
arrangement of the Holland scales in Figure 2, which should be read
clockwise on either solution, conforms to the RIASEC ordering. Comparing the distances of adjacent types with the alternating types, and
alternating types with opposite types, shows that all of the 54 comparisons were in the predicted direction. In summary, the configuration in Figure 2 is the best estimate of the relationships among Holland's
six types. The calculus assumption is an exact theoretical specification
of these empirical relations.
    Holland, in his writings, often depicts the six types forming an equi-
lateral hexagon. His use of a hexagon rather than a circle came about
because "Roe had a circle, so we called the resulting configuration a hexagon" (Weinrach, 1980, p. 408; it should be noted that

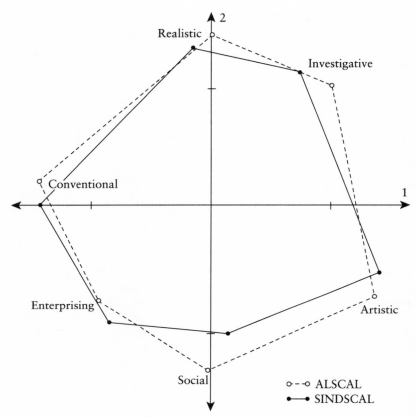

Figure 2   ALSCAL and SINDSCAL solutions for the 60 RIASEC
correlation matrices

straight-line distances in a circle [chords] and a hexagon are identical). The hexagonal structure (or a circle with equidistant points around the circumference), however, adds an additional constraint on the calculus assumption: The distances are equal between scale points within adjacent categories, alternating categories, and opposite categories. Thus, Holland's structural hypothesis has taken three forms: the simple circular arrangement hypothesis, the calculus assumption, and the hexagonal hypothesis. Investigators have often mistakenly reported that findings support the strong hexagonal hypothesis when, in fact, their analyses have been directed at assessing a weak form of the calculus assumption (simple circular arrangement) or the calculus assumption itself.

Prediger's Structural Hypothesis

Although Holland's model is a two-dimensional structure, the nature of these dimensions has been rarely investigated. An exception has been Prediger's (1976, 1982) proposal that two bipolar dimensions of work tasks, Data/Ideas and Things/People, account for the hexagonal hypothesis of occupations and interests. (Incidentally, Prediger's dimensions are very similar to factors [e.g., Cottle, 1950; Strong, 1943; Thurstone, 1931] identified in initial studies of interest structure.) The Data-Ideas and Things-People dimensions have become a core component of the American College Testing Program (1988) career guidance services. The ACT World-of-Work Map uses these dimensions to plot the full range of DOT occupations grouped in 23 job families and to plot a person's similarity to these job families.

As shown in Table 4, Prediger has specified the coordinates for the six interest categories to satisfy the requirements of an equilateral hexagon. The Things-People dimension has the Things pole anchored by the Realistic category and the opposite end of the dimension, People, is anchored by Social. The Data-Ideas dimension has the Data axis intersecting the midpoint between the Enterprising and Conventional categories and the Ideas axis intersecting the midpoint between the Investigative and Artistic categories. With the specification of coordinate axes, the hexagon is precisely defined.

Results and Discussion The ALSCAL and SINDSCAL results discussed above, when brought to bear on Prediger's theory-based dimensions, prove valuable here as well (see Table 4 and Figure 2). An important feature of these analyses, and the basis for comparison between the empirical axes and theory-based axes, is that the INDSCAL axes are uniquely determined, given the data sets. A unique orientation suggests, as discussed by Arabie, Carroll, and DeSarbo (1987), that the INDSCAL axes are the preferred orientation because arbitrary rotation usually leads to a different pattern of source weights and, thus, a reduction in goodness of fit. This does *not* suggest that another set of axes obtained by rotation or a more general model that allows correlated dimensions might be more substantively interpretable. (See Arabie et al., 1987, pp. 44–45, for a discussion of the IDIOSCAL model.) A rotation of the INDSCAL axes to theory-driven axes, if possible, would imply only that the stretched or shrunk object spaces are along axes other than theory-driven axes, not that these rotated axes could not account for the object placement (L. J. Hubert, personal communication, 1989). Because orthogonal rotation of the INDSCAL axes will not improve the fit to the theory-driven axes, because the present set of axes conform closely to Prediger's, and because several other orientations resulted in a loss of explained variance, I have assumed that the coordinate axes displayed in Figure 2 are uniquely determined.

Substantial support for Prediger's hypothesized placement of these dimensions seemed to be provided by the ALSCAL and SINDSCAL solutions (see Table 4 and Figure 2) with one exception: the Conventional category. Instead of being located between axis 1, the Data pole, and axis 2, the Things pole, the Conventional category simply anchors the negative end of axis 1. (Prediger's labels are being used for the sake of clarity.) Another deviation, albeit minor, is the distance between opposite types: The AC distance is considerably greater than the RS and the IE distances, whereas the RS and IE distances are approximately equal. Nevertheless, the ALSCAL axes, for example, show that axis 1, which intersects the Realistic and Social categories, coincides exactly with the hypothesized Things-People dimension, whereas axis 2 deviates somewhat, approximately 10 degrees, from the hypothesized Data-Ideas dimension. In summary, the empirical axes are a good approximation to Prediger's theory-based dimensions, suggesting that the hypothesized nature of these dimensions, that is, preferences for working with things or people and preferences for working with data or ideas may account for how individuals respond to the RIASEC items.

Inspection of Figure 2 shows that the configurations approximate Holland's theoretical model, a symmetrical (or equilateral) hexagon. For a more precise evaluation of the hexagonal hypothesis, a constrained analysis was applied to the 60 data sets. The stimulus space was specified with the Data-Ideas and Things-People numerical coordinates (Prediger, 1982, p. 262, see Table 4). The difference between the two solutions was relatively small: The ALSCAL constrained analysis accounted for 69% of the variance, compared with 77% found in the unconstrained analysis. Whether a loss of approximately 9% of the accountable variance or the finding that the Conventional category anchors the Data pole are of practical importance can only be evaluated through further research: studies, for example, that assess the effect of these discrepancies on the accuracy of congruence predictions.

It should be emphasized that the orientation of the ALSCAL (or the SINDSCAL) axes represents a solution defined in terms of the variance accounted for and not necessarily the substantive properties of the circular model. The fact that attribute vectors such as Data/Ideas and Things/People may closely fit these coordinate axes does not preclude the study of alternative properties (e.g., Holland's theory-based attributes that differentiate opposite-interest types) that may underlie the circular model. Certainly, two perpendicular coordinate axes are more parsimonious and therefore more scientifically preferable to three attribute vectors or two nonperpendicular attribute vectors (see Rosenberg & Sedlak, 1972). But most circular models, like Holland's structure-of-interest model, present alternative perspectives or inter-pretations of the interrelationships among points; hence, mapping more than two properties on a two-dimensional space may serve important functions. Multiple attribute vectors fitted to the circular structure-of-interest, for example, would assist us in better understanding the stimu-lus-response properties of interest inventories and could be used to develop occupational classifications and methods to locate a client's vocational interests on circular models. The latter suggestion is best exemplified in Prediger's (1976, 1981) research that is the basis of the ACT World-of-Work Map (American College Testing Program, 1988).

Evaluating Measure-Hexagon Fit

Holland's RIASEC model has had a profound influence on the field of interest measurement. Since the 1970s, beginning with the incorpora-tion of Holland scales in the *Strong* (Campbell & Holland, 1972; Hansen & Johansson, 1972), developers of interest inventories have either suggested that scale scores from their measures can be trans-lated to Holland scales (e.g., Zytowski & Kuder, 1986) or have devel-oped alternative measures (Harrington & O'Shea, 1982; Johansson, 1986) presumed to assess Holland's typology. Attempts to evaluate the claims that these alternative measures are, in fact, measuring Holland's constructs take a number of forms, the most frequent, and a necessary first step, being studies correlating the presumed Holland scales with the VPI or SDS scales. Evidence also necessary to buttress such claims is the demonstration that the internal relations among presumed Holland scales fit the calculus assumption or hexagonal hypothesis.

Overall, the evidence from the latter studies—the fit of a measure's internal relations to the hexagonal model—has been difficult to sum-marize, based as they are on individual studies using a variety of samples and methodologies. One possible way to compare the configural fit across studies or RIASEC measures is to examine the multidimensional scaling source weights, sometimes called subject or dimension weights. The source weight on a dimension when the dimensions are uncorrelated is the correlation of the distances between stimulus coor-dinates on that dimension and the corresponding pairwise disparities in the source's data. The sum of the squared source weights, referred to as the RSQ values in the ALSCAL solution, gives the proportion of the variance of that source's optimally scaled data that is accounted for by the dimensions. But as Arabie, Carroll, and DeSarbo (1987) caution, sources with identical or similar RSQs do not necessarily have

Table 5   Mean Source Weights for RIASEC Measures From the ALSCAL
Constrained Solution of 60 Correlation Matrices

		Dimension Weights			
Measure	n	Data/Ideas	People/Things	Relative Salience	RSQ
Holland	32	.58	.57	1.02	.70
VPI	20	.59	.58	1.00	.71
SDS	12	.56	.56	1.05	.65
Strong	14	.70	.53	.77	.78
SVIB	3	.71	.51	.72	.78
SCII	11	.69	.53	.79	.78
UNIACT	4	.71	.48	.70	.75
CAI-V & -E	4	.50	.55	1.12	.56
CAI-V	2	.46	.57	1.25	.54
CAI-E	2	.54	.54	.99	.58
CDM	4	.45	.56	1.28	.52

Note. Total number of sources is 58 due to elimination of the ACT *Vocational Interest Profile* sources.
VPI = *Vocational Preference Inventory*, SDS = *Self-Directed Search*, SVIB = *Strong Vocational Interest Blank*, SCII = *Strong-Campbell Interest Inventory*, UNIACT = *Unisex Edition of ACT Interest Inventory*, CAI-V = *Career Assessment Inventory Vocational Edition*, CAI-E = *Career Assessment Inventory Enhanced Edition*, and CDM = *Career Decision-Making Inventory*.

solutions that are identical or similar. Nonetheless, RSQ values can be loosely taken to indicate the goodness of fit of the source's data to the ALSCAL solution.

Results   With this cautionary note, Table 3 displays the RSQ values for the 60 sources (studies) from the unconstrained and constrained ALSCAL solutions. One immediate observation is that there is considerable variation in the goodness of fit among RIASEC measures. To evaluate the measure-model fit, several analyses using the weights from the constrained solution (recall that this solution was constrained using Prediger's coordinate axes) were conducted.

Table 5 shows the mean source weights, relative salience values, and RSQ values for the RIASEC measures; the mean relative salience and RSQ values are plotted in Figure 3. Figure 3, a method to represent source weights (see Coxon, 1982; Young, 1978), displays the RIASEC measures by the relative salience (ratio) of the People-Things dimension to the Data-Ideas dimension (horizontal axis) and by the RSQ, amount of variation explained (vertical axis; the ACT

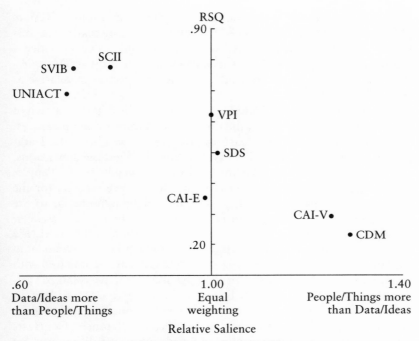

Figure 3 Mean source weight plot for the RIASEC measures

Note. SCII = *Strong-Campbell Interest Inventory*, SVIB = *Strong Vocational Interest Blank*, UNIACT = *Unisex Edition of ACT Interest Inventory*, VPI = *Vocational Preference Inventory*, SDS = *Self-Directed Search*, CAI-E = *Career Assessment Inventory Enhanced Edition*, CAI-V = *Career Assessment Inventory Vocational Edition*, and CDM = *Career Decision-Making Inventory*.

Vocational Interest Profile was excluded from these analyses, reducing the number of data points to 58.) Inspection of the mean RSQ values in Table 5 and Figure 3 shows that the best fit to the hexagon came from the *Strong* and *Unisex Edition of ACT Interest Inventory* (UNIACT) scales. Scales of both editions of the *Career Assessment Inventory* (CAI-E, CAI-V) and the *Career Decision-Making Inventory* (CDM) show a relatively poor fit. The VPI and SDS display an intermediate measure-model fit relative to the other measures.

Planned contrasts were conducted to provide a more precise evaluation of the measure-model fit. For these contrasts, the measures, with the exception of the UNIACT and CDM, were grouped and labeled: Holland (VPI, SDS), *Strong* (the *Strong Vocational Interest Blank*, SVIB, and *Strong-Campbell Interest Inventory*, SCII, editions), and CAI (CAI-V, CAI-E). The Holland measures were considered a benchmark measure for the RIASEC model and thus were contrasted with the other four RIASEC measures—the *Strong*, UNIACT, CAI, and CDM. The mean RSQ values for these contrasts are shown in Table 5. Results based on the RSQ values showed that only the *Strong* scales, $F(1, 53)$ = 3.87, $p < .05$, when compared with the Holland scales, provided a significantly better fit to the hexagon model, whereas the CDM scales, $F(1, 53)$ = 5.28, $p < .03$, showed a significantly poorer fit relative to the Holland scales.

Examination of Table 5 and Figure 3 also reveals that the pattern of the relative salience given to the dimensions differs among measures: The *Strong* and UNIACT measures give greater weight to the Data-Ideas dimension, the Holland measures equally weight the dimensions, and the CAI and CDM measures give greater weight to the People-Things dimension. Contrasts comparing the relative weights for the Holland measures (incidentally, an equal weight hypothesis) to the four other measures confirm three of these four observed differences: *Strong* ($F = 10.20$, $p < .002$), UNIACT ($F = 6.30$, $p < .02$), CAI ($F = .63$, $p = .43$), and CDM ($F = 4.20$, $p < .05$). Evidently, the increment in explained variance for the *Strong* and UNIACT scales, compared with the Holland measures—and, possibly, the decrement in explained variance for the CDM—is primarily accounted for by the Data-Ideas dimension. Between-measure comparisons on the source weights for the People-Things dimension showed no significant differences. Contrasts on the Data-Ideas source weights showed significant differences for the *Strong* scales, $F(1, 53)$ = 13.90, $p < .001$, and UNIACT scales, $F(1, 53)$ = 6.12, $p < .02$, when compared with Holland scales. In summary, the *Strong* and UNIACT scales are arguably better in differentiating the Data-Ideas dimension than the Holland, CAI, and CDM scales.

The observed variation among the sources could be due also to subject variables and/or an interaction between measures and subject variables. Sex differences have been implicated in the fit between measures and Holland's model, with women showing a poorer measure-model fit (Rounds, Davison, & Dawis, 1979). The present data set (25 sources for males and 24 sources for females), however, shows no significant sex differences for goodness of fit (RSQ values), $F(1, 48)$ = .79, $p = .38$, or for the relative salience of the dimensions, $F(1, 48)$ = 1.52, $p = .22$. Tests of the moderating effect of sex on measure-model fit using the Holland and Strong sources were also nonsignificant for these weight indices. Although sex differences have been found in item-response comparisons, and basic interest and general interest theme scale-score comparisons (Hansen, 1978; Holland & Gottfredson, 1976), the present findings indicate that these level differences are not reflected in the structural relations among RIASEC scales.

One critical issue that affects the interpretation of the present findings concerns the independence of the sources. The present data come from a limited group of investigators that usually includes the test authors or students and colleagues of these authors and, in a number of instances, the sources are from the same study. The data collected by the same research group may be more similar than are data collected by independent investigators. The results, for example, may depend on the sampling methodology used by a research group (e.g., Center for Interest Measurement Research, American College Testing Program). Such nonindependence would make significance testing problematic and also raise questions about the validity of the results. It is possible that the sources may be more appropriately conceptualized as measure-sampling units, and the evaluation of measures may be, instead, an evaluation of the quality of the research data collected by a particular research group. In terms of the present results, additional sources from independent investigators are needed before the possible confounding influence of research centers or groups can be evaluated.

Roe's Structural Hypothesis

Roe's circular order hypothesis has attracted relatively little attention. Much of the research has been conducted by Meir (Meir, 1973; Meir, Bar, Lahav, & Shalhevet, 1975; Meir & Ben-Yehuda, 1976), who has examined the fit of the internal relationships among scores on a Hebrew interest inventory (*Ramak*; Meir & Barak, 1974) to Roe's order hypothesis. In each study, the structure was tested with Israeli subjects by means of the Guttman-Lingoes Smallest Space Analysis technique. Rounds and Zevon (1983) reviewed these studies and concluded that the multidimensional scaling research by Meir and his colleagues provided no support for Roe's hypothesized interest configurations. On the contrary, each study has found a different circular ordering of the interest fields and different scale point clusters.

The question of the adequacy of the *Ramak* as a measure of Roe's eight interest fields is one possible explanation for the lack of fit between the *Ramak* data and Roe's circular model. Inasmuch as Roe's hypothesized circular model is culturally determined, another plausible explanation concerns the diversity and breadth of American occupations in comparison with Israeli occupations. Neither of these explanations, however, received support from Gati's (1979) Smallest Space Analysis of the *Vocational Interest Inventory* (VII; Lunneborg, 1975) scale correlations based on 235 male and female American university students (see also Lunneborg & Lunneborg's, 1975, principal components analysis of the VII matrix) or Knapp, Knapp, and Buttafuoco's (1978) study of changes in interests assessed by the *California Occupational Preference System* (COPS) for 1,243 junior and senior high school students. Aside from the *Ramak,* the VII and COPS appear to be the only instruments based on Roe's system. Gati has presented a spatial arrangement of Roe's fields that is identical to Meir's (1973) arrangement of Te-Sc-Od-AE-Sv-GC-Or-Bu (Technology, Science, Outdoor, Arts and Entertainment, Service, General Cultural, Organization, Business Contact), whereas Knapp and Knapp's (1984) research has suggested a Te-Od-Bu-Or-GC-AE-Sv-Sc arrangement, findings that question the adequacy of Roe's model.

Parallelism of Roe's and Holland's Models

As a result of the apparent similarity of Holland's and Roe's models, Holland (1976) and Lunneborg (1975, 1981) have suggested a parallelism between components of these models. Specifically, the following types and fields are hypothesized to represent similar interest areas: Holland's Realistic (R) and Roe's Technology (Te) and Outdoor (Od); Holland's Investigative (I) and Roe's Science (Sc); Holland's Artistic (A) and Roe's General Cultural (GC) and Arts and Entertainment (AE); Holland's Social (S) and Roe's Service (Sv); Holland's Enterprising (E) and Roe's Business Contact (Bu); and Holland's Conventional (C) and Roe's Organization (Or).

The evidence for this hypothesized parallelism is not particularly compelling. Meir and Ben-Yehuda (1976) displayed a two-dimensional spatial representation with four scale clusters defining two orthogonal dimensions: SC and Od opposing E, C, Bu, and Or; and Te, R, and I opposing AE, A, GC, Sv, and S. In spite of the apparent correspondence between fields, the parallel fields are not always nearest to each other: Bu lies nearer to C than to E, and Od lies nearer to S than to R. A reanalysis (Fitzgerald & Hubert, 1987; Gati, 1979) of Lunneborg and Lunneborg's (1975) correlations of Roe and Holland scales also shows disagreement with the parallel field hypothesis. Gati reported that Or is between Bu and E, that C is nearer to E than to Or, and that S is nearer to GC than Sv, whereas Fitzgerald and Hubert found that the Od appeared as an isolate between the science cluster (Sc, I) and the artistic cluster (AE, A) and that GC was in the social cluster (Sv, S) rather than the artistic cluster (AE, A). These results are not unexpected because there have been consistent findings of disagreement between Roe's theoretical and the empirical ordering of interest fields.

Gati's Structural Hypothesis

Because of the less than perfect fit of the data to circular interest models, Gati (1979) has proposed a hierarchical representation of Holland's and Roe's interest categories. These hierarchical models are simple partitions: (R, I), (A, S), and (E, C) for Holland and (Te, Od, Sc), (AE),

(Sv, GC), and (Bu, Or) for Roe. Gati (1979, 1982) presented the hierarchical model as a competitive structure to the circular model, arguing that his model fits the empirical relations among the interest fields more adequately than either Holland's or Roe's models. The results and the logic on which the hierarchical model depend have been questioned (Rounds & Zevon, 1983), but Hubert and Arabie (1987) provided the most damaging critique. They demonstrated that Gati's model is only a simple refinement of a circular interest model in which Holland's and Roe's interest categories are not considered equally spaced along the circle. Thus, this hierarchical model generates an ordering of the interest fields that is congruent with and readily obtainable from the circular interest model.

DISCUSSION

Over the last 15 years, there has been increasing consensus in the vocational literature (Borgen, 1986) that the internal relations of interest scales are best represented by Holland's circular order conjecture. In the analyses presented, configural verification and dimensional representation of Holland's model, goals well suited to multidimensional scaling procedures, were pursued by using results (correlation matrices) from individual studies. Overall, this methodological approach to synthesizing the results of individual studies was successful in evaluating structural hypotheses and moderator variables. The findings provide impressive support for Holland's structural hypothesis with measures that are presumed to assess the RIASEC types. The evidence not only supports the simple order hypothesis, but also supports Holland's stronger structural hypothesis, the calculus assumption. On the other hand, Roe's structural hypothesis has faired poorly, with as many empirical orderings of her fields as there have been proposed measures. Second, the findings show that two dimensions can be mapped on the Holland model that are similar in location to Prediger's theory-based coordinate axes. Although these findings are not sufficient support for the labels given to the dimensions, it is apparent that research should focus on these dimensions for explanations of the circular arrangement of interests.

One advantage in using three-way scaling was the contribution of the source weights to understanding how characteristics of these sources relate to the overall fit. The findings, for example, showed that the RIASEC measures differentially contribute to the source-model goodness of fit that has implications about the use of these measures in vocational counseling. It appears that the internal relations for at least five measures presumed to assess RIASEC interest types—*Strong* (SVIB and SCII), UNIACT, VPI, and SDS—demonstrate an adequate fit to Holland's model. But not all attempts to construct alternative forms have been as successful as these five measures, with the *Career Assessment Inventory—Vocational Edition* (CAI-V) and the CDM showing a relatively poor measure-model fit. A detailed discussion of the differences among these measures is beyond the scope of this chapter, but it is worth noting that the relative salience of the Data-Ideas dimension seems to be related to RIASEC summary code distributions. RIASEC summary codes for the *Strong* and UNIACT measures, when compared with Holland measures, are more evenly distributed across the six categories. For the Holland measures, a greater proportion of Social codes for women and Realistic codes for men are found (Harmon & Zytowski, 1980; Holland, 1985b, 1985c; Prediger & Johnson, 1979). Although there are many hypotheses that can be compared in this way, the main purpose here is to suggest the advantages of this particular strategy in analyzing multiple data sources. (Since this chapter was written, additional research [Rounds & Tracey, 1993; Rounds, Tracey, & Hubert, 1992; Tracey & Rounds, 1993; Tracey & Rounds, 1994] has been conducted that develops and expands several of the ideas presented here.)

STRUCTURE OF BASIC INTERESTS

In *Making Vocational Choices: A Theory of Vocational Personalities and Work Environments,* Holland (1985a) claims that evidence for the RIASEC arrangement for vocational interests is substantial. When viewed from the perspective of interest measures developed to assess the six types (general interest hypothesis), the evidence (especially the data presented above) indeed provides a strong case. But the major support for this claim and the basis of Holland's generalization to vocational interests comes from two studies (Cole, 1973; Cole & Hanson, 1971) examining the internal relations among scales that not only assess Holland interest categories, but that also were developed to measure a wide variety of occupational interests and basic interests. In this section, I will bring the same structural questions examined above about general interests to bear on the domain of basic interest dimensions.

Cole's Studies

In an analysis of interest patterns of men, Cole and Hanson (1971) applied a spatial configuration technique, a variation of principal components, separately to correlations of 50 SVIB Occupational Scales (Campbell, 1966), 22 SVIB Basic Interest Scales (Campbell, Borgen, Eastes, Johansson, & Peterson, 1968), 23 KOIS Occupational Scales (Kuder, 1966), and 9 *Minnesota Vocational Interest Inventory* (MVII)

Basic Interest Scales (Clark, 1961). Cole (1973) then replicated her analysis on interest inventories developed for women: 27 SVIB Occupational Scales (Strong, 1959), 19 SVIB Basic Interest Scales (Campbell, 1971), and 9 KOIS Occupational Scales (Kuder, 1966). Cole argued that the configurations of the scales for men and women across the various inventories were similar and conform to Roe's and Holland's circular configurations. A review of the results, however, leaves some doubt that the data, especially for women, are quite as supportive as claimed. In contrast to her report on the structure of men's interest, Cole (1973) did not classify the scales for women into Holland's system and plot their mean spatial locations, leaving the interpretation in the eye of the beholder. Taking account of such differences, one notes several discrepancies from the Holland ordering for the women's scales: The spatial configuration for the SVIB Occupational Scales shows that some scales, such as Nurse, Occupational Therapist, and Elementary Teacher, usually coded Social, are located between Realistic and Conventional and opposite to Artistic scales. For the SVIB Basic Interest Scales, Enterprising scales (Law/Politics, Public Speaking) are grouped with Medical Science and Sports near the solution's origin.

Reevaluation of Cole's Findings

A more elaborate test of the structure of basic interest scales is clearly called for, especially because Cole's conclusions are often cited in support of Holland's model and have shaped much of the current thought about the structure of interests. Interest inventories have also undergone considerable revision since Cole's paper (Borgen, 1986). One important change is that males and females are now scored on the same set of basic interest scales, allowing a direct comparison of the interest configurations of men and women. The last 15 years has also seen an increase in the number and variety of basic scales scored in interest inventories.

A replication of Cole's study was performed using internal relations of Basic Interest Scales from the *Strong-Campbell Interest Inventory* (SCII) and the *Jackson Vocational Interest Survey* (JVIS). One purpose of the study was to assess the fit of basic interest configurations to the circular structure proposed by Holland. Another purpose was to compare the basic interest configurations of men and women. Correlation matrices of the scales for men and women in each of the interest inventories were separately submitted to a nonmetric multidimensional scaling analysis (SYSTAT; Wilkinson, 1986). The matrices for the 23 SCII Basic Interest Scales based on samples of 300 men and 300 women were obtained from Hansen and Campbell (1985, p. 38) and those for the 26 JVIS basic interest (work role) scales based on 779 men and 600 women were from Jackson (1977, p. 42).

Table 6   Stress Values for Two- and Three-Dimensional Solutions

Measure	No. of Scales	Female		Male	
		2	3	2	3
JVIS	26	.13	.07	.11	.06
SCII	23	.21	.10	.20	.12

Note. JVIS = *Jackson Vocational Interest Survey*; SCII = *Strong-Campbell Interest Inventory.*

Results

Table 6 shows the stress values (Kruskal formula 1) for two and three dimensions by gender and measure. The badness of fit values for the SCII scales indicate that three dimensions rather than two dimensions may more adequately represent the relation among the scales, a finding also reported by Cole (1973; Cole & Hanson, 1971). For the JVIS scales, a two-dimensional representation seems to be the best fit. Because one purpose of this analysis is to examine the circular structure of basic interests, a two-dimensional instead of a three-dimensional solution for the SCII Basic Interest Scales is displayed. The configurations (Figures 4 through 7) have been oriented by instrument in the same general way to simplify visual comparison. Configural comparisons (ordering of basic interest scales) will take precedence over dimensional comparisons. Dimensional comparisons and interpretations, however, are proposed when the MDS axes conform to existing models or clarify differences among solutions.

JVIS Solutions   Figures 4 and 5 depict the solutions for males and females derived from correlations among their respective responses to 26 scales of the JVIS. One immediate observation is that the scales form semicircles at both ends of Dimension 1. This is partially due to the JVIS forced-choice format in which items from similar scales emphasizing science and mastery of nonpersonal aspects of the environment are paired with items from scales involving interpersonal activities.

Jackson (1977, pp. 43–44) has grouped these scales into eight general interest themes: (a) Logical (Mathematics, Physical Science, Engineering), (b) Practical (Nature-Agriculture, Family Activity, Creative Arts, Skilled Trades, Personal Service), (c) Inquiring (Life Sciences, Medical Service, Social Science), (d) Expressive (Performing Arts, Creative Arts, Author-Journalism), (e) Helping (Elementary Education, Social Service, Teaching), (f) Communicative (Technical Writing, Author-Journalism), (g) Enterprising (Professional Advising, Human Relations Management, Finance, Law, Supervision, Business, Sales),

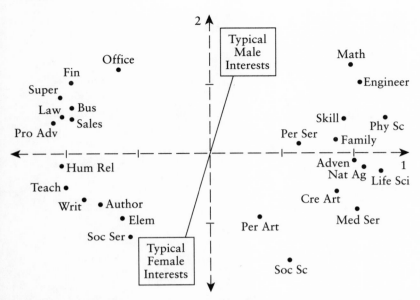

Figure 4 Two-dimensional scaling solution for males obtained from the JVIS Basic Interest Scale correlations with the gender-difference variable imbedded as a directed line

Note. Cre Art = Creative Arts, Per Art = Performing Arts, Math = Mathematics, Phy Sc = Physical Science, Engineer = Engineering, Life Sci = Life Sciences, Soc Sc = Social Science, Adven = Adventure, Nat Agr = Nature-Agriculture, Skill = Skilled Trades, Per Ser = Personal Service, Family = Family Activity, Med Ser = Medical Service, Teach = Teaching, Soc Ser = Social Service, Elem = Elementary Education, Fin = Finance, Bus = Business, Office = Office Work, Super = Supervision, Hum Rel = Human Relations Management, Pro Adv = Professional Advising, Author = Author-Journalism, and Writ = Technical Writing.

Based on correlations from *Manual for the Jackson Vocational Interest Survey,* by D. N. Jackson, 1977, p. 42.

and (h) Conventional (Office Work, Sales, Business, Supervision). Notice that several scales belong to more than one general interest theme: Business, Sales, and Supervision belong to both the Enterprising and Conventional themes; Creative Arts defines the Practical and Expressive themes. Overall, the general interest theme groupings appear to be a reasonable way to summarize the scale configurations: Most scales are located nearer to the scales that define the general interest theme than to scales that define other themes. Two exceptions occurred: Social Science in the female solution was not located near the scales that define the Inquiring theme. Author-Journalism was located in both solutions near Technical Writing, a location important for the definition of the Communicative theme; neither Author-Journalism nor Technical Writing were located near the Expressive theme scales as expected.

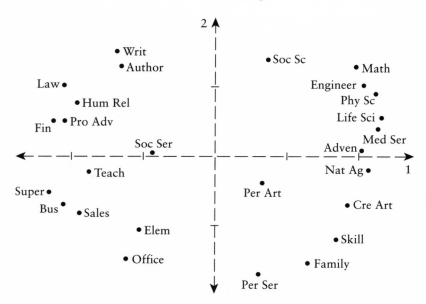

Figure 5 Two-dimensional scaling solution for females obtained from the JVIS Basic Interest Scale correlations

Note. Cre Art = Creative Arts, Per Art = Performing Arts, Math = Mathematics, Phy Sc = Physical Science, Engineer = Engineering, Life Sci = Life Sciences, Soc Sc = Social Science, Adven = Adventure, Nat Agr = Nature-Agriculture, Skill = Skilled Trades, Per Ser = Personal Service, Family = Family Activity, Med Ser = Medical Service, Teach = Teaching, Soc Ser = Social Service, Elem = Elementary Education, Fin = Finance, Bus = Business, Office = Office Work, Super = Supervision, Hum Rel = Human Relations Management, Pro Adv = Professional Advising, Author = Author-Journalism, and Writ = Technical Writing.

Based on correlations from *Manual for the Jackson Vocational Interest Survey,* by D. N. Jackson, 1977, p. 42.

As can be seen from Figures 4 and 5, the ordering of Jackson's themes approximates Holland's theoretical ordering—but for men only, not for women. The RIASEC ordering can only be approximated because several general interest themes (e.g., Logical and Practical) are not directly translatable to Holland categories. (The JVIS scales are assigned Holland codes below to evaluate the order hypothesis directly.)

The most notable finding that affects a circular order hypothesis is that these solutions show considerable gender differences in the location of basic interest groupings. Beginning in the upper right quadrant and moving clockwise on the JVIS solutions, the following shifts in the order of scales from Figure 4 to Figure 5 occur: The Practical theme scales are grouped between the Logical and Inquiring scales for men; for women, the Practical scales shift to the lower right quadrant, ordering themselves in a broad circular arrangement between the Inquiring and Conventional scales. The Social Science scale, located near the positive end of Dimension 2 for women, is located at the opposite end for men. The Helping scales for men are found next to the Communicative scales; for women, the Helping scales are located between the Conventional and Enterprising scales, primarily due to the shift of the Social Service scale. Finally, the Conventional and Communicative scale groups are located in reverse order for women and men.

Overall, the shifts in scales result in a configuration for women that locates most professional interests or complex job activities (e.g., Law, Author-Journalism, Social Science, Mathematics, Engineering) in the upper half of the configuration, toward the positive end of Dimension 2, and the skilled and semiskilled interests or less complex job tasks (Sales, Office Work, Personal Service, Skilled Trades) in the lower half, the negative end of Dimension 2. Thus, the level of the task, or the task complexity, may influence preferences for women, but, in this case, not for men. On the other hand, the JVIS configuration for men has basic interests more often endorsed by males (e.g., Finance, Business) in the upper half, toward the positive pole of Dimension 2, and basic interests more often endorsed by females (e.g., Social Service, Social Science) in the lower half of the configuration.

SCII Solutions   The SCII Basic Interest Scale configurations for men and women are given in Figures 6 and 7. In both figures, the Artistic and Enterprising scales are tightly grouped together, whereas the opposite is true for the Realistic scales. The RIASEC scale groups, which will be discussed later in this chapter, are presented later in Table 8. For women, the Realistic scales are scattered throughout the spatial representation, whereas for men, these scales form a broad semicircle, beginning at the positive pole of Dimension 2 and ending at the negative end of the same dimension.

Similar to the JVIS solutions, the configuration of SCII Basic Interest Scales approximates Holland's RIASEC ordering for men but not for women. And once again, gender differences are evident: For men, the Social scales are grouped between the Artistic scales and the center of the configuration, whereas for women, the Social scales are clearly located opposite the Artistic scales and adjacent to the Realistic and Enterprising scales. A somewhat unexpected finding for women is the location of the Adventure scale: It is grouped with the Artistic scales. In comparison, the Adventure scale is found near the Athletics and Military scales for men.

A level dimension for women similar to that found in the JVIS solution seems to account for the spatial variation among the basic interest scales. Rank ordering the scales on Dimension 1 (reading from left to right in Figure 7) shows that the activities and occupations vary from writing, mathematics, science, and law to nature-agriculture, athletics, social service, domestic activities, and office practices. Similar

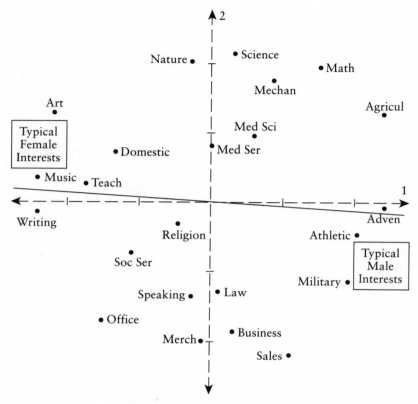

Figure 6   Two-dimensional scaling solution for males obtained from
the SCII Basic Interest Scale correlations with the gender-
difference variable imbedded as a directed line

Note. Agricul = Agriculture, Adven = Adventure, Military = Military Activities,
Mechan = Mechanical Activities, Math = Mathematics, Med Sci = Medical Science,
Med Ser = Medical Service, Music = Music/Dramatics, Teach = Teaching, Soc Ser =
Social Service, Domestic = Domestic Activities, Religion = Religious Activities,
Speaking = Public Speaking, Law = Law/Politics, Merch = Merchandising,
Business = Business Management, and Office = Office Practices.

Based on correlations from *Manual for the SVIB-SCII Strong-Campbell Interest Survey* (4th ed.),
by J. C. Hansen and D. P. Campbell, 1985, p. 38.

to the Occupational Level scale of the SVIB (Campbell, 1971), Dimension 1 for women could be considered a measure of the socioeconomic level of the individual's interests.

Gender Differences   If the SCII Dimension 1 for women suggests a
level interpretation, the same dimension for men shown in Figure 6
suggests a gender interpretation, with the interests typically associated with men and women anchoring the two opposing ends. To test
this latter interpretation, the difference between mean basic interest
scale endorsements for the Men- and Women-in-General samples (Hansen

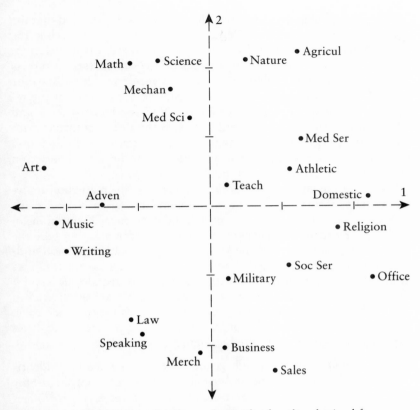

Figure 7 Two-dimensional scaling solution for females obtained from the SCII Basic Interest Scale correlations

Note. Agricul = Agriculture, Adven = Adventure, Military = Military Activities, Mechan = Mechanical Activities, Math = Mathematics, Med Sci = Medical Science, Med Ser = Medical Service, Music = Music/Dramatics, Teach = Teaching, Soc Ser = Social Service, Domestic = Domestic Activities, Religion = Religious Activities, Speaking = Public Speaking, Law = Law/Politics, Merch = Merchandising, Business = Business Management, and Office = Office Practices.

Based on correlations from *Manual for the SVIB-SCII Strong-Campbell Interest Survey* (4th ed.), by J. C. Hansen and D. P. Campbell, 1985, p. 38.

& Campbell, 1985, Table 5.1, p. 37) were regressed onto the MDS stimuli coordinates for the male and female solutions. Table 5.1 in the SCII manual (Hansen & Campbell, 1985) displays mean scores for the 23 Basic Interest Scales by sex. Taking the difference between scale scores for men and women, an array of 23 scores is formed, with men scoring the highest (mean difference in parenthesis) on, for example, Mechanical Activities (6.6), Military Activities (6.2), and Athletics (6.2) and women scoring the highest on, for example, Music/Dramatics (–6.2), Art (–7.0), and Domestic Activities (–8.2).

The regression analysis for men ($R = .89$, $p < .001$) showed that the vector representing gender differences in interests fits very well in the space, whereas for women ($R = .14$, $p > .05$), there was no relationship between this variable and the basic interest representation. As depicted in Figure 6, the gender difference vector was fitted into the basic interest representation for men using an application of the regression weights (direction cosines are .997 for Dimension 1 and –.074 for Dimension 2). Notice that this vector almost coincides with Dimension 1. Thus, it appears that gender differences typically found in SCII scale score comparisons are reflected in the spatial variation among basic interests for men, but not for women.

Given the above findings, I decided to replicate the regression analysis on the coordinates of the JVIS configuration. Again, a gender-difference variable was defined by taking the differences between mean basic interest scale endorsements for males and females, but here the JVIS norm group was used (Jackson, 1977, p. 8). The regression findings were similar to those for the SCII: The multiple correlation was moderate for males ($R = .74$, $p < .001$) and low for females ($R = .56$, $p < .05$), indicating that stereotypic gender interests are implicated in the configuration for males. The direction cosines for the male basic interest coordinates are .246 for Dimension 1 and .969 for Dimension 2, generating the vector plotted in Figure 4.

Gender Similarities   Although gender differences have been identified, correlation of the male and female basic interest coordinates for each measure indicates that there are also similarities between women and men in the basic interest representations: Dimension 1 for the JVIS ($r = .99$) and Dimension 2 for SCII ($r = .95$). This can be seen in Table 7. Furthermore, examination of these dimensions across measures shows a similar configuration of interest scales, that is, a dimension that could be labeled Things/People or Investigative/Enterprising, although neither label seems to capture the variety of interests. More specifically, interests in pure and applied science and nature define one pole, and business contact and verbal interests define the other end of the dimension (cf. Waller, Lykken, & Tellegen's ECSCAL plot of occupational interests in this volume). When viewed as a Things-People dimension, the types of interests have more in common with Strong's (1943) formulations of things and people than Prediger's (1982) proposal.

A closer inspection of the Things-People dimension across the four solutions (see Figures 4 through 7) shows almost identical circular ordering between adjacent groups of scales defining each end of the dimension. The scales, for example, that reference the broad area of scientific interests are ordered (the order within groupings may vary): Mathematics; Engineering, Mechanical; Physical Science, Science; and

Table 7 Correlations of Male and Female Stimulus Coordinates
for the SCII and JVIS

	Male		Female	
Dimension	1	2	1	2
Male				
1	—	.00	.17	−.20
2	.00	—	−.16	.95
Female				
1	.99	−.04	—	.00
2	.03	.13	.00	—

Note. SCII, *Strong-Campbell Interest Inventory* correlations are above the diagonal; JVIS, *Jackson Vocational Interest Inventory* correlations are below the diagonal.

Life Science, Nature, Nature-Agriculture. The arrangement of these scales reflects a research and applications dimension extending from symbols and nonverbal languages (mathematics) and inanimate objects (engineering, physics) to plants and animals (biology, nature). The verbal and business contact scales also display a consistent arrangement: Technical Writing, Author-Journalism, Writing; Professional Advising, Human Relations Management, Law, Law/Politics, Public Speaking; and Merchandising, Business Management, Business, Sales. These scales appear to be ordered on a continuum from activities involving negotiating, recommending, and advising to those involving managing, supervising, coordinating, and selling. The similar arrangements of interest scales for both genders and both measures indicate that it may be possible to develop a more elaborate and definitive model of the structure of interests using basic interest scales. Such a model for basic interests, however, awaits a better understanding of the influence of gender on vocational preferences.

Evaluating Holland's Order Hypothesis

Scaling the SCII and JVIS correlation matrices indicates that several interest scales and RIASEC categories deviate from Holland's order hypothesis. Because of the number of scales and the nature of these deviations, it is difficult to determine precisely whether these departures are sufficient to reject the circular order hypothesis or to determine which of the categories deviate from the RIASEC order.

Given the above, two methodologies were used to evaluate whether the circular order hypothesis is manifest in the scaling solutions. The first methodology involved simply plotting the mean scale values for the basic interest scales representing the six Holland categories. Table 8 presents the RIASEC classification of the SCII and JVIS Basic

Table 8   Basic Interest Scales for the SCII and JVIS Grouped
           by Holland Category

Strong-Campbell Interest Inventory	*Jackson Vocational Interest Inventory*
Realistic (R)	
Agriculture	Nature-Agriculture
Nature	Engineering
Adventure	Adventure
Mechanical Activities	Skill Trades
Military Activities	
Investigative (I)	
Science	Physical Sciences
Mathematics	Mathematics
Medical Science	Life Science
Medical Service	Medical Service
	Social Sciences
Artistic (A)	
Music/Dramatics	Performing Arts
Art	Creative Arts
Writing	Technical Writing
	Author-Journalism
Social (S)	
Teaching	Teaching
Social Service	Social Service
Athletics	Elementary Education
Domestic Activities	Family Activity
Religious Activities	
Enterprising (E)	
Public Speaking	Human Relations Management
Law/Politics	Law
Merchandising	Professional Advising
Sales	Sales
Business Management	Business
	Supervision
	Personal Service
Conventional (C)	
Office Practices	Office Work
	Finance

Note. SCII = *Strong-Campbell Interest Inventory*; JVIS = *Jackson Vocational Interest Survey.*

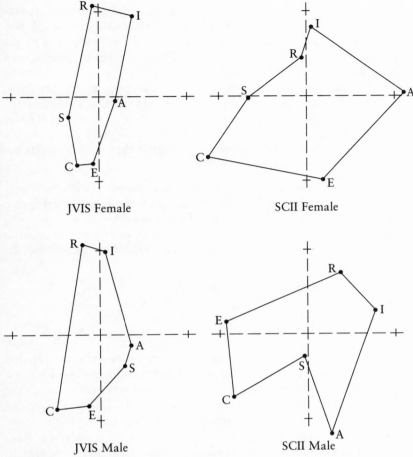

Figure 8 Spatial configuration of Basic Interest Scales categorized
by Holland's classification for the JVIS and SCII by gender

Note. R = Realistic, I = Investigative, A = Artistic, S = Social, E = Enterprising, and
C = Conventional.

Interest Scales. The SCII scale classification comes from Hansen and
Campbell (1985). I assigned the JVIS scales to the Holland categories.

Mean Planar Locations Figure 8 gives the mean spatial locations for
each category by scaling solution. (To facilitate comparisons between
solutions, the configurations have been reoriented with the Realistic
and Investigative categories defining the positive end of Dimension 2,
and categories are connected by lines according to their circular

arrangement.) Overall, the Holland categories depart from the hypothesized circular order for three of the four of the configurations shown in Figure 8. The configural fit to Holland's order hypothesis using the number and type of departures as an index of fit is better for men than for women. For the men, the departures involve an order reversal of adjacent categories (Conventional and Enterprising) for the SCII, whereas the expected RIASEC order occurs for the JVIS. For the women, the departures involve the Social category: A RIAECS order is shown for the SCII and JVIS configurations. In both cases, the Social category is located opposite the Artistic type and between the Conventional and Realistic types.

Combinatorial Data Analysis   Hubert and Arabie (1989) have suggested a more precise method for evaluating conjectures of order within correlation matrices. Their strategy finds the best least squares fit of the partitioned similarities matrix (here, the basic interest correlation matrix partitioned by Holland categories), defined by maximizing the usual squared multiple correlation:

$$R^2 = 1 - \text{Sum}(r_{ij} - \hat{r}_{ij})^2 / \text{Sum}(r_{ij} - \bar{r})^2$$

$$\text{where} \quad r_{ij} = \text{similarity value (correlation)}$$
$$\bar{r} = \text{average similarity value}$$
$$\hat{r}_{ij} = \text{fitted value.}$$

Under an unrestricted analysis, the similarity values are compared with fitted values defined by the average within and across cell values. In a restricted analysis, the fitted values are constrained to satisfy the particular hypothesis under consideration (here Holland's circular RIASEC order). The comparison of the unrestricted R^2 with the restricted R^2 provides an estimate of the fit of RIASEC ordering. Random permutations of the ordered objects are used to test the significance of the restricted R^2.

Application of Hubert and Arabie's procedure to the SCII correlation matrices for women and men shows that Holland's order conjecture does rather poorly. The unrestricted R^2—at .50 for women and .46 for men—was small in both cases, suggesting that the fit for RIASEC partitions is less than satisfactory. A good fit, relative to the unconstrained analysis, was found when circular order constraints were applied: Restricted R^2 was .46 for women and .43 for men, both with p values less than .01. Nevertheless, a good fit was also found when linear constraints were applied to the matrices: R^2 was .46 for women and .44 for men. These minor differences in the magnitude of R^2 for the circular and linear constrained analyses suggest that even though Holland's ordered hypothesis cannot be rejected, a linear order hypothesis is just as viable as the circular order conjecture for representing the internal relations of basic interest scales.

DISCUSSION

The research bases of the circular structure of interest models comes from studies of the relations of Holland's six categories and indicates that two dimensions do an adequate job of summarizing the variance. Although Cole's studies extended the research base to basic interests, the research presented herein raises serious questions about Cole's conclusion that basic interests for men and women are organized in a two-dimensional space according to Holland's circular structure of interest. The present findings indicate a poor fit of basic interests to Holland's model.

The results also clearly show that there are structural similarities and differences between men and women in their vocational interests. Three dimensions emerged across the four data sets. The first dimension found across measures and gender samples contrasts an interest in things versus people. The second dimension found for configurations based on data for female samples was interpreted as a measure of the complexity of work tasks or a dimension that contrasts professional interests versus skilled and semiskilled interests. The third dimension found for configurations based on data for male samples was interpreted as a measure of preference for activities and occupations stereotypically associated with men versus those stereotypically associated with women. Gender differences in the structure of interests implies that men and women perceive these interests (in activities, occupations) along different dimensions or attend and respond to different aspects of these interests. It also implies that the meaning of interest scales and categories may differ for women and men. For instance, culturally constructed expectations for and of women may well explain why the pursuit of artistic interests (or an artistic occupation) may be perceived by women to be more adventurous than social.

The basic interest configurations are consistent with previous findings that Roe's circular arrangement of interests is incorrect. Roe's hypothesis indicates that Outdoor interests are located between Technical and Science and that General Culture is located between Science and Arts and Entertainment. Contrary to Roe's model, the basic interest configurations show that Outdoor is located between Science and Arts and that General Culture (a measure of verbal interest and probably also encompassing interests that are entrepreneurial) is located between Service and Business Contact. In fact, Lunneborg and Lunneborg (1975) reported exactly this ordering of Roe's categories.

For a variety of reasons, neither the Holland Realistic nor Conventional themes fared well in the analysis. The Conventional theme was not well represented by basic interest scales, with one SCII scale and two JVIS scales classified into this theme. It might be noted that Jackson avoided the problems created by Holland's too-narrow definition by assigning interests typically thought of as Enterprising (sales, business, supervision) to this category, which he also called Conventional (compare also Roe's Organizational category). The SCII Realistic scales were scattered throughout the interest space and do not seem to define a coherent category. Jackson's strategy was to develop a Practical theme that included basic interest scales referencing Realistic scales but also other interests that would be found in Holland's Social (Family Activity) and Enterprising (Personal Service) categories. However, neither Holland's nor Jackson's approach have fully taken account of the broad domain of semiskilled and skilled occupational activities. A more elaborate differentiation than either has proposed is called for and would necessarily have an impact on the circular structure of interests.

DOES THE SUM OF THE PARTS EQUAL THE WHOLE?

Does the whole equal the sum of its parts? Do six general interest themes equal the whole of basic interests? An evaluation of vocational interest structural hypotheses suggest that these questions remain open to further discussion and examination. As I have argued, this discussion would be facilitated by a basic interest catalog and research measures to assess basic interests, important benefits of which would include the development and interpretation of general interest factors. Jackson (1977), commenting on the importance of basic interest factors, has said:

> ...(t)he emergence of the larger number of themes in the JVIS as contrasted with fewer previously is no doubt attributable to the existence of a larger number of Basic Interest scales, as well as the JVIS method of scale development, resulting in greater scale independence. (p. 24)

Jackson's larger number of themes (general interest factors), however, is not a major departure from Holland's types or Roe's interest categories or, for that matter, Strong's occupational families. Table 9 displays Holland's types, Roe's categories, Jackson's general interest theme factors, and Strong's occupational families (the labels are from Super & Crites, 1962, who credit Darley, 1941). Reading down the columns, the categories have been ordered according to the results of the present investigation. (Note that Table 9 is illustrative for males only; results for females were so divergent from the Holland hypothesized order that further study is needed.) Reading across the classifications, the interest categories have been listed in terms of content similarity. The irregularities in the horizontal alignments represent an

Table 9 Hypothesized Order and Similarity of General Interest Categories

Holland (1973)	Roe (1956)	Strong (1943)	Jackson (1977)
			Logical
Realistic	Technical	Technical	
			Practical
		Physical Science	
Investigative	Science		
		Biological Science	
	Outdoor		
			Inquiring
Artistic	Arts/Entertainment		Expressive
Social	Service	Social Welfare	Helping
	General Culture	Linguistic	Communicative
			Enterprising
Enterprising	Business Contact	Business Contact	
	Organizational		Conventional
Conventional		Business Detail	

attempt to approximate variations in levels of generality of the Roe, Strong, and Jackson categories with respect to the Holland classifications.

Table 9 suggests several observations about the categories and their order. What is gained from the generality and simplicity of Holland's categories is lost in favor of precision, a bandwidth-fidelity trade-off. Measures of categories as broad as "realistic" may have their advantages, but given that two-thirds of the occupations in the *Dictionary of Holland Occupational Codes* (Gottfredson & Holland, 1989) are coded Realistic, they certainly do not help much to clarify a client's occupational interests. As the present results for the basic interest scales suggest, when more narrow-band categories are proposed, they do not necessarily line up in the relations of adjacency suggested by Holland's categories.

For example, content analysis of Holland's VPI Realistic scale indicates that it is composed of skilled and semiskilled occupational titles. The occupations involve work in the outdoors with plants and animals (hunting and fishing guide, tree surgeon, fish and wildlife specialist), craft technology or skilled trades (airplane mechanic, auto mechanic, electrician, electronic technician, machinist), vehicle operation (bus driver, locomotive engineer), quality control (construction inspector), engineering technology (surveyor). In the circular structure of interests, therefore, Outdoor and Technical should be adjacent categories, but the present findings have shown that Outdoor seems to be located between Investigative and Artistic.

To take another example, content analysis of Holland's VPI Artistic scale indicates that it is composed of occupational titles related to music (musician, concert singer, composer, music arranger, symphony conductor), the visual arts (commercial artist, portrait artist, cartoonist, sculptor/sculptress [sic]), and literary, language, or writing occupations (poet, author, freelance writer, journalist, playwright). The expected structural order places the performing arts and the literary arts adjacent to one another, but the findings presented here indicate that the verbal interest categories (e.g., Roe's General Culture and Jackson's Communicative) tend to be located between the Social and Enterprising categories, whereas the performing arts are located as expected between Investigative and Social.

The separate existence of a linguistic or verbal interest category, like Roe's General Culture or Jackson's Communicative factor, has had a long tradition in interest measurement. A verbal interest factor was initially identified in Thurstone's (1931) and Strong's (1943) factor analytic studies. Kuder (1939), using a deductive scale construction strategy, developed the Literary scale for the *Kuder Preference Record*. Verbal interest, however, has been defined in two ways: interest in creative and original writing (e.g., writing by poets and novelists) and interest in writing and editing reports, manuals, and articles (e.g., writing by technical writers and journalists). Although both types of writing consist of an interest in the use of words and in the manipulation of verbal concepts, the latter bread-and-butter writing interests seem to be more highly related to Enterprising interests (e.g., public speaking, law, public relations) than are creative writing interests (Holdsworth & Cramp, 1982; see also Lunneborg's, 1981, discussion of General Cultural). Interests in creative writing are more similar to performing and visual art interests.

However, this is not to suggest that in other instances the broad- and narrow-band categories do not converge. Holland's Investigative type and Roe's Science category, for example, are subdivided by Jackson into Logical and Inquiring factors, a distinction that may roughly parallel Strong's (1943) occupational families of Physical Science and Biological Science. These categories are found in the expected order.

As Jackson pointed out, we need to build broad-band categories from studies of more narrow-band categories such as basic interests. Thus, the mixed review discussed here may tend to support the suspicion that six categories may not constitute the best representation of the vocational interest domain. What I have wanted to suggest is that broad-band interest categories have tended to travel too far from the original and still unattainable goals of vocational interest research: to identify basic interests and to build therefrom structures of more generalized categories that will prove useful to both the vocational client and the vocational researcher. Recent factor analytic research has expanded enormously the number and types of interests identified. Scrutiny of the available research indicates that a catalog of such material as has been provided thus far could be begun and would indeed prove useful. In his assessment of Jackson's and Lunneborg and Lunneborg's multivariate work, Borgen (1986) has pointed out that the "simpler models have clearly earned a place in both theory and practice, but these lessons of greater complexity of multivariate structure should also be applied where it is feasible" (p. 102). The question then becomes, as Borgen also notes, one of evaluating the trade-offs. It has been my intention to acknowledge fully the significant virtues and efficacies of Holland's and Roe's models, but also to argue that there are compelling reasons to modify the structure in the pursuit of greater accuracy, with the hope that by doing so we will also retain the parsimony and utility such models have provided.

Preparation of this chapter was supported in part by a National Academy of Education Spencer Fellowship. I would like to thank Lawrence Hubert for his suggestion that I use combinatorial data analysis and for his assistance in its application. This chapter has benefited from the comments and critiques of John Holland, Lenore Harmon, Lawrence Hubert, Dale Prediger, Terence Tracey, and Lynda Zwinger. Thanks are also due to Elizabeth Droz for the literature search and data preparation.

REFERENCES

American College Testing Program. (1968). *The ACT Guidance Profile manual.* Iowa City, IA: Author.

American College Testing Program. (1988). *Interim psychometric handbook for the 3rd edition ACT career planning program.* Iowa City, IA: Author.

Arabie, P., Carroll, J. D., & DeSarbo, W. S. (1987). *Three-way scaling and clustering.* Beverly Hills, CA: Sage.

Athanasou, J. A. (1982, February). *Factor analysis of male and female responses on the Vocational Interest scales of the Vocational Preference Inventory.* Paper presented at the Australian Council for Educational Research, Melbourne.

Athanasou, J. A., O'Gorman, J., & Meyer, E. (1981). Factorial validity of the Vocational Interest scales of the Holland Vocational Preference Inventory for Australian high school students. *Educational and Psychological Measurement, 41,* 523–527.

Borgen, F. H. (1986). New approaches to the assessment of interests. In W. B. Walsh & S. H. Osipow (Eds.), *Advances in vocational psychology: Vol. 1. The assessment of interest* (pp. 31–54). Hillsdale, NJ: Erlbaum.

Brookings, J. B., & Bolton, B. (1986). Vocational interest dimensions of adult handicapped persons. *Measurement and Evaluation in Counseling and Development, 18,* 168–175.

Bull, P. E. (1975). Structure of occupational interests in New Zealand and America on Holland's typology. *Journal of Counseling Psychology, 22,* 554–556.

Burisch, M. (1986). Methods of personality inventory development—a comparative analysis. In A. Angleitner & J. S. Wiggins (Eds.), *Personality assessment via questionnaires: Current issues in theory and measurement* (pp. 109–120). Berlin: Springer-Verlag.

Campbell, D. P. (1966). *Manual for the Strong Vocational Interest Blank for men and women.* Stanford, CA: Stanford University Press.

Campbell, D. P. (1971). *Handbook for the Strong Vocational Interest Blank.* Stanford, CA: Stanford University Press.

Campbell, D. P. (1977). *Manual for the Strong-Campbell Interest Inventory* (2d ed.). Stanford, CA: Stanford University Press.

Campbell, D. P., Borgen, F. H., Eastes, S., Johansson, C. B., & Peterson, R. A. (1968). A set of Basic Interest Scales for the Strong Vocational Interest Blank for men. *Journal of Applied Psychology Monographs, 52,* (6, Pt. 2).

Campbell, D. P., & Hansen, J. C. (1981). *Manual for the SVIB-SCII* (3d ed.). Stanford, CA: Stanford University Press.

Campbell, D. P., & Holland, J. L. (1972). A merger in vocational interest research: Applying Holland's theory to Strong's data. *Journal of Vocational Behavior, 2,* 353–376.

Cattell, R. B. (1950). *Personality: A systematic theoretical and factual study.* New York: McGraw-Hill.

Clark, K. E. (1961). *The vocational interests of nonprofessional men.* Minneapolis: University of Minnesota Press.

Cole, N. S. (1973). On measuring the vocational interests of women. *Journal of Counseling Psychology, 20,* 105–112.

Cole, N. S., & Hanson, G. R. (1971). An analysis of the structure of vocational interests. *Journal of Counseling Psychology, 18,* 478–486.

Cooley, W. W., & Lohnes, P. R. (1971). *Multivariate data analysis.* New York: Wiley.

Cottle, W. C. (1950). A factorial study of the Multiphasic, Strong, Kuder, and Bell inventories using a population of adult males. *Psychometrika, 15,* 25–47.

Coxon, A. P. M. (1982). *The user's guide to multidimensional scaling.* Exeter, NH: Heinemann Educational Books.

Crabtree, P. D., & Hales, L. W. (1974). Holland's hexagonal model applied to rural youth. *Vocational Guidance Quarterly, 22,* 218–223.

Darley, J. G. (1941). *Clinical aspects and interpretation of the Strong Vocational Interest Blank.* New York: The Psychological Corporation.

Davison, M. L. (1985). Multidimensional scaling versus components analysis of test intercorrelations. *Psychological Bulletin, 97,* 94–105.

Dawis, R. V. (1980). Measuring interests. In D. A. Payne (Ed.), *New directions for testing and measurement: Recent developments in affective measurement.* San Francisco: Jossey-Bass.

Droege, R. C., & Hawk, J. (1977). Development of a U.S. Employment Service interest inventory. *Journal of Employment Counseling, 14,* 65–71.

Fitzgerald, L. F., & Hubert, L. J. (1987). Multidimensional scaling: Some possibilities for counseling psychology. *Journal of Counseling Psychology, 34,* 469–480.

Fleishman, E. A., & Quaintance, M. K. (1984). *Taxonomies of human performance: The description of human tasks.* Orlando, FL: Academic Press.

Folsom, C. H., Jr. (1971). *The validity of Holland's theory of vocational choice.* Unpublished doctoral dissertation, University of Maine, Orono.

Fouad, N. A., Cudeck, R., & Hansen, J. C. (1984). Convergent validity of the Spanish and English forms of the *Strong-Campbell Interest Inventory* for bilingual Hispanic high school students. *Journal of Counseling Psychology, 31,* 339-348.

French, J. W., Ekstrom, R. B., & Price, L. A. (1963). *Kit of reference tests for cognitive factors.* Princeton, NJ: Educational Testing Service.

Gati, I. (1979). A hierarchical model for the structure of vocational interests. *Journal of Vocational Behavior, 15,* 90-106.

Gati, I. (1982). Testing models for the structure of vocational interests. *Journal of Vocational Behavior, 21,* 164-182.

Gottfredson, G. D., Holland, J. L., & Holland, J. E. (1978). The seventh revision of the Vocational Preference Inventory. *JSAS Catalog of Selected Documents in Psychology, 8,* 98. (Ms. No. 1783).

Gottfredson, G. D., & Holland, J. L. (1989). *Dictionary of Holland occupational codes* (2d ed.). Odessa, FL: Psychological Assessment Resources.

Guilford, J. P., Christensen, P. R., Bond, N. A., & Sutton, M. A. (1954). A factor analytic study of human interests. *Psychological Monographs, 68* (4, Whole No. 375).

Hansen, J. C. (1978). Sex differences in vocational differences: Three levels of exploration. In C. K. Tittle & D. G. Zytowski (Eds.), *Sex-fair interest measurement: Research and implications* (pp. 69-76). Washington, DC: U.S. Government Printing Office.

Hansen, J. C. (1984). The measurement of vocational interests: Issues and future directions. In S. D. Brown & R. W. Lent (Eds.), *Handbook of counseling psychology* (pp. 99-136). New York: Wiley.

Hansen, J. C., & Campbell, D. P. (1985). *Manual for the SVIB-SCII Strong-Campbell Interest Inventory* (4th ed.). Palo Alto, CA: Consulting Psychologists Press.

Hansen, J. C., & Johansson, C. B. (1972). The application of Holland's vocational model to the Strong Vocational Interest Blank for women. *Journal of Vocational Behavior, 2,* 479-493.

Hanson, G. R., Prediger, D. J., & Schussel, R. H. (1977). *Development and validation of sex-balanced interest inventory scales* (ACT Research Report No. 78). Iowa City, IA: American College Testing Program.

Harmon, L. W., & Zytowski, D. G. (1980). Reliability of Holland codes across measures for adult females. *Journal of Counseling Psychology, 27,* 478-483.

Harrington, T. F., & O'Shea, A. J. (1982). *The Harrington-O'Shea Career Decision-Making System manual.* Circle Pines, MN: American Guidance Service.

Holdsworth, R., & Cramp, L. (1982). SHL *Occupational Interest Inventories: Manual and user's guide.* Esher, UK: Saville & Holdsworth.

Holland, J. L. (1958). A personality inventory employing occupational titles. *Journal of Applied Psychology, 42,* 336-342.

Holland, J. L. (1965). *Manual for the Vocational Preference Inventory* (6th rev.). Palo Alto, CA: Consulting Psychologists Press.

Holland, J. L. (1972). *The Self-Directed Search: Professional manual.* Palo Alto, CA: Consulting Psychologists Press.

Holland, J. L. (1973). *Making vocational choices: A theory of careers.* Englewood Cliffs, NJ: Prentice-Hall.

Holland, J. L. (1975). *Manual for the Vocational Preference Inventory.* Palo Alto, CA: Consulting Psychologists Press.

Holland, J. L. (1976). Vocational preferences. In M. D. Dunnette (Ed.), *Handbook of industrial and organizational psychology.* Chicago: Rand McNally.

Holland, J. L. (1979). *The Self-Directed Search: Professional manual.* Palo Alto, CA: Consulting Psychologists Press.

Holland, J. L. (1985a). *Making vocational choices: A theory of vocational personalities and work environments* (2d ed). Englewood Cliffs, NJ: Prentice-Hall.

Holland, J. L. (1985b). *Manual for the Vocational Preference Inventory.* Odessa, FL: Psychological Assessment Resources.

Holland, J. L. (1985c). *The Self-Directed Search: Professional manual.* Odessa, FL: Psychological Assessment Resources.

Holland, J. L., & Gottfredson, G. D. (1976). Sex differences, items revisions, validity, and the Self-Directed Search. *Measurement and Evaluation in Guidance, 8,* 224–228.

Holland, J. L., Whitney, D. R., Cole, N.S., & Richards, J. M., Jr. (1969). *An empirical occupational classification derived from a theory of personality and intended for practice and research* (ACT Research Report No. 29). Iowa City, IA: American College Testing Program.

Hubert, L., & Arabie, P. (1987). Evaluating order hypotheses within proximity matrices. *Psychological Bulletin, 102,* 172–178.

Hubert, L., & Arabie, P. (1989). Combinatorial data analysis: Confirmatory comparisons between sets of matrices. *Applied Scholastic Models and Data Anaylsis, 5,* 273–325.

Jackson, D. N. (1977). *Manual for the Jackson Vocational Interest Survey.* Port Huron, MI: Research Psychologists Press.

Johansson, C. B. (1976). *Manual for the Career Assessment Inventory.* Minneapolis: National Computer Systems.

Johansson, C. B. (1986). *Career Assessment Inventory: The enhanced version.* Minneapolis: National Computer Systems.

Knapp, R. R., & Knapp, L. (1984). *Manual for the COPS Interest Inventory.* San Diego: Educational and Industrial Testing Service.

Knapp, R. R., Knapp, L., & Buttafuoco, P. M. (1978). Interest changes and the classification of occupations. *Measurement and Evaluation in Guidance, 11,* 14–19.

Kuder, F. G. (1939). *Kuder Preference Record—Form A.* Chicago: University of Chicago Bookstore.

Kuder, F. G. (1966). *Kuder Occupational Interest Survey general manual.* Chicago: Science Research Associates.

Kuder, F. G. (1977). *Activity interests and occupational choice.* Chicago: Science Research Associates.

Lamb, R. R., & Prediger, D. J. (1981). *Technical report for the Unisex Edition of the ACT Interest Inventory (UNIACT).* Iowa City, IA: American College Testing Program.

Lubinski, D., & Thompson, T. (1986). Functional units of human behavior and their integration: A dispositional analysis. In T. Thompson & M. D. Zeiler (Eds.), *Analysis and integration of behavioral units* (pp. 275–314). Hillsdale, NJ: Erlbaum.

Lunneborg, C. E., & Lunneborg, P. W. (1975). Factor structure of the vocational interest models of Roe and Holland. *Journal of Vocational Behavior, 7,* 313–326.

Lunneborg, P. W. (1975). *Manual for the Vocational Interest Inventory.* Seattle: University of Washington, Educational Assessment Center.

Lunneborg, P. W. (1981). *The Vocational Interest Inventory (VII) manual* (2d ed.). Los Angeles: Western Psychological Services.

Meehl, P. E. (1986). Trait language and behaviorese. In T. Thompson & M. D. Zeiler (Eds.), *Analysis and integration of behavioral units* (pp. 315–334). Hillsdale, NJ: Erlbaum.

Meir, E. I. (1973). The structure of occupations by interests—A smallest space analysis. *Journal of Vocational Behavior, 3,* 21–31.

Meir, E. I., Bar, R., Lahav, G., & Shalhevet, R. (1975). Interest inventories based on Roe's classification modified for negative respondents. *Journal of Vocational Behavior, 7,* 127–133.

Meir, E. I., & Barak, A. (1974). A simple instrument for measuring vocational interests based on Roe's classification of occupations. *Journal of Vocational Behavior, 4,* 33–42.

Meir, E. I., & Ben-Yehuda, A. (1976). Inventories based on Roe and Holland yield similar results. *Journal of Vocational Behavior, 8,* 269–274.

Power, P. G., Holland, J. L., Daiger, D. C., & Takai, R. T. (1979). The relation of student characteristics to the influence of the Self-Directed Search. *Measurement and Evaluation in Guidance, 12,* 98–107.

Prediger, D. J. (1976). A world-of-work map for career exploration. *Vocational Guidance Quarterly, 24,* 198–208.

Prediger, D. J. (1981). Getting "ideas" out of the DOT and into vocational guidance. *Vocational Guidance Quarterly, 29,* 293–305.

Prediger, D. J. (1982). Dimensions underlying Holland's hexagon: Missing link between interests and occupations? *Journal of Vocational Behavior, 21,* 259–287.

Prediger, D. J., & Johnson, R. W. (1979, May). *Alternatives to sex-restrictive vocational interest assessment* (ACT Research Report No. 79). Iowa City, IA: American College Testing Program.

Pruzansky, S. (1975). *How to use SINDSCAL: A computer program for individual differences in multidimensional scaling.* Murray Hill, NJ: AT & T Bell Laboratories.

Roe, A. (1956). *The psychology of occupations.* New York: Wiley.

Roe, A., & Klos, D. (1969). Occupational classification. *Counseling Psychologist, 1,* 84–89.

Rose, H. A., & Elton, C. F. (1982). The relation of congruence, differentiation, and consistency to interest and aptitude scores in women with stable and unstable vocational choices. *Journal of Vocational Behavior, 20,* 162–174.

Rosenberg, S., & Sedlak, A. (1972). Structural representations of implicit personality theory. In L. Berkowitz (Ed.), *Advances in experimental social psychology* (Vol. 6, pp. 235–297). New York: Academic Press.

Rounds, J. B., Jr. (1981). The comparative and combined utility of need and interest data in the prediction of job satisfaction (Doctoral dissertation, University of Minnesota, 1981). *Dissertation Abstracts International 42,* 4920-B.

Rounds, J. B., Jr., Davison, M. L., & Dawis, R. V. (1979). The fit between Strong-Campbell Interest Inventory General Occupational Themes and Holland's hexagonal model. *Journal of Vocational Behavior, 15,* 303–315.

Rounds, J. B., Jr., & Dawis, R. V. (1979). Factor analysis of Strong Vocational Interest Blank items. *Journal of Applied Psychology, 64,* 132–143.

Rounds, J. B., Jr., Dawis, R. V., & Lofquist, L. H. (1979). Life history correlates of vocational needs for a female adult sample. *Journal of Counseling Psychology, 26,* 487–496.

Rounds, J. B., Jr., Shubsachs, A. P., Dawis, R. V., & Lofquist, L. H. (1978). A test of Holland's environmental formulations. *Journal of Applied Psychology, 63,* 609–616.

Rounds, J. B., & Tracey, T. J. (1993). Prediger's dimensional representation of Holland's RIASEC circumplex. *Journal of Applied Psychology, 78,* 875–890.

Rounds, J., Tracey, T. J., & Hubert, L. (1992). Methods for evaluating vocational interest structural hypotheses. *Journal of Vocational Behavior, 40,* 239–259.

Rounds, J. B., & Zevon, M. A. (1983). Multidimensional scaling research in vocational psychology. *Applied Psychological Measurement, 7,* 491–510.

Strong, E. K., Jr. (1943). *Vocational interests of men and women.* Stanford, CA: Stanford University Press.

Strong, E. K., Jr. (1959). *Strong Vocational Interest Blank manual.* Palo Alto, CA: Consulting Psychologist Press.

Super, D. E., & Crites, J. O. (1962). *Appraising vocational fitness by means of psychological tests* (rev. ed.). New York: Harper.

Tellegen, A. (1991). Personality traits: Issues of definition, evidence, and assessment. In D. Cicchetti & W. Grove (Eds.), *Thinking clearly about psychology: Essays in honor of Paul Everett Meehl.* Minneapolis: University of Minnesota Press.

Thurstone, L. L. (1931). A multiple factor study of vocational interests. *Personnel Journal, 3,* 198–205.

Tracey, T. J., & Rounds, J. (1993). Evaluating Holland's and Gati's vocational interest models: A structural meta-analysis. *Psychological Bulletin, 113,* 229–246.

Tracey, T. J., & Rounds, J. (1994). An examination of the structure of Roe's eight interest fields. *Journal of Vocational Behavior, 44,* 279–296.

Tuck, B. F., & Keeling, B. (1980). Sex and cultural differences in the factorial structure of the Self-Directed Search. *Journal of Vocational Behavior, 16,* 105–114.

U.S. Department of Labor. (1979). *Guide for occupational exploration.* Washington, DC: U.S. Government Printing Office.

Wakefield, J. A., & Doughtie, E. B. (1973). The geometric relationship between Holland's personality typology and the Vocational Preference Inventory. *Journal of Counseling Psychology, 20,* 513–518.

Weinrach, S. G. (1980). Have hexagon will travel: An interview with John Holland. *Personnel and Guidance Journal, 58,* 406–414.

Wigington, J. H. (1983). The applicability of Holland's typology to clients. *Journal of Vocational Behavior, 23,* 286–293.

Wilkinson, L. (1986). *SYSTAT: The system for statistics.* Evanston, IL: SYSTAT.

Young, F. W., Takane, Y., & Lewyckyj, R. (1978). Three notes on ALSCAL. *Psychometrika, 43,* 433–435.

Zytowski, D. G., & Kuder, F. (1986). Advances in the Kuder Occupational Interest Survey. In W. B. Walsh & S. H. Osipow (Eds.), *Advances in vocational psychology: Vol. 1. The assessment of interest* (pp. 31–54). Hillsdale, NJ: Erlbaum.

Chapter 9

Occupational Interests, Leisure Time Interests, and Personality

Three Domains or One? Findings From the Minnesota Twin Registry

Niels G. Waller
University of California, Davis

David T. Lykken and Auke Tellegen
University of Minnesota

INTRODUCTION

Occupational interests and aptitudes have justifiably dominated the field of vocational assessment. However, with the growing impetus to assimilate strictly vocational phenomena and concepts into more comprehensive psychological frameworks (e.g., Dawis & Lofquist, 1984), connections between vocation-related and other individual difference variables become important issues of contemporary vocational psychology. The relation between personality and occupational interests is an obvious case in point. Although Holland (1985) has declared that interests are part of the personality domain, empirical research in this area has not been plentiful (Borgen, 1986). In a broader framework, leisure time interests and their relations to occupational interests and personality are additional relevant concerns. Also important— in all individual differences research—are questions of genetic and environmental influences.

In this chapter, we report findings from correlational, factor-analytic, and multidimensional scaling studies of basic dimensions of occupational and leisure time interests: studies of the relations among these two types of interest variables and between these variables and personality. Because our sample includes several hundred twin pairs from the Minnesota Twin Registry, we also report estimates of the stability and heritability of these interest variables.

Subjects

Data were collected by mail from a large sample of middle-aged twins and their spouses, participants in the Minnesota Twin Registry (Lykken, Bouchard, McGue, & Tellegen, 1990), a birth record-based registry of twins born in Minnesota from 1936 through 1955, most of whom still reside in the upper Midwest portion of the United States. The sample included 1,728 men and 2,286 women. The mean age of the subjects at the time of testing was 39.45 (*SD* = 11.29) and 37.60 (*SD* = 10.38) years for males and females, respectively. About two-thirds of the sample were twins, including a total of 768 pairs who were concordant in providing complete test data; 65% of the pairs were female, and 55% were monozygotic (MZ) pairs. All dizygotic (DZ) twins were same-sex pairs. The questionnaires were also administered to 33 pairs of adult MZ twins (MZA twins) and 34 pairs of DZ (DZA) twins who had been separated in infancy and reared apart. This sample is more fully described in Tellegen et al. (1988).

Instruments

Study participants were sent a test booklet that contained several inventories tapping various domains of psychological functioning. In this chapter, we focus on the interrelatedness of three of these domains: (a) occupational interests, (b) personality, and (c) leisure time interests. This section presents a brief description of the measures used in the study.

Occupational Interests Inventory   A 100-item questionnaire was developed to measure the domain of occupational interests. In developing this instrument, we reviewed the interest literature with the goal of identifying the major factors of this sphere. The results of this review suggested that 15 to 25 factors, varying in breadth, can be reliably identified (for reviews of this literature, see Alley & Matthews, 1982; Guilford, Christensen, Bond, & Sutton, 1954; Holland, 1959; Roe, 1956; Rounds & Dawis, 1979). One hundred items were written to tap the broader factors from this review. In contrast to the college-oriented, white-collar bias of many popular interest inventories (cf. Alley & Matthews, 1982), some 40% of our items refer to jobs that do not require post–secondary education.

An objective of our study was to obtain a model of occupational interests that was not confounded by the individual's particular talents, abilities, education, or status needs. Subjects were therefore asked to pretend that each occupation "provides you with the same income and the same respect in the community. Then rate each activity—Like, Indifferent, Dislike—strictly according to how much you think you would enjoy that type of work and those working conditions. Pretend all jobs yield equal pay, equal status."

Personality Questionnaire   The *Multidimensional Personality Questionnaire* (MPQ; Tellegen, 1982), a factor-analytically derived, 300-item, true/false measure of normal-range personality functioning, was used to assess 11 lower-order personality constructs with the following scale names: (a) Wellbeing, (b) Social Potency, (c) Achievement, (d) Social Closeness, (e) Stress Reaction, (f) Alienation, (g) Aggression, (h) Control, (i) Harmavoidance, (j) Traditionalism, and (k) Absorption. The scales of the MPQ are relatively independent of one another and have high internal consistencies (Tellegen, 1982). Furthermore, recent work by Reise and Waller (1990), using an item response theory paradigm, has shown that the MPQ scales provide an impressive amount of statistical information—and therefore provide precise measurement—across a wide range of the trait continuum. These properties make the MPQ a desirable instrument for exploring relations between personality and interests.

Leisure Time Interest Inventory   A 120-item questionnaire describing a wide variety of leisure time activities was developed to measure the domain of leisure time interests. These activities ranged from "going fishing" and "nightlife: bars, nightclubs, discos, etc." to "volunteer work" and "taking a college course in some subject of interest" to "going on a camera safari in Africa, Borneo, the desert, or the Amazon basin" to "getting involved in controversial issues." Most of the items were stated rather generally—for example, "Risky pastimes: hang gliding, mountain climbing, surfing, etc."—a practice that yields a richer item content at the risk of conflating unrelated attributes.

Because our objective was to explore the relations among expressed *interests*, rather than current practices, subjects were asked, "How often would you engage in each of the following leisure time activities if you had the time and the money to do what you want?... Remember, when considering each item, pretend you are not limited by time, or money, or by age or health. Assuming that you *could* do any of these things, how often do you think that you *would* do them." Responses were obtained on a five-point scale labeled: "never—seldom—sometimes—frequently—often as possible."

Scaling of Item Responses

In both interest inventories, but especially with the *Leisure Time Interest* inventory (LTI), there was marked variation from subject to subject in the use of the available response categories. Moreover, most items in both inventories correlated positively with most other items— that is, there was a strong common factor in both item-covariance matrices. Without prejudging whether this factor reflected a kind of response set that might be relatively independent of item content, or a psychologically significant variable related to breadth of interest, we decided to measure this factor separately in both interest inventories and to rescale the items in order to remove its effect. We reasoned that a subject who used the highest rating of 5 only, say, 8 times, was expressing relatively stronger enthusiasm for those 8 items than a subject who used this highest rating 30 times. Although the latter person might truly be more interested in a greater number of activities than the former person, that difference in average interest could be easily assessed, for example, from the mean ratings. Our rescaling of the items was intended to bring out more clearly our subjects' relative interests for, and discriminations between, items or item clusters. An ideal subject, reacting to the 120 LTI items in such a way as to maximally differentiate his or her reactions to the 120 leisure time activities, would use each of the five response categories an equal number of times, that is, 120/5 = 24 times each. For such a subject having a rectangular distribution of response category usage, the five response categories were assigned the values .1, .3, .5, .7, and .9, with the high and low ratings equidistant from the mean or middle scale value.

Therefore, we designed an ipsative scaling procedure that "rectangularizes" each individual's distribution of 120 item responses and, in effect, computes within-subject percentile scores expressed as proportions. For a subject who seldom uses high ratings, response categories 4 and 5 receive values further from the mean, say, .8 and .95, instead of .7 and .9, respectively. If that same subject overuses the low-end categories, then responses of 1 and 2 might be assigned scale values of, say, .2 and .36, instead of .1 and .3, respectively.

The algorithm to accomplish this scaling was as follows. The scale value for the lowest category was set equal to $(K1/2)/120$, where $K1 = $ that subject's number of uses of Category 1. The scale value for the second response category was set equal to $(K1 + K2/2)/120$, the third to $(K1 + K2 + K3/2)/120$, and so on. Thus, the scaled values represent the midpoints of intervals on the response scale, where the width of the interval is proportional to that subject's frequency of using that response category. That individual's mean response, equal to $(K1 + 2K2 + 3K3 + 4K4 + 5K5)/120$, was retained as a separate variable.

The variance of scale usage was also retained as a variable, expressed as a proportion of the maximum possible variance given N scale values and that subject's mean (Vmax = $-M^2 + N^*M - (N - 1)$). In the case of the LTI inventory, factor analysis of these scaled responses, together with the mean and the variance, yielded much clearer and more interpretable factors than did the analyses of the unscaled scores.

THE STRUCTURE OF OCCUPATIONAL AND LEISURE TIME INTERESTS

Interest Inventories

A series of exploratory factor analyses was performed separately on the item intercorrelations for the occupational and leisure time inventories in an effort to uncover the structure of these item sets. In these analyses, principal axis factoring was employed with subsequent orthogonal (varimax) and oblique (oblimin) rotations. In each domain, the items were analyzed separately by gender. In the case of the LTI inventory, the factor analyses of the ipsatized items that resulted in the clearer factor structure is the one reported here. In the case of the occupational inventory, ipsatization followed the factor analysis, though it rescaled the computation of factor scores.

For the occupational interest items, seventeen congruent factors appeared for the female and male samples, while 18 congruent factors emerged from the analyses of the leisure time items. Because the oblique and orthogonal solutions from these analyses were quite similar, we chose to interpret the orthogonal solutions because of the mathematical simplicity of these latter structures. Factor-based scales were constructed by unit weighting the items loading most strongly on each factor.

Table 1 displays the names of the 17 occupational interest factors found in these analyses, as well as a typical item from each factor.

Inspection of Table 1 suggests that the 17 factors span the major dimensions of vocational interest that have been identified in the literature (e.g., Alley & Matthews, 1982; Guilford, Christensen, Bond, & Sutton, 1954; Rounds & Dawis, 1979). Furthermore, a Blue Collar factor, a dimension not well represented in the literature, was also clearly identifiable in our analysis. In general, the occupational interest factors represent broad areas of interests, such as interests in people (Personal Service, Medical) or things (Arts & Crafts, Farmer), though some factors, such as our Military factor, clearly represent more narrowly defined domains.

Table 1   Seventeen Occupational Interest Factors

Factor	Sample Item
Blue Collar	Skilled trades (appliance repair, auto mechanic, carpenter, electrician, plumber, etc.)
Writer	Novelist, scriptwriter, playwright
Politics	Elected public official (legislator, mayor, alderman, etc.)
Medical	Physician (general practice)
Athletics	Professional athlete (basketball, baseball, football, hockey, etc.)
Explorer-Scientist	Physical scientist (astronomer, chemist, geologist, physicist, etc.)
Numbers Person	Bookkeeper, accountant, auditor
Personal Service	Hairdresser, barber, cosmetician, masseur, etc.
Commissioned Sales	Selling (real estate, machinery, cars and trucks, etc.)
Religion	Missionary, medical missionary, evangelist, etc.
Animals	Veterinarian (horses, farm animals, zoo animals)
Food Service	Caterer; manager of a cafeteria, restaurant, bakery
Arts & Crafts	Maker of hand-worked items (pottery, embroidery, jewelry, carvings, lace, etc.)
Farmer	Farmer (wheat, corn, soybeans, etc.)
Performing Arts	Performing artist (actor, singer, dancer, etc.)
Law	Trial lawyer, defense attorney, district attorney
Military	Commissioned officer in one of the armed services

Table 2 displays the names and typical items for the 18 leisure time interest factors. As can be seen in the table, the leisure time interest factors vary more widely among themselves in content specificity than do the occupational interest factors. For example, the Intellectual Interests and the Passive Entertainment factors clearly represent broad areas of interests and behaviors. Other factors, however, such as the Police Calls–Fires and Gambling factors refer to highly specific interests.

A comparison of the occupational and leisure time interest factors reported in Tables 1 and 2 suggests that several themes are common to the two domains. For example, factors representing interests in athletics, politics, religion, and the arts are clearly identifiable in both sets of analyses. This observation led us to ask whether these *cross-domain* factors relate to one another in a meaningful fashion. To answer

Table 2   Eighteen Leisure Time Interest Factors

Factor	Sample Item
Intellectual interests	Reading or rereading literary classics
Politics	Working with others on political or social issues
Socializing	Getting together with a lively group of friends and acquaintances
Hunting-Fishing	Hunting small game, rabbits, squirrels, etc.
Sierra Club	Backpacking, hiking, camping out
Religion	Doing work for your church or synagogue
Husbandry	Rebuilding, repairing things (furniture, clothes, cars, machines, etc.)
Domestic	Working with fabrics, yarn (sewing, knitting, crocheting, tailoring, etc.)
Passive Entertainment	Watching TV adventure or comedy programs
Fitness	Jogging or running for exercise
Gambling	Betting on the horses, dog races, etc.
Police Calls–Fires	Going to fires
The Arts	Attending live theater or musicals
Foreign Travel	Going on a cruise ship to interesting places
Reading	Reading mystery or detective novels
Sports Fan	Attending sporting events (ballgames, races, hockey, etc.)
Swinger	Nightlife (bars, nightclubs, discos, etc.)
Danger Seeking	Risky pastimes (hang gliding, mountain climbing, surfing, etc.)

this question, we conducted a rational analysis of the items from these factors.

A close inspection of the items from the cross-domain factors suggested the following model. Several of the factors from the two domains define opposite poles of an active–passive or producer–consumer dimension. For example, consider the two athletics factors, Athletics (occupational) and Sports Fan (leisure time). In our analyses of the occupational interest items, we uncovered an Athletics factor, which was defined by the desire to be a professional athlete. This factor can be viewed as falling on the active pole of a dimension that has the more passive leisure time Sports Fan factor defining the opposite end. Similarly, our occupational Writer factor, which is characterized by the activities of writing novels, scripts, or plays, falls on the producer end of a dimension that has the more consumer-oriented Reading leisure time factor loading on the consumer pole.

To elucidate the empirical ties between these domains, we correlated the factor scores on the 17 occupational and 18 leisure time interest factors for our 4,014 subjects. This analysis enabled us to determine, among other things, whether individuals high on the occupational interest factors of Politics, Religion, or Athletics, for example, also scored high on the corresponding leisure time interest factors. Table 3 presents the results from this analysis.

Several aspects of Table 3 warrant comment. First, note that many of the occupational interest and leisure time interest factors correlate substantially with one another, with some of the correlations being more predictable than others. For example, individuals who said they would enjoy religious occupations also expressed an interest in religious leisure time activities. Furthermore, many of these same people said that they would not enjoy such hedonistic activities as Gambling or being a Swinger. On the other hand, other relations were less predictable and are therefore more heuristic. For example, a number of individuals who scored high on our occupational interest factor Explorer-Scientist also scored high on our leisure time interest factor Danger Seeking.

Correlations of Interests With Personality

It is well known that two variables, A and B, can correlate with one another because A influences B, B influences A, or because A and B are both influenced by a third variable, C, or any combination of these. It is conceivable that occupational interest and leisure time interests are a reflection of more fundamental variables, such as personality traits. Indeed, one might predict this to be the case, insofar as contemporary models of occupational interests, such as Holland's hexagonal model of vocational choice (Holland, 1959), are formulated in personological terms. To explore this question, we correlated the scores from the 11 lower-order MPQ scales with the factor scores from the occupational and leisure time interest factors.

Table 4 reports the correlations among the rescaled occupational interest factors and the 11 personality scales. As can be seen in the table, few strong relations exist between these two domains, as measured by our scales. Specifically, only two MPQ scales, Social Potency and Harmavoidance, relate strongly to the occupational interest factors Social Potency to Politics, Sales, and Law, and negatively to Personal Service; while Harmavoidance relates strongly to the factors Numerical and Personal Service, and negatively to Explorer-Scientist. Furthermore, several of the MPQ scales—Wellbeing, Achievement, Stress Reaction, Alienation, Control, Traditionalism, and Absorption— have no correlations greater than .30 with any of the interest

Table 3   Relations Among 17 Occupational Factors and 18 Leisure Time Interest Factors

Occupational Interest Factors	Leisure Time Interest Factors																	
	I	P	S	H-F	SC	R	H	D	PE	F	G	PC	A	FT	RD	SP	SW	DS
Blue Collar	-.25	-.17	-.21	**.62**	**.30**	-.13	**.40**	-.35	-.14	-.06	.16	.29	-.47	-.08	-.27	**.39**	.10	.23
Writer	**.48**	.29	.01	-.36	-.16	-.03	-.19	.02	-.10	-.02	-.16	-.24	**.34**	.10	.29	-.28	-.07	-.05
Politics	.28	**.58**	.22	-.16	-.27	.02	-.23	-.18	-.10	-.00	.08	-.09	.04	.04	.06	-.04	.03	-.00
Medical	.13	.03	.08	-.30	-.06	.05	-.15	.22	.06	.09	-.18	-.07	.22	.07	.13	-.27	-.11	-.06
Athletics	-.19	.01	.02	.26	.06	-.19	-.08	-.38	-.16	**.39**	.22	-.01	-.26	-.03	-.17	**.45**	.12	.20
Scientist	.18	.02	-.22	.13	**.39**	-.29	.08	-.15	-.36	.12	-.14	-.14	.08	.25	-.03	-.15	-.03	**.34**
Numbers	-.06	-.15	.07	-.19	-.25	.19	-.03	.22	.28	-.04	-.01	.02	-.02	-.13	.14	-.04	-.06	-.26
Personal Service	-.04	-.18	.14	-.45	-.20	-.07	-.18	**.57**	**.42**	-.08	-.26	-.02	.24	-.13	.15	-.25	-.16	-.38
Sales	-.04	.15	.16	.13	-.19	-.07	-.00	-.27	-.03	-.03	**.41**	.02	-.23	-.01	-.11	.16	.11	.03
Religious	.19	.10	.03	-.22	-.14	**.68**	-.11	.20	.02	-.11	-.32	-.03	.23	-.09	.03	-.15	-.32	-.23
Animals	-.11	-.18	-.19	.17	**.51**	-.14	.07	.06	-.07	.02	-.10	.00	-.07	.04	-.05	-.00	-.04	.06
Food Service	-.17	-.20	.15	-.24	-.20	.11	-.11	**.41**	**.35**	-.10	-.01	.01	.07	-.11	.11	-.08	.07	-.29
Arts & Crafts	.10	-.18	-.09	-.29	.02	-.00	.23	**.42**	.05	-.11	-.27	-.20	**.43**	.05	.12	-.34	-.14	-.17
Farmer	-.17	-.18	-.20	**.35**	**.36**	.05	.20	.05	-.06	-.08	-.01	.08	-.24	-.09	-.16	.15	-.07	-.00
Performing Arts	.13	.05	.15	-.45	-.23	-.00	-.27	.18	.10	.05	-.15	-.21	**.59**	.07	.15	-.32	.05	-.10
Law	.08	.29	.08	.06	-.11	-.18	-.10	-.31	-.16	.04	.23	.02	-.11	.12	.02	.05	.12	.19
Military	-.04	.01	-.05	.28	-.00	-.02	.08	-.25	-.05	-.07	.14	.17	-.25	.00	-.08	.22	.06	.07

Note. Correlations ≥ .30 in boldfaced type.
Leisure time interest factors are as follows: I = Intellectual Interests, P = Politics, S = Socializing, H-F = Hunting-Fishing, SC = Sierra Club, R = Religion, H = Husbandry, D = Domestic, PE = Passive Entertainment, F = Fitness, G = Gambling, PC = Police Calls–Fires, A = Arts, FT = Foreign Travel, RD=Reading, SP = Sports, SW = Swinger, and DS = Danger Seeking.

Table 4   Relations Among 17 Occupational Interest Factors and 11 MPQ Scales (*N* = 4,014)

Occupational Interest Factors	MPQ Scales										
	WB	SP	ACH	SC	SR	AL	AGG	CN	HA	TRAD	ABS
Blue Collar	-.07	-.12	.05	**-.30**	-.07	.16	.21	-.07	-.25	.11	-.17
Writer	.04	.21	.02	.02	-.01	-.15	-.10	.03	.00	-.27	.16
Politics	.09	**.46**	.11	.16	-.11	-.08	.02	.01	-.04	-.14	.00
Medical	.03	.01	-.02	.16	-.00	-.12	-.11	.04	.07	-.11	.08
Athletics	.07	.17	.04	.04	-.12	-.01	.17	-.07	-.18	-.03	-.07
Scientist	.01	.06	.03	-.15	-.13	-.10	.03	-.03	**-.38**	-.27	.14
Numbers	-.07	-.26	.01	-.00	.12	.02	-.12	.16	.31	.19	-.12
Personal Service	-.00	**-.32**	-.18	-.00	.20	-.00	-.29	.08	**.47**	.16	.05
Sales	.09	**.30**	.11	.06	-.08	.03	.14	-.01	-.03	.06	-.09
Religion	.01	-.10	-.07	.09	.00	-.06	-.25	.11	.22	.26	.00
Animals	-.01	-.14	-.05	-.06	-.03	.00	-.00	-.02	-.09	-.03	.03
Food Service	-.02	-.22	-.13	.11	.17	.06	-.10	.02	**.33**	.11	-.01
Arts & Crafts	-.03	-.20	-.07	-.02	.10	-.01	-.16	.06	.16	-.05	.16
Farmer	-.01	-.20	-.00	-.17	.00	.08	.01	-.04	-.03	.16	-.05
Performing Arts	-.01	.10	-.11	.20	.11	-.08	-.10	-.03	.12	-.15	.22
Law	.06	**.37**	.17	-.00	-.10	-.04	.16	-.02	-.21	-.14	-.01
Military	-.03	.08	.05	-.12	-.02	.08	.17	-.02	-.11	.10	-.11

Note. Correlations ≥ .30 are in boldfaced type. However, correlations of .10 are highly significant for *N* = 4,000.
MPQ Scales are as follows: WB = Wellbeing, SP = Social Potency, ACH = Achievement, SC = Social Closeness, SR = Stress Reaction, AL = Alienation, AGG = Aggression, CN = Control, HA = Harmavoidance, TRAD = Traditionalism, and ABS = Absorption.

dimensions. Note, however, that even the small correlations are statistically significant with this large sample and that most of them make intuitive sense. Thus, Aggression is correlated negatively with Medical, Personal Service, Religion, and Artistic occupational interests, and positively with Blue Collar, Athletics, Commissioned Sales, Law, and Military leisure time interests. Absorption is negatively correlated with Blue Collar and positively correlated with Writer, Explorer-Scientist, Arts & Crafts, and Performing Arts. Costa, McCrae, and Holland (1984) report sizable correlations between the Extraversion scale of the NEO personality inventory and two of Holland's vocational scales, Enterprising and Social, which accords with our findings for the Social Potency scale of the MPQ. Costa et al. also found occupational interest correlations with the NEO Openness scale that resemble the correlates of the MPQ Absorption scale.

Table 5 reports the correlations among the rescaled leisure time interest factors and the MPQ scales. Once again, Social Potency and Harmavoidance are the two personality traits that relate most strongly with expressed interests in the leisure time interest factors. Once again, patterns of low but significant correlations make sense and help delineate the nature of the variables. Thus, interest in being a Swinger correlates positively with the MPQ scales Alienation and Aggression, while it correlates negatively with the scales Control and Traditionalism.

Multidimensional Scaling

Our analyses of the occupational interest inventory data reliably identified 17 lower-order factors. Furthermore, these factors were found to have few strong relations with the personality constructs measured by the MPQ. Although popular models of vocational interests (e.g., Holland, 1959) are formulated on personological terms, our data suggest that the domains of vocational interests and personality are relatively independent of one another. Nevertheless, two personality traits, Social Potency and Harmavoidance, do correlate strongly and systematically with several of the interest dimensions. We therefore included these variables in the following analysis.

To explore the higher-order structure of the occupational interest domain, a nonmetric multidimensional scaling of the occupational interest factor scales and the two MPQ scales was performed. We note that the scores for each of our factorial interest scales are not true factor scores; they were obtained by selecting "marker" items and simply summing the item scores. Although factor scales of this type are highly correlated with the factors they represent—unlike the factors themselves—they are not necessarily uncorrelated. The scale intercorrelations may even be substantial, reflecting systematic

Table 5   Relations Among 18 Leisure Time Interest Factors and 11 MPQ Scales

Leisure Time Interest Factors	MPQ Scales										
	WB	SP	ACH	SC	SR	AL	AGG	CN	HA	TRAD	ABS
Intellectual Interests	.05	.10	.05	-.04	-.11	-.21	-.21	.16	.01	-.23	.06
Politics	.09	.38	.13	.09	-.14	-.10	.00	.01	-.11	-.19	.02
Socializing	.11	.16	-.04	.49	-.03	-.05	-.03	-.03	.14	.02	-.04
Hunting–Fishing	-.00	.06	.06	-.18	-.09	.13	.29	-.13	-.31	.10	-.11
Sierra Club	.00	-.05	.01	-.19	-.08	-.00	.05	-.07	-.27	-.08	.07
Religion	.03	-.18	-.06	.13	.02	-.03	-.31	.16	.33	.49	-.09
Husbandry	.03	-.05	.21	-.19	-.07	.09	.02	.03	-.12	.09	-.02
Domestic	.02	-.31	-.07	.05	.13	-.04	-.29	.11	.38	.09	.06
Passive Entertainment	-.13	-.30	-.22	.06	.24	.07	-.06	.07	.40	.17	-.13
Fitness	.05	.04	.03	.07	-.13	-.15	-.01	.02	-.11	-.11	-.02
Gambling	-.03	.16	.02	.00	.01	.11	.26	-.16	-.11	-.01	-.10
Police Calls–Fires	-.08	-.07	-.04	-.04	.10	.15	.17	-.07	-.03	.18	-.09
The Arts	.01	.03	-.04	.09	.05	-.09	-.18	.04	.12	-.15	.28
Foreign Travel	.03	.13	.00	.01	-.07	-.11	.00	-.02	-.15	-.12	.07
Reading	.00	-.06	-.05	-.01	.04	-.09	-.12	.08	.11	-.13	.03
Sports Fan	-.03	-.01	-.03	-.07	-.02	.13	.19	-.06	-.03	.16	-.22
Swinger	-.11	.13	-.02	-.00	.10	.18	.32	-.20	-.14	-.20	.02
Danger Seeking	.01	.22	.14	-.16	-.10	.06	.26	-.22	**-.62**	-.20	.09

Note. Correlations ≥ .30 are in boldfaced type.
MPQ Scales are as follows: WB = Wellbeing, SP = Social Potency, ACH = Achievement, SC = Social Closeness, SR = Stress Reaction, AL = Alienation, AGG = Aggression, CN = Control, HA = Harmavoidance, TRAD = Traditionalism, and ABS = Absorption.

patterns of secondary item factor loadings (i.e., item factorial complexity). Analysis of the scale correlations are of interest because they may reveal meaningful general or higher-order dimensions.

Multidimensional scaling (MDS) is an attractive complement to factor analysis for exploring the structure of a data set. Although still not widely employed in this area of psychological research, MDS has been used several times to study the structure of vocational interests. For example, several researchers (see Rounds & Zevon, 1983, for a review) have used MDS to investigate Holland's model of vocational choice. General reviews of MDS have recently appeared (e.g., Davison, 1983; Kruskal & Wish, 1978; MacCallum, 1988), and reviews specific to counseling psychology (Fitzgerald & Hubert, 1987; Rounds & Zevon 1983) are available.

Two different scaling programs were applied to the correlations among the 17 occupational interest variables and the MPQ Social Potency and Harmavoidance scales, namely, the SYSTAT scaling module (Wilkinson, 1988) and Ecscal (Tellegen, 1989). With SYSTAT, two- and three-dimensional solutions were attempted, using the nonmetric option that optimizes an ordinal (monotonic) relation between the scaled distances and the observed correlations. The fit of the two-dimensional solution was only modest (stress formula 1 = .26), whereas extraction of a third dimension resulted in a degenerate case. Ecscal produced a configuration with a reasonably good fit (as measured by its own fit index; see discussion that follows). Judged visually, the two-dimensional SYSTAT and Ecscal plots are rather similar, and only the latter will be discussed. First, inasmuch as it is a new procedure, the following is an informal characterization of some of Ecscal's basic features.

Ecscal: A Nonmetric Multidimensional Scaling Algorithm   Like other scaling methods, Ecscal (an acronym for element-centered scaling) is a procedure for generating a spatial map from a matrix of similarities (e.g., correlations, rated similarities or dissimilarities, co-occurrences) among objects (e.g., psychological variables, colors, concepts, foods). The map is to show these objects at distances representing the original similarities.

Ecscal's particular method is thoroughly nonmetric, more so than other available approaches. As we will describe, its iterative process— which does not even start with a metrically derived configuration— directly optimizes a monotonic fit of the scaled distances to the input data.

Ecscal is specifically designed to generate distances that reflect the "viewpoints" of the objects or elements included in the similarity matrix. Accordingly, Ecscal is responsive only to comparative magnitudes of similarity values occurring in the *same row* of the similarity matrix because each row fully represents one object's "outlook" on all other objects, and because each object is represented by a row. In other words, only same-row similarity relations need to be considered.

More precisely, Ecscal seeks to place *n* objects in a Euclidean space at relative distances that duplicate, as well as possible, the within-pair ranks of the $n(n - 1)/2$ pairs of values in each row of an $n \times n$ matrix of observed object similarities. Its procedure is designed to maximize a basically straightforward quantity: the total net number of same-row similarity pairs whose within-pair ranks are correctly represented by the relative lengths of the corresponding pairs of derived distances. To summarize, Ecscal is a program for placing the members of a set of objects in a Euclidean space (of specified dimensionality) in a configuration approximating one that reproduces the largest possible net number of same-row, within-pair ranks found in the matrix of observed object similarities.

To give an illustration, suppose we want to scale in two dimensions the correlations among five variables. Using the 5×5 intercorrelation matrix as input, Ecscal will place the five objects (variables in this case) as points in two-dimensional space. Starting from a simple initial configuration or setting, it will move the five objects in a sequence in which each step increases the net number of correctly reproduced pairwise similarity orderings. Thus, if in row 1 of the matrix, $r12 = .50$ and $r13 = .40$, then Ecscal will correctly reproduce the pairwise ordering $(r12, r13)$ if it moves object 2 closer to object 1 than to object 3.

In our example (provided there are no ties), a maximum of $(5 \times 4) /2 = 10$ correlation pairs can be rank ordered correctly in any row of the matrix, and a total of $5 \times 10 = 50$ pairs in the total matrix. Note, incidentally, that among the similarity pairs in row *i* are 4 pairs containing the correlation of variable *i* with itself, which is presumably the highest in row *i*; for example, row 1 includes pairs (r_{11}, r_{12}), (r_{11}, r_{13}), (r_{11}, r_{14}), and (r_{11}, r_{15}). The inclusion of self similarities permits representation of our assumption that each object is more similar to itself than to any other object and invites a corresponding spatial separation of each object from every other object in the scaling solution.

Suppose now that in our example the final scaling solution reproduces 8 pairwise similarity orderings correctly and 2 incorrectly in row *i* of the matrix. Then the net number of correct rank orderings in row *i* is computed to be $8 - 2 = 6$. The corresponding *representation value* of element *i* equals $(8 - 2)/10 = .60$. The representation value of object *i*, then, is the net proportion in row *i* of the similarity matrix of all untied similarity pairs whose within-pair rank orderings are correctly reproduced. The *average* of all object representation values is Ecscal's index of fit alluded to earlier. It turns out that the numerator of the representation value formula is the same as that of gamma, Goodman and Kruskal's (1954) rank-order correlation index. Like gammas, representation values range from −1 to 1, though in a good solution, no objects should have a negative representation value. Unlike the widely used stress formulas, the representation value is unambiguous because it is a direct measure of goodness of monotonic fit. An object's representation value can also be viewed as its *nonmetric communality.*

Another distinctive feature of Ecscal is that it places objects in a *discrete,* rather than a continuous, space. In the two-dimensional case, it utilizes an $m \times m$ grid and limits the possible locations of the objects to the midpoints of the $m \times m$ cells of the grid. The procedure starts out with a coarse 3×3 grid and, in one of its options, places all objects initially at the origin, which is defined as the midpoint of the center cell of the grid. Objects are then moved in a predetermined heuristic order, each object being moved tentatively to a number of different adjacent cells to identify moves that would improve the fit (i.e., increase the net number of correctly rank-ordered, same-row similarity pairs). If such moves are found, the one that most improves the fit is implemented, which transfers the object in question to a new location; otherwise, the object is not moved this time around. This process continues until no further moves result in fit improvement. At that point, the scale coordinates of each object are multiplied by 2; for example, the coordinates of an object placed in the upper right-hand cell are changed from 1, 1 to 2, 2. Because objects continue to be moved to adjacent cells, doubling the coordinates has the effect of superimposing a finer grid—a 5×5—upon the evolving scale configuration. The objects can now be deployed over a more densely spaced set of cell midpoints and are moved about again until additional moves no longer improve the fit. The process of grid refinement followed by object moves is repeated until further refinement fails to improve the fit. The program then terminates its fitting process, computes and prints the individual and average object representation values, standardizes and prints the final object coordinates, and plots the configuration.

Ecscal Scaling of Occupational Interests Figure 1 shows the two-dimensional Ecscal plot of the 17 occupational interests plus the Social Potency and Harmavoidance (labeled Safety Mindedness in Figure 1) variables based on their intercorrelations. The average object representation value of this solution is .82, with the individual values ranging from .59 to .96, a rather good outcome. The figure also shows the results of a factor analysis. We have found that embedding factor-analytic simple structures in scaling solutions can be illuminating; it provides a mutual check on both dimensional structures and calls attention to incongruities. The procedure is analogous to Shepard and Arabie's method of embedding clustering results in scaling solutions (Shepard & Arabie, 1979).

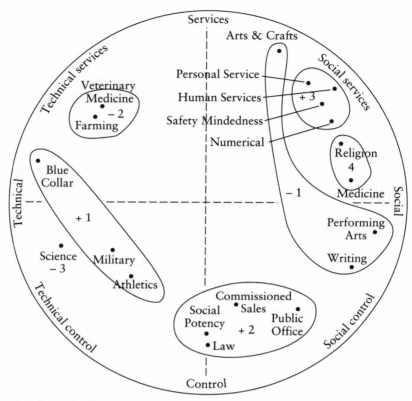

Figure 1   Two-dimensional Ecscal plot of 17 occupational interests factors and two MPQ scales

When scaling and factor-analytic structures are shown in the same figure, one also can hardly ignore their differing functions. Factor-analytic results give us a indication of what kind of scales, as well as how many, are needed to measure adequately a person's major characteristics in a given domain. This psychometrically essential information concerns variance sources and cannot be adequately recovered from a scaling solution (Davison, 1985). A scaling solution, on the other hand, can capture essential ordinal features of a similarity structure in a reduced (low dimensional) space and display these features as an easily apprehended visual-spatial configuration.

We will now take a closer look at the details of our results, starting with the factor analysis. The four-factor solution was chosen inasmuch as the eigenvalue slope of the principal components indicated four major dimensions. Factor 1 opposes "tough" and stereotypically masculine occupations to interest in occupations involving artistic activities. Factor 2 opposes Social Potency and interest in cosmopolitan, socially enterprising occupations to interest in farming and caring for animals. Factor 3 opposes interest in science to a combination of Harmavoidance (Safety Mindedness in Figure 1) and interest in social service occupations that are presumably seen as relatively unadventurous. Factor 4 seems to represent interest in professional-level helping occupations.

Figure 1 shows how well the factor-analytic and scaling results comport with one another. We assigned each variable as a marker to the rotated factor on which it received its highest loading. Closed curves were drawn around each set of same-signed markers of the same factor. Because three of the four factors are bipolar, the enclosed subsets number seven. Figure 1 shows that the enclosed areas tend to be relatively compact, distinct, and nonoverlapping, and that the opposite-signed markers of the same factor tend to be far apart, all indications that the scaling and factor-analytic structures are generally congruent and mutually supportive. The one exception (also found in the SYSTAT solution) is a marker of the artistic pole of Factor 1, namely, Arts & Crafts, which the scaling program moved far away from the other two markers—Writing and Performing Arts—stretching their enclosing curve. Inspection of the correlations reveals that unlike Writing and Performing Arts, Arts & Crafts is negatively correlated with all four of the socially assertive positive markers of Factor 2, shown at the bottom of the figure. The scaling process was more sensitive to these differential correlation features than the factor analysis, which seems to reflect our respondents' view that Arts & Crafts has a distinctly less socially assertive quality than Performing Arts and Writing.

Turning to the most salient features of the scaling solution, the dotted lines represent a rotation of the original scale vectors to mark what seem to be meaningful major dimensions. We labeled the horizontal dimension Social versus Technical because it clearly contrasts interpersonally oriented with technically and physically oriented occupations. The vertical dimension impresses us as a control-manipulation-mastery versus service-provision-care vector, and we named it Control versus Service. This schema invites comparison with others, particularly the two-dimensional interest structure of the widely used Unisex Edition of the *ACT Interest Inventory* (UNIACT; Lamb & Prediger, 1981). The two UNIACT dimensions are thought to be the general dimensions underlying Holland's (1985) and Roe's (1956) basic interest types. One dimension, People versus Things, contrasts Holland's Social and Realistic occupations. The second dimension, Ideas versus Data, pits arts and sciences against a variety of managerial, financial, and record keeping business occupations, thus contrasting the Holland Artistic and Investigative occupations with the Enterprising and Conventional ones.

Our Social versus Technical and UNIACT's People versus Things dimensions seem very similar, but our Control versus Service dimension clearly differs from the UNIACT Ideas versus Data dimension. No single global scheme is likely to be sufficient for capturing the major interest variations in all populations. For example, developmental differences may be important. The UNIACT dimension may reflect distinctive characteristics of not only its descriptors but also of the precollege population on which it was developed. Our own general dimensions necessarily reflect the character of our broadly based primary factor scales and our large adult population sample. They provide a partially new perspective that may prove heuristically fruitful in exploring individual's vocational attitudes and the perceptions underlying them.

The Heritability and Stability of Interests

A total of 768 pairs of Minnesota Registry twins were concordant in providing complete test data. Of these concordant pairs, 240 were asked to retake the *Occupational Interests Inventory* and the *Leisure Time Interest Inventory* between two to three years after the first administration; complete returns were obtained from both members of 198 pairs, 53 MZ and 52 DZ female pairs plus 49 MZ and 33 DZ male pairs. These data allowed us to investigate both the heritability and the stability of occupational and leisure time interests.

Quadratic regressions on age were computed for the interest scales separately by sex, and norms were constructed to permit the scale scores to be converted to age- and sex-corrected *t*-scores with a mean of 50 and *SD* of 10. This procedure partials out the effects of age and sex on the intraclass correlations and subsequent heritability estimates (see McGue & Bouchard, 1984, for a justification of this procedure).

Tables 6 and 7 report the MZ and DZ intraclass correlations, heritabilities (h^2), and test-retest stabilities for the occupational interest and leisure time interest scales from this sample. The heritabilities were computed via Falconer's formula: twice the difference between the MZ and DZ correlations. This method provides valid estimates of heritability when the data satisfy the following assumptions: (a) assortative mating is absent, (b) genetic effects are purely additive, and (c) gene-environment interaction is minimal. Even when these assumptions are not entirely valid, minor violations of the assumptions should not vitiate the general conclusions. However, when the MZ correlations are more than twice the value of the corresponding DZ correlations, the MZ correlation itself is the best estimate of heritability (these estimates are shown in parentheses in the tables). We do not present these data as final estimates of heritability, but only as evidence that genetic factors significantly influence expressed interests.

Table 6 Heritabilities and Test-Retest Stabilities for 17 Occupational Interest Factors

Factors	Males				Females				MZA
	MZ	DZ	h^2	Test-retest MZ & DZ	MZ	DZ	h^2	Test-retest MZ & DZ	h^2
N of Pairs:	148	119			273	228			33
Blue Collar	.65	.40	.50	.86	.55	.21	(.55)	.80	.53
Writer	.56	.21	(.56)	.80	.49	.28	.42	.75	.03
Politics	.43	.18	(.43)	.78	.46	.20	(.46)	.65	.44
Medical	.42	.15	(.42)	.76	.42	.15	(.42)	.68	-.04
Athletics	.51	.11	(.51)	.83	.46	.23	.46	.72	.53
Scientist	.41	.19	(.41)	.69	.39	.40	(.00)	.79	.59
Numbers	.41	.17	(.41)	.76	.44	.27	.34	.80	.49
Personal Service	.33	.22	.22	.69	.47	.21	(.47)	.72	.18
Sales	.52	.07	(.52)	.72	.38	.24	.28	.61	.03
Religion	.56	.28	.56	.76	.50	.21	(.50)	.73	.52
Animals	.52	.12	(.52)	.75	.49	.15	(.49)	.77	.36
Food Service	.27	.20	.14	.65	.44	.17	(.44)	.65	.11
Arts & Crafts	.38	.18	(.38)	.73	.37	.20	.34	.66	.40
Farmer	.47	.29	.36	.74	.44	.23	.42	.78	.60
Performing Arts	.54	.32	.44	.78	.56	.22	(.56)	.73	.64
Law	.36	.12	(.36)	.75	.41	.05	(.41)	.70	.33
Military	.31	.01	(.31)	.69	.19	.10	.18	.57	.17

Note. Parenthetical figures refer to estimates based on MZ correlations.

Table 7   Heritabilities and Test-Retest Stabilities for 18 Leisure Time Interest Factors

| | Males | | | | Females | | | | MZA |
	MZ	DZ	h^2	Test-retest MZ & DZ	MZ	DZ	h^2	Test-retest MZ & DZ	h^2
Factors N of Pairs:	148	119			273	228			33
Intellectual Interests	.57	.20	(.57)	.80	.59	.27	(.59)	.76	.54
Politics	.46	.20	(.46)	.70	.42	.27	.30	.70	.16
Socializing	.50	.14	(.50)	.67	.39	.21	.36	.70	.42
Hunting-Fishing	.67	.39	.56	.87	.48	.26	.44	.75	.42
Sierra Club	.51	.26	.50	.70	.56	.24	(.56)	.79	.53
Religion	.52	.36	.32	.83	.63	.28	(.63)	.82	.57
Husbandry	.63	.17	(.63)	.80	.41	.08	(.41)	.68	.65
Domestic	.47	.25	.44	.73	.46	.21	(.46)	.83	.46
Passive Entertainment	.51	.13	(.51)	.68	.52	.18	(.52)	.75	.46
Fitness	.49	.13	(.49)	.79	.56	.23	(.56)	.71	.41
Gambling	.61	.33	.56	.83	.45	.35	.20	.78	.48
Police Calls–Fires	.49	.15	(.49)	.74	.44	.28	.32	.66	.77
The Arts	.50	.18	(.50)	.78	.47	.21	(.47)	.76	.22
Foreign Travel	.27	-.05	(.27)	.52	.43	.11	(.43)	.57	.17
Reading	.45	.07	(.45)	.69	.46	.18	(.46)	.72	.16
Sports Fan	.51	.34	.34	.87	.46	.22	(.46)	.75	.59
Swinging	.43	.15	(.43)	.75	.45	.20	(.45)	.77	.47
Danger Seeking	.39	.26	.26	.63	.43	.14	(.43)	.75	.46

Note. Parenthetical figures refer to estimates based on MZ correlations.

The data reported in Tables 6 and 7 illustrate that the twin intercorrelations and test-retest stabilities for the interest scales were quite similar for both sexes. For example, the median MZ correlations for the occupational interest scales were .43 and .44 for the male and female subjects, respectively. The median DZ correlations were .18 and .21 for males and females, respectively. The median test-retest stabilities were .75 and .72. Within-pair correlations for MZ twins reared apart (MZA) directly estimate broad heritability without relying on the assumptions of the Falconer formula. It is noteworthy that 4 of the 17 occupational interest scales yield negligible MZA correlations (.13 or less), whereas 8 of them yield substantial correlations, ranging from .41 to .65. The average MZA correlation for the occupational interest scales was .35, in contrast to .14 for 34 DZA pairs. The average MZA correlation for the 18 leisure time interest scales was .45, versus .18 for the DZA twins.

The data for the leisure time interest scales mirror almost exactly the pattern of relations found for occupational interests. The median MZ correlation was .50 for the males and .46 for the females. The median DZ correlations were .19 and .18 for males and females, respectively; the median test-retest stabilities were .75 for both sexes.

As might be expected, less stable interests (e.g., Military or Foreign Travel) are associated with lower MZ correlations. Put another way, it is the stable component of interest variance that sets the upper limit for heritability. It may be that some of these interests are less stable because they are, in fact, less *traited,* that is, relatively large numbers of people do not have well-defined attitudes toward some of these occupations or activities.

Figure 2 presents multiple box-and-whisker plots (Tukey, 1977) for the MZ and DZ twin correlations for both the occupational interest and leisure time interest scales for both sexes. The boxes envelop the middle 50% of the distributions, whereas the whiskers represent the distribution tails. These plots nicely illustrate that the MZ co-twins are quite a bit more similar to one another than are the DZ co-twins, suggesting that individual differences in interests are due, in part, to hereditary factors. The plots also show that the average within zygosity twin correlations are very similar both across sex and across interest domains.

In summary, our data provide additional support to the growing body of literature suggesting that expressed interests are both heritable (Carter, 1932; Grotevant, Scarr, & Weinberg, 1977; Nichols, 1978; Roberts & Johansson, 1974; Vandenberg & Kelly, 1964; Vandenberg & Stafford, 1967) and stable over time (Hansen & Stocco, 1980; Hansen & Swanson, 1983; Strong, 1951; Swanson & Hansen,

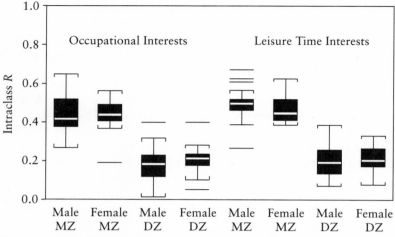

Figure 2   Multiple boxplots for MZ and DZ intraclass correlations for
17 occupational interest and 18 leisure time interest factors

1988). In our sample, for example, approximately 50% of the variance—and two-thirds of the stable variance—of the occupational interest and leisure time interest scales could be attributed to genetic factors. Thus, the role of genetic factors in the development and maintenance of expressed interests appears to be of about equal magnitude as it is in the domain of personality (Tellegen et al., 1988).

DISCUSSION

In this chapter, we have explored relations among three domains of individual differences: (a) occupational interests, (b) leisure time interests, and (c) personality. Although each of these domains has been explored in the past—sometimes in great detail—our work represents one of the few attempts to look at these domains simultaneously in a large sample.

Because of our design and our inclusion of twin data, we were able to consider questions that few researchers are given the opportunity to ask. For example, Hansen (1984) notes that

> most major theorists [of occupational interests] (Berdie, 1944; Darley & Hagenah, 1955; Strong, 1943; Super, 1949) have included five determinants of interests in their theories: (a) Interests arise from environmental and/or social influences; (b) Interests are genetic; (c) Interests are personality traits; (d) Interests are motives, drives, or needs; (e) Interests are expressions of self-concept. (p. 100)

Our data allowed us to examine the veracity of three of these statements.

Are interests largely genetic or environmental? When we looked at the role of heredity in the expression of interests, we found that more than half of the stable variance on many of these traits was attributable to genetic factors. Thus, the proposition that "interests are genetic" was clearly supported by our data. However, the fact that less than half of the variance of some traits for one or both sexes could be accounted for by genetic factors also suggests that "interests arise from environmental...influences." Rather than frame the question in either-or terms, psychologists should instead ask, What are the complementary roles of genetic and environmental factors in the development and maintenance of interests?

Are interests personality traits? Our data suggest that the answer to this question is no. When we correlated the 17 occupational interest and 18 leisure time interest scales with the 11 personality scales of the MPQ, we found that only two personality scales, Social Potency (dominance) and Harmavoidance, related strongly to the interest dimensions. Other researchers have reached similar conclusions. Hansen (1984, p. 117), for example, notes that "for the most part, correlational studies between interest scores and personality scores have been extremely disappointing."

Our data show that many occupational interest and leisure time interests are stable, genetically influenced person variables that are relatively independent of personality. Thus, although genetic factors account for at least 50% of the stable variance in both the domains of personality (Tellegen et al., 1988) and interests, our data suggest that these genetic factors are not the same in the two domains. This brings us back to the title of this chapter. Are occupational interests, leisure time interests, and personality three domains or one? Our findings largely indicate the former. Nevertheless, in the following discussion, we reason that personality factors are relevant to leisure time interests and occupational interests, and to vocational choice.

First, our data do show several clear associations between personality and interests, involving especially the Social Potency and Harmavoidance traits. These correlations not only tell us that certain occupational interests are directly trait related, but also indicate that respondents' *perceptions* of these occupations tend to be consensual. Our respondents must have been in some agreement that a political job calls for assertiveness and entails visibility, that scientific pursuits are adventurous and exciting, and that social service occupations tend to be less socially assertive and less physically adventurous than other vocations. Without shared occupational perceptions of this sort, no correlations with personality could have been obtained.

The numerous low correlations between personality and interests are more ambiguous. It may be that certain interests are not relevant to personality, as we defined it with our inventory, *or* that the occupations in question are perceived differently by different people. The low personality correlates of the Medical and Military occupational interests scales, for example, may reflect differences among respondents in how important they believe the social service, achievement, job security, or prestige features of these occupations are. Attitudes toward most occupations are formed without direct job experience and may reflect idiosyncratic appraisals. If these idiosyncratic appraisals are personality related, additional substantial correlations between occupational interests and personality traits should be demonstrable. One could ask respondents to rate their interest not only in occupation O but also in various specific activities actually required for occupation O. Personality correlates may be stronger for a composite based on the O-relevant activities than for the direct ratings of O itself, which may reflect idiosyncratic perceptions. On the other hand, the job perceptions that are more consensual may also be the more accurate ones, perhaps underlying more realistic preferences. But we know of no data in this area and we may underestimate the influence of inaccurate stereotypes (e.g., "scientists' lives are full of excitement").

In any case, vocational psychologists undoubtedly encounter clients whose job preferences are inappropriate, either because their job perceptions or their self-perceptions are inaccurate, or both. Corrective vocational information can be usefully augmented with systematic assessments of personality characteristics and of leisure time interests and activities. One can think of examples: Someone who is a good chef might think of starting a nouvelle cuisine restaurant. But this person might not realize that one's own appetite for risk taking and long hours are not quite strong enough for this competitive line of work, or that one's conscientiousness and affiliativeness could be real assets in a more social-service–oriented career. A would-be psychiatric social worker, though motivated to work with people, might in the long run be temperamentally more suited for a less bureaucratic and more entrepreneurial occupation. A would-be experimental chemist, though genuinely interested in the sciences, may have underestimated the patience required for repetitive laboratory work.

So far in our discussion, the problem of improving the fit of people and vocations has been posed too simply as merely one of making better choices, of choosing jobs or people better. To be sure, obvious examples of this can be added to the earlier ones; shy people are generally not well suited for sales jobs; highly stress-reactive people are generally not ideal for high-pressure managerial positions. But we also find in the same occupation people with very different personalities doing very well: Some successful salespersons are ebullient extroverts and some are soft-spoken; although most successful psychologists like people, some don't; not all successful lawyers are aggressive; and a few happy Trappist monks are loquacious. These distinctive traits influence the particular work roles people undertake. Workers often find, or fashion, or are ultimately provided, a niche in their job environment that is personality congruent, that is, conducive to personal fulfillment and job stability. Insofar as people's jobs are in fact structured in accordance with their personalities, we encounter in the work sphere (including areas of low correlations between personality variables and measured occupational interests) a process of trait-situation matching (Tellegen, 1989; Waller, Benet, & Farney, 1994), resulting in person-environment correlation (Buss, 1984) and, thus, also in gene-environment covariation. Whether a particular person-environment fit is adaptive or dysfunctional or lacking, personality assessment can help clarify not only the what of vocational preference and choice but also the how of vocational adjustment.

REFERENCES

Alley, W. E., & Matthews, M. D. (1982). The vocational interest career examination: A description of the instrument and possible applications. *The Journal of Psychology, 12,* 169–193.

Borgen, F. H. (1986). New approaches to the assessment of interests. In W. B. Walsh & S. H. Osipow (Eds.), *Advances in vocational psychology: Vol. 1. The assessment of interests* (pp. 83–125). Hillsdale, NJ: Erlbaum.

Buss, D. M. (1984). Toward a psychology of person-environment (PE) correlation: The role of spouse selection. *Journal of Personality and Social Psychology, 47,* 361–377.

Carter, H. D. (1932). Twin similarities in occupational interests. *Journal of Educational Psychology, 23,* 641–655.

Costa, P. T., Jr., McCrae, R. R., & Holland, J. L. (1984). Personality and vocational interests in an adult sample. *Journal of Applied Psychology, 69,* 390–400.

Davison, M. L. (1983). *Multidimensional scaling.* New York: Wiley.

Davison, M. L. (1985). Multidimensional scaling versus components analysis of test intercorrelations. *Psychological Bulletin, 97,* 94–105.

Dawis, R. V., & Lofquist, L. H. (1984). *A psychological theory of work adjustment: An individual differences model and its applications.* Minneapolis: University of Minnesota Press.

Fitzgerald, L. F., & Hubert, L. J. (1987). Multidimensional scaling: Some possibilities for counseling psychology. *Journal of Counseling Psychology, 34,* 469–480.

Goodman, L. A., & Kruskal, W. H. (1954). Measures of association for cross-classifications. *Journal of the American Statistical Association, 49,* 732–764.

Grotevant, H., Scarr, S., & Weinberg, R. (1977). Patterns of interest similarity in adoptive and biological families. *Journal of Personality and Social Psychology, 33,* 667–676.

Guilford, J. P., Christensen, P. R., Bond, N. A., Jr., & Sutton, M. A. (1954). A factor analysis study of human interests. *Psychological Monographs, 68,* Whole No. 375.

Hansen, J. C. (1984). Measurement of vocational interests: Issues and future directions. In S. Brown & R. Lent (Eds.), *Handbook of counseling psychology* (pp. 99–136). New York: Wiley.

Hansen, J. C., & Stocco, J. L. (1980). Stability of vocational interests of adolescents and young adults. *Measurement and Evaluation in Guidance, 13,* 173–178.

Hansen, J. C., & Swanson, J. L. (1983). Stability of interests and the concurrent and predictive validity of the 1981 Strong-Campbell Interest Inventory for college majors. *Journal of Counseling Psychology, 30,* 194–201.

Holland, J. L. (1959). A theory of vocational choice. *Journal of Counseling Psychology, 6,* 35–44.

Holland, J. L. (1985). *Making vocational choices: A theory of vocational personalities and work environments* (2d ed). Englewood Cliffs, NJ: Prentice Hall.

Kruskal, J. B., & Wish, M. (1978). *Multidimensional scaling. Sage University paper series on quantitative applications in the social sciences* (No. 07–011). Beverly Hills, CA: Sage.

Lamb, R. R., & Prediger, D. J. (1981). *Technical report for the Unisex Edition of the ACT Interest Inventory* (UNIACT). Iowa City, IA: American College Testing.

Lykken, D. T., Bouchard, T. J., McGue, M., & Tellegen, A. (1990). The Minnesota twin family registry: Some initial findings. *Acta Geneticae Medicae et Gemellologiae, 39,* 35–70.

MacCallum, R. (1988). Multidimensional scaling. In J. R. Nesselroade & R. T. Cattell (Eds.), *Handbook of multivariate experimental psychology: Perspectives on individual differences* (2d ed., pp. 421–445). New York: Wiley.

McGue, M., & Bouchard, T. J., Jr. (1984). Adjustment of twin data for the effects of age and sex. *Behavior Genetics, 14,* 325–343.

Nichols, R. C. (1978). Twin studies of ability, personality, and interests. *Homo, 29,* 158–173.

Reise, S. P., & Waller, N. G. (1990). Fitting the two-parameter model to personality data. *Applied Psychological Measurement, 14,* 45–58.

Roberts, C. A., & Johansson, C. B. (1974). The inheritance of cognitive interest styles among twins. *Journal of Vocational Behavior, 4,* 237–243.

Roe, A. (1956). *The psychology of occupations.* New York: Wiley.

Rounds, J. B., & Zevon, M. A. (1983). Multidimensional scaling research in vocational psychology. In M. L. Davison (Ed.), *Special Issue: Applied Psychological Measurement, 7,* 491–510.

Rounds, J. B., & Dawis, R. V. (1979). Factor analysis of Strong Vocational Interest Blank items. *Journal of Applied Psychology, 64,* 132–143.

Shepard, R. N., & Arabie, P. (1979). Additive clustering: Representation of similarities as combinations of discrete overlapping properties. *Psychological Review, 86,* 87–123.

Strong, E. K., Jr. (1951). Permanence of interest scores after 22 years. *Journal of Applied Psychology, 35,* 89–91.

Swanson, J. L., & Hansen J. C. (1988). Stability of vocational interests over 4-year, 8-year, and 12-year intervals. *Journal of Vocational Behavior, 33,* 185–202.

Tellegen, A. (1982). *Brief manual of the Multidimensional Personality Questionnaire.* Unpublished manuscript, University of Minnesota, Minneapolis.

Tellegen, A. (1988). *Ecscal: A nonmetric discrete-dimensional scaling program.* Unpublished manuscript, University of Minnesota, Minneapolis.

Tellegen, A. (1989). Personality traits: Issues of definition, evidence, and assessment. In D. Cicchetti & W. Grove (Eds.), *Thinking clearly about psychology: Essays in honor of Paul Everett Meehl.* Minneapolis: University of Minnesota Press.

Tellegen, A., Lykken, D. T., Bouchard, T., Wilcox, K., Segal, N., & Rich, S. (1988). Personality similarity in twins reared apart and together. *Journal of Personality and Social Psychology, 73,* 1031–1039.

Tukey, J. W. (1977). *Exploratory Data Analysis.* Reading, MA: Addison-Wesley.

Vandenberg, S. G., & Kelly, L. (1964). Heredity components in vocational preferences. *Acta Geneticae Medicae et Gemellologiae, 13,* 266–277.

Vandenberg, S. G., & Stafford, R. E. (1967). Heredity influences on vocational preferences as shown by scores of twins on the Minnesota Vocational Interest Inventory. *Journal of Applied Psychology, 51,* 17–19.

Waller, N. G., Benet, V., & Farney, D. L. (1994). Modeling person-situation correspondence over time: A study of 103 evangelical disciple-makers. *Journal of Personality, 62,* 177–197.

Wilkinson, L. (1988). *SYSTAT: The System for Statistics.* Evanston, IL: SYSTAT.

Part Four

New Areas
of Research

The field of individual differences has focused on what are usually called *dispositional variables*—attributes of individuals that are predictive of (that "predispose one to") certain classes of behavior. These attributes are not often inferrable from ordinary everyday behavior and must be elicited by tests in order to be evaluated. Perhaps because of the early and continuing success of psychological tests as instruments for measuring individual differences, and the accompanying spectacular development of the statistical theory of psychological measurement, individual differences researchers have for the most part focused their attention and energy on the "traditional" topics discussed in Part 3.

But there are always innovators. Part 4 of this volume is devoted to two "nontraditional" individual differences topics. In Chapter 10, Stanley Strong discusses interpersonal behavior. He presents a novel theory of the demand (need) and supply (scarcity) of emotional and material resources in an interpersonal exchange. Strong presents experimental evidence for his theory and supports various theoretical implications with numerous citations from the social psychological literature. It is differences in beliefs about the exchange that results in individual differences in interpersonal behavior, Strong concludes, adding that such beliefs are better inferred from behavior in standardized situations (such as tests) than from self-reporting.

In Chapter 11, James Jenkins, Winifred Strange, and Linda Polka explore speech perception in a nonnative language. They ask the question, Do nonnative speakers "hear with an accent" as well as speak with an accent? The conclusion of Jenkins, Strange, and Polka is yes. Describing a series of experiments, they examine the identification and discrimination of speech sounds familiar to speakers of American English that are confused by nonnative listeners (/r/ and /l/ sounds as they are heard by Japanese listeners) and the origins of such confusion in perceptual reorganization in infants (occurring at about the end of the first year, when infants are also learning to produce the first speech sounds). They find that training directed at improving the perception of /r/ and /l/ in nonnative speakers yields only modest improvement. They also discuss how individual differences—in addition to stimulus materials, criterial tasks, and orienting tasks—affect the perception of nonnative speech sounds.

Chapter 10

Interpersonal Influence Theory
The Situational and Individual Determinants of Interpersonal Behavior

Stanley R. Strong
Virginia Commonwealth University

RESOURCE EXCHANGE IN SOCIAL INTERACTION

People are social animals. They spend most of their lives interacting with others. The most startling fact of biological evolution is the emergence of Homo sapiens as social creatures, creatures eminently equipped to wrest survival from the physical environment through collective action. The difference between the Neanderthal and Homo sapiens was not cranial size but the cranial organization that gave Homo sapiens superior abilities to communicate with one another. Experts surmise that these superior abilities supported complex and effective collective action among Homo sapiens, an effectiveness that may have contributed to the rapid extinction of the Neanderthal (Bailey, 1987).

People are inclined to affiliate with others. Through collective action, people generate the materials and conditions that facilitate their survival and growth. Effective group action requires specialization of member contributions and coordination of their efforts. To maintain the members' contributions to the group, the fruits of the group's effort must be distributed among them. Affiliation with others, highly developed abilities to communicate with others, and the complex and structured systems of social exchange thus allowed are endemic to the human condition.

Like other living creatures, people act on their environment to render it hospitable to their needs. Their environment is largely composed of other people whose actions control most of the materials and conditions—the resources—they need to survive and grow. Thus, much of human behavior is intended to influence others to behave hospitably to one's needs. People form, maintain, and alter relationships with others whom they perceive to control resources they need. In relationships, people exchange behaviors intended to influence each other in order to adopt and maintain behaviors that are hospitable to their needs. Each tailors his or her interpersonal (social) behavior to the opportunities and dangers that the other's behavior poses to need fulfillment.

In interpersonal interactions, people negotiate the resources they will make available to each other and the needs to be fulfilled through their relationship. They exchange resources as they reach consensus about the structure of their relationship. People base their behaviors on their impressions of the resources they and the other control and the needs they and the other have. Their vulnerability to each other's influence is a joint function of (a) their needs that correspond to (i.e., that can be fulfilled by) the resources they perceive the other to control and (b) the needs they perceive the other to have that correspond to the resources they control. People influence each other's behavior by affecting each other's impressions of resources and needs. Interpersonal behaviors convey information about the person's characteristics and about the person's perception of the other's characteristics. The information is intended to affect the other's impressions of resources and needs, thereby influencing the other's behavior.

Emotional Resources

The basic human need is to affiliate with fellow creatures and exchange emotional resources such as liking, care, support, and affection. The need for affiliation is part of our heritage as mammals. The most important evolutionary change from reptiles to mammals was the emergence of extended care for and affiliation with offspring. Primate social systems are based on kinship and arise from brain structures that equip mammals with affiliative emotions (Bailey, 1987). The power of affiliation needs in human behavior is intensified by people's reliance on collective action to generate material resources for survival and growth. The need for and exchange of emotional resources is the glue that forms and maintains social groups. People are intrinsically inclined to seek, respond to, and exchange positive affiliation behaviors. Negative or hostile behaviors deny emotional resources and threaten the successful formation or continuance of social groups.

Thus, people are highly responsive to hostile behaviors such as indifference, rejection, and harm. Such behaviors threaten their affiliation needs and threaten the formation or continuation of needed social groups.

Material Resources

Effective group action requires that the contributions of group members be specialized and coordinated and that the benefits of collective action be distributed among the members. The highly developed cortex of the human brain, a heritage of primate evolution, allows people to communicate with one another in complex ways. Communication abilities enable humans to form highly structured and complex social groups. The specialization and coordination of individual contributions to group activities are shaped and maintained by the distribution of the material resources collective action generates.

The distribution of material resources in social groups is closely related to the perceived value of member contributions to the success of group efforts. Coordination skills and scarce contributions that are critical to group success are highly valued, whereas contributions that are less scarce or critical are less valued. Members who coordinate activities or make critical and scarce contributions receive favorable shares of the material resources the group generates. Those who offer more common contributions are less favored. The result is the emergence of status hierarchies in human groups. High status (dominant) members coordinate activities, control the distribution of material resources, and make scarce and critical contributions. Low status (submissive) members contribute their energies and efforts to more common activities in obedience to dominant members.

When people are forming relationships, the first order of business is to determine the structure of their relationship in terms of their contributions to and benefits from group effort. The relationship structure that evolves reflects the participants' perceptions of the material resources each controls. Material resources are the materials, skills, abilities, and knowledge required to accomplish the purposes underlying the formation of the relationship. As a working consensus emerges, the relationship is consummated and maintained through the exchange of material and emotional resources. At any point, one or both participants may become dissatisfied with the structure of the relationship and launch efforts to change the other's impression of the distribution of resources in the relationship. If a new working consensus is not achieved, the relationship may be abandoned. In any case, relationships are maintained only as long as they serve the needs of their members.

CLASSIFICATION OF INTERPERSONAL BEHAVIOR

Interpersonal behaviors are intended to manage other people's impressions of the distribution of emotional and material resources and needs in relationships. They carry information about the emotional resources I offer and need and the ones you offer and need, and about the material resources I have or need and that you have or need. The basic information about emotional resources identifies the extent to which I offer (or give) emotional resources. The messages vary from "I give" to "I do not give" and define the emotional resource dimension of interpersonal behavior. The basic information about material resources identifies the extent to which I control scarce resources. The messages vary from "I have (I control)" to "I need (I do not control)" and define the scarce material resource dimension of interpersonal behavior.

The emotional and scarce material resource dimensions are orthogonal and define the Cartesian plane presented in Figure 1. The emotional resource dimension is the horizontal axis presented at the bottom of the figure, and the material resource dimension is the vertical axis presented on the left side of the figure. Each point on the plane represents a different combination of basic information about resources and needs in the relationship. The other messages on the plane expand the implicit meaning of the combinations of basic messages; they provide additional information about the distribution of emotional and scarce material resources in the relationship. For example, the implicit meaning of the combination of the basic messages "I do not give emotional resources" and "I need scarce material resources" is conveyed in the message "You do not need (or want) scarce material resources"; the combination "I give emotional resources" and "I have scarce material resources" is expanded with "You need scarce material resources."

In Figure 1, interpersonal behaviors classified toward the poles of the emotional resource axis focus on information about the distribution of emotional resources and needs. Behaviors that inform the other that "I give emotional resources" are classified as *ingratiation,* whereas those that inform the other that "I do not give emotional resources" are classified as *intimidation* (Jones & Pittman, 1982). Within ingratiation, *nurturant behaviors* additionally inform the other that "You need emotional resources," whereas *cooperative behaviors* add "I need emotional resources." Within intimidation, *critical behaviors* add "I do not need emotional resources," whereas *distrustful behaviors* add "You do not want emotional resources."

Behaviors classified toward the poles of the scarce material resource axis in Figure 1 focus on information about the distribution of material resources and needs. Those that inform the other that "I have

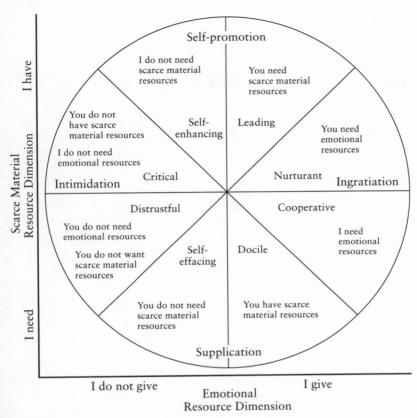

Figure 1   Resource messages of interpersonal behaviors

scarce material resources" are classified as *self-promotion,* whereas those that inform the other that "I need scarce material resources" are classified as *supplication* (Jones & Pittman, 1982). Within self-promotion, *leading behaviors* add "You need scarce material resources," whereas *self-enhancing* behaviors add "I do not need scarce material resources." Within supplication, *docile behaviors* add "You have scarce material resources," whereas *self-effacing behaviors* add "You do not need scarce material resources."

Figure 2 presents representative behaviors that embody the information about resources and needs within each class of interpersonal behavior (Strong & Hills, 1986). Behaviors on the right side of the classification model attempt to influence the other's impressions by presenting positive information about the distribution of resources and

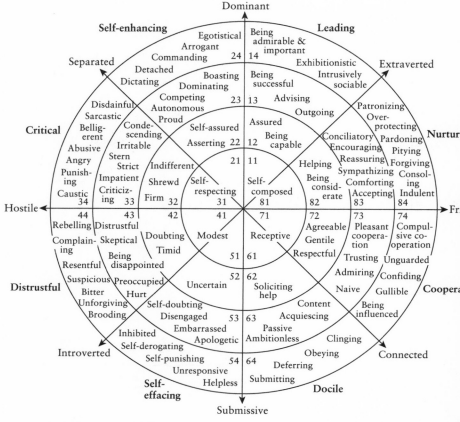

Figure 2   Classification of interpersonal behaviors

From *Interpersonal Communication Rating Scale,* by S. R. Strong and H. I. Hills, 1986, Department of Psychology, Virginia Commonwealth University. Unpublished work.

needs within a positive emotional climate. They propose the exchange of contributions and benefits in a context of liking, consideration, appreciation, care, support, respect, and affection. Behaviors on the left side of the model attempt to influence impressions through the negation and denial of aspects of resources and needs in a context of indifference, self-denigration, dislike, disdain, bitterness, rejection, and withdrawal. They attempt to induce the other to alter the distribution of contributions and benefits not only by denying certain resources and needs but also by threatening the existence of the relationship. The behaviors threaten withdrawal if proposed changes are not accepted. The threat to abandon the relationship intensifies the impact of demands for change.

DETERMINANTS OF INTERPERSONAL BEHAVIOR

Interpersonal behaviors are attempts to influence the other's impressions of the distribution of material and emotional resources and needs in relationships. They also embody the exchange of resources that facilitate fulfillment of participants' needs. The interpersonal behaviors a person employs reflect one's impression of the opportunities and dangers for need fulfillment present in a relationship. Thus, the two categories of determinants of interpersonal behavior are (a) the features of a relationship that influence a person's perception of the distribution of resources and needs in the relationship and (b) the characteristics of the person that define features of relationships as opportunities or dangers.

The features of relationships that influence a person's perception of the distribution of resources and needs are the behaviors the other employs and the extent and nature of one's own and the other's dependence on the relationship. The characteristics of the person that define features of relationships as opportunities or dangers are needs and beliefs about how features of relationships relate to need fulfillment. Individual differences in interpersonal behavior are a function of differences in these beliefs.

The Other's Interpersonal Behavior

If the proposed classification of interpersonal behaviors in terms of the information they present about resources and needs is valid, then the relative perceptual and behavioral impacts of interpersonal behavior on interactants should systematically reflect the structure of the classification model. Strong et al. (1988) tested this proposition in an experiment in which one of the participants in two-person groups persistently employed behaviors from one of the eight classes of interpersonal behaviors presented in Figure 2 (shown in bold-faced type in the figure). College women volunteered to participate in a study advertised as "an investigation"of how women negotiate consensus in a creative story construction task. Each subject was paired with a confederate subject who was trained to follow a scripted role containing a high frequency of one of the eight classes of behaviors. The subjects worked together for 16 minutes to generate stories for two *Thematic Apperception Test* (TAT) cards. They were instructed to develop a story for each card individually and then share their stories and create and agree on the most creative story for each card. After the experimental interactions, subjects described their perceptions of their partner (the confederate) using the *Impact Message Inventory* (IMI; Perkins, et al., 1979). The interactions were videotaped and the behaviors of the participants were coded into the eight classes of interpersonal behaviors using the *Interpersonal Communication Rating Scale* (Strong & Hills, 1986).

Item responses on the IMI are scored on 15 scales that form a circumplex pattern along status and affiliation dimensions. The scales are combined into four cluster scores, one for each pole of the dimensions. To determine the relative perceptual impacts of the eight interpersonal behaviors, the differences in perceptual impact of each behavior, as opposed to the impact of the other seven behaviors, were assessed with a priori contrasts in an analysis of variance of each cluster score. For each behavior, the F values on the dominant and submissive cluster scores were combined, as were those on the friendly and hostile cluster scores. The results of these operations were two values for each behavior that indicated its relative perceptual impact on the IMI status and affiliation dimensions. These values were used as coordinates on the status and affiliation dimensions, and vectors drawn from the origin to the point on the plane defined by the coordinates graphically depicted the relative perceptual impacts of the behaviors.

Figure 3 presents the relative perceptual impact vectors of the eight interpersonal behaviors. The direction of each vector indicates the relative effect of the confederates' behavior on the subjects' perception of the confederates. The length of the vector indicates the intensity of the effect. The relative positions of the perceptual impact vectors correspond exactly to the positions of the behaviors relative to one another in the model. The vectors reveal that the perceptual impacts on the status dimension were strongest for the most hostile behaviors. It was proposed earlier that the threat to abandon the relationship conveyed in behaviors on the left side of the model intensified the impact of demands for change in the distribution of material resources in the relationship. The greater perceptual impacts of hostile behaviors on the status dimension is consistent with that proposition.

Strong et al. (1988) organized the ratings of the women's behaviors in each interaction in confederate stimulus/subject response pairs. They eliminated the data pairs in which the confederate stimulus was not classified in the category of behavior emphasized in the confederate's role. They then determined for each subject/confederate pair the proportion of the subject's total responses that were classified in each of the eight behavior categories and transformed the proportions into a normally distributed variable. They determined the effect of each confederate behavior relative to the effects of the other seven behaviors with a priori contrasts in an analysis of variance for each subject behavior. The analyses resulted in eight F ratios for each confederate behavior that indicated its relative impact on each subject response behavior.

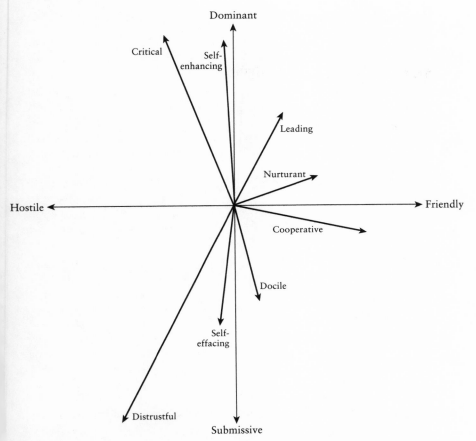

Figure 3 Relative perceptual impact vectors of interpersonal behaviors

To generate status and affiliation dimension coordinates of the behaviors' relative impacts on subjects' response behaviors, the eight F ratios for each confederate behavior were linearly combined twice using the geometric properties of the classification model. One combination weighted the F ratios to derive a coordinate for the status dimension; the other combination weighted the F ratios to derive a coordinate for the affiliation dimension. Vectors drawn from the origin to the point on the plane defined by the status and affiliation coordinates graphically depicted the direction and intensity of each confederate behavior's relative impact on the subjects' overall response behavior.

Figure 4 presents the relative behavioral impact vectors of the eight interpersonal behaviors. The direction of each resultant vector

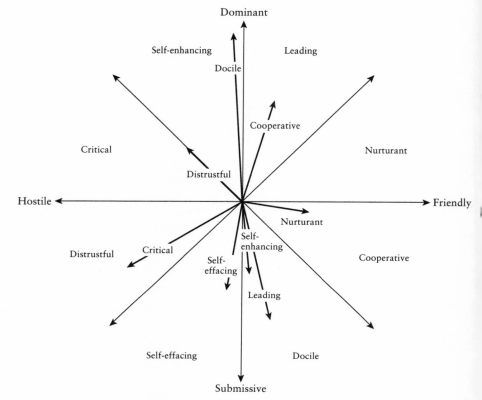

Figure 4   Relative behavioral impact vectors of interpersonal behaviors

indicates the bias or underlying thrust the confederate behavior generated in the overall pattern of subject response behavior (subject behaviors encouraged and, inversely, discouraged). The length of each vector indicates the strength of the resultant effect. As can be seen in Figure 4, behavioral effects systematically reflected the structure of the model. Submissive behaviors encouraged dominant responses and discouraged submissive responses. Dominant behaviors encouraged submissive responses and discouraged dominant responses. Friendly behaviors encouraged friendly responses and discouraged hostile responses. Hostile behaviors encouraged hostile responses and discouraged friendly responses. The only exception to this pattern was for self-effacing behaviors. Self-effacing behaviors encouraged self-effacing responses. Other research (Gergen & Taylor, 1969; Gruszkos, 1986) suggests that this inversion of expected effect was a consequence of the subjects' instructions to cooperate and achieve consensus.

The overall pattern of behavioral impacts corresponds closely to the expected effects of the behaviors' resource messages presented in the model. The pattern is also consistent with the major hypothesis of interpersonal theory, *complementarity* (Carson, 1969; Kiesler, 1983; Strong, 1986). Complementarity proposes that responses to another's behavior in an interaction will be reciprocal on the status dimension (submissive behaviors encourage dominant behaviors and vice versa) and correspondent on the affiliation dimension (friendly beget friendly, and hostile, hostile). However, the relationships Strong et al. (1988) observed between specific behaviors did not conform well to complementarity. Of the 24 significant relationships they reported between specific confederate and subject behaviors, only seven conformed to the expectations of complementarity. In a review of research on interpersonal behavior, Orford (1986) concluded that complementarity as a guide to the exchange of specific behaviors in relationships is faulty at best. Different behaviors result in different effects in different relationships.

Strong et al. (1988) concluded that, while how a person behaves toward another profoundly influences how the other behaves toward the person,

> a specific interpersonal behavior does not impel a specific response from the other. Rather, the person's behavior...biases the other's responses in a particular direction, a direction that is evident in the other's overall pattern of responses but may not be apparent in specific responses. (p. 809)

The behaviors a person employs profoundly and systematically influence the other's behavior.

Relationship Dependence

The impact of another's behavior on a person's behavior is qualified by the person's perception of his or her own and the other's dependence on the relationship. People form, alter, and maintain relationships to obtain the emotional and material resources they need. A person's dependence on a relationship is a function of how critical the resources it provides are to the person's needs and the extent to which the resources cannot be obtained in other relationships. A person is highly dependent on a relationship when the resources it provides are critical and cannot be obtained readily through another relationship. A person is less dependent on a relationship when the resources it provides are not very important or when they can be obtained readily through another relationship. Because people have strong needs for emotional resources and are highly dependent on social groups to meet their material needs, their behavior is constrained by needs to be liked and receive approval.

The more dependent a person is on a relationship, the more inclined the person is to behave in ways that maintain the other's participation in the relationship. The person is inclined to give emotional resources and conform his or her contributions to the other's needs. Such behaviors are efforts to enhance the other's satisfaction with the relationship and thus maintain the other's continued participation in it. However, relationships are never one sided. The other participates in the relationship to service the other's own needs. Thus, the other is dependent at some level on the person's continued participation in the relationship. Dependence on the person inclines the other to give emotional resources and conform contributions to the person's needs. The effect of relationship dependence on interpersonal behavior is a function of the person's perception of the extent and relative degree of his or her own and the other's dependence on the relationship. Interpersonal behavior is a function of interdependence.

Interdependence has the following effects on interpersonal behavior:

- *When a person perceives his or her own dependence to be high and the other's dependence to be low, the person gives emotional resources and conforms contributions to the needs of the other.* As described above, these behaviors are intended to encourage the other to maintain the relationship. The person avoids disputes about the exchange of material resources in the relationship as long as she or he perceives the needed resources may be received through the relationship.

- *When a person perceives his or her own dependence to be low and the other's dependence to be high, the person exchanges emotional and material resources with the other as long as the other conforms to his or her wishes.* The person does not hesitate to threaten to abandon the relationship if the other does not fully conform. These behaviors reflect the person's perception that the other is easily replaced. The person gives the minimum resources the other wants only as long as the other fully satisfies the needs the person seeks to fulfill in the relationship. If the other's behavior is not fully satisfactory, the person counts on the other's greater dependence to render him or her responsive to demands for change.

- *When a person perceives both his or her own and the other's dependence to be low, the person gives emotional resources and conforms to the other's wishes as long as the exchange is satisfactory.* However, with minimal dissatisfaction, the person threatens to abandon the relationship. Because the person perceives little dependence on the relationship, little dissatisfaction is tolerated before demanding change in the exchange. If the other is likewise less dependent on the relationship, it dissolves. If the other is more dependent than the person had perceived, the other conforms to the demands, and the person changes his or her perception of the interdependence balance in the relationship. Because relationships with little interdependence dissolve readily in face of dissatisfaction, those that continue are marked with satisfactory exchanges of emotional and material resources. The resources in any case are easily found in other relationships or are not particularly important to either party.

- *When a person perceives both his or her own and the other's dependence to be high, the person gives emotional resources and conforms to the other's wishes as long as the exchange is reasonably satisfactory.* However, with moderate dissatisfaction, the person demands changes by threatening to abandon the relationship. These behaviors reflect the person's efforts to maintain an important relationship, but also his or her perception that the other's high dependence renders the other vulnerable to demands for change. If both perceive the other to be highly dependent and both are themselves highly dependent, dissatisfaction leads to strident and caustic efforts to induce the other to change within a relationship both are reluctant to abandon. Such relationships spawn behavioral dysfunction. Both participants, such as two partners or parent and child, are trapped in persistent and caustic behavioral exchanges that debilitate both self and other.

Three factors affect dependence on a relationship: (a) the resources the other controls that facilitate fulfillment of needs, (b) the availability of alternative relationships that could provide the same resources as the current relationship, and (c) accountability and responsibility to people outside the relationship.

Resources the Other Controls   All people control resources valuable to others. Because of people's intrinsic need to affiliate, the other's emotional resources are valuable to them. Beyond this, effective group action requires a diversity of material resource contributions, not only coordination and critical specialized skills, but also a host of less specialized skills that nearly anyone can contribute. Armies need the contributions of foot soldiers as much as those of generals. Families need lawn mowers, dishwashers, grocery shoppers, child care providers, housecleaners, garbage emptiers, and cooks as much as they need coordinators and income generators. The nature of the needs to be met in a relationship determines the nature and diversity of resource contributions needed from members.

Although all people have resources of value to others, all resources are not of equal value. Our needs impart value to the other's resources. We seek and enter relationships only with people who control the specific resources that fulfill the specific needs that motivate our search for relationships. In addition, some resources are more scarce and critical to group success than others. Knowledge of social psychology and skill in imparting that knowledge to others is more scarce than the skills of sitting still, listening, taking notes, reading books, and taking tests. Skills that allow one to bring home a large paycheck are more scarce than skills that allow one to bring home a small paycheck. Skills in determining the tasks necessary to accomplish a group goal and coordinating the specialized efforts of group members are more scarce than skills in moving dirt with shovels, putting parts on a machine, typing reports, and so on. Although all of the skills are necessary for group success, some are more scarce and more critical to group success.

The level of our dependence on another is a joint function of (a) how critical the resources the other controls are to our survival, growth, and well-being and (b) the scarcity of the resources the other controls. The other's dependence on us is a function of the same features in the resources we control. The structure of a relationship reflects the members' perceptions of the relative criticalness and scarcity of the resources each controls:

- A person who perceives the other's resources to be more critical and scarce than his or her own is more dependent and will tend to employ submissive behaviors.

- A person who perceives the other's resources to be less critical and scarce than his or her own is less dependent and will tend to employ dominant behaviors.

- A person who perceives his or her own and other's resources to be of equal value will tend to employ a mixture of behaviors, none of which are extremely dominant or submissive.

In laboratory group experiments, subjects' perceptions of the relative values of member resources to group goals have been manipulated by providing such information directly or by controlling one member's behavior such as to imply possession (or lack of possession) of valuable resources. Simpson and Strong (1987) told subjects paired with confederates in a creativity story construction task that either they or the confederate was more creative and thus should lead.

Subjects complied more with the confederate's ideas when they believed the confederate was more creative (and the leader) than when they thought they were the more creative (and the leader). Jones and Jones (1964) found that subjects conformed to the opinions of other subjects who were appointed leaders and were to evaluate them. Fleischer and Chertkoff (1986) found that when they told pairs of subjects that one of them had strong abilities relevant to their task, that member was usually accepted as the leader. Gintner and Lindskold (1975) demonstrated the same effect in larger groups. People who talk a lot in groups tend to be selected as leaders. Bavalas, Hastorf, Gross, and Kite (1965) found that when they induced members who talked little initially to talk a lot, these members were seen as the leaders of the groups. In the Strong et al. (1988) study, subjects responded to confederate self-enhancing, leading, and nurturant stimuli with docile and cooperative responses. Subjects responded to confederate docile and cooperative stimuli with nurturant and leading responses.

In a field correlational study, Howard, Blumstein, and Schwartz (1986) explored the relationships of a number of indices of social power to the use of influence tactics by members of couples in committed relationships. They asked subjects to identify the behaviors their partners employed when the partner "wants you to do something you do not want to do." They found that members who reported themselves to have less income, be less physically attractive, and be more dependent than their partners, and those who were partners of men were perceived by their partners to use more supplication (plead, cry, act ill, helpless) and manipulation (hints, flattery, seductiveness, reminding of past favors). On the other hand, they found that men were seen to use more disengagement (sulk, make the partner feel guilty, leave the scene). Cowan, Drinkard, and MacGavin (1984) asked sixth-, ninth-, and 12th-grade children to list "how I get my way" with their friends, mothers, and fathers. With their friends, they reported using direct, bilateral, strong, and bargaining strategies. With their fathers, they reported using indirect, unilateral, weak, positive affect, asking, and eliciting reciprocation strategies. Similarly, Raush and his colleagues (Raush, 1965; Raush, Dittmann, & Taylor, 1959a; Raush, Dittmann, & Taylor, 1959b; Raush, Farbman, & Llewellyn, 1960) found that boys in in-patient treatment and matched "normal" boys tended to use dominant behaviors with each other and submissive behaviors with adult staff members.

When people are uncertain of their partner's resources, they are inclined to employ supplication. The women in the Strong et al. (1988) study employed more self-effacing and docile behaviors in the first half of the interactions than in the second half. People are also inclined to employ supplication when they perceive their partner to control superior resources that the partner is likely to withdraw or that the partner is likely to become hostile in response to displeasure with the person's behavior. Carlsmith, Lepper, and Landauer (1974) found that children obeyed adults whom they perceived to be threatening more than ones they perceived as nice. Strong et al. found that subjects employed more docile, distrustful, and critical responses to critical confederate stimuli than to other stimuli. The critical responses suggest that the subjects did not entirely accept the confederates' assertions of superiority carried in their critical behaviors. The literature on self-handicapping can be understood partially as self-effacing behaviors intended to forestall criticism from others (Kolditz & Arkin, 1982; Smith, Snyder, & Handelsman, 1982). Weiner, Amirkhan, Folkes, and Verette's (1987) study of the excuses people give for broken social contracts shows that people are well aware of, and readily use, the responsibility avoiding features of self-effacing behavior. The value of supplication in the face of criticism (and potential criticism) is suggested by Strong et al.'s finding that subjects were more likely to employ nurturant behavior in response to confederate supplication than to any other confederate behavior.

Alternative Relationships   With varying levels of difficulty and cost, all relationships can be replaced. The resources potentially available through one relationship can be obtained through another. However, establishing another relationship entails costs. It takes effort to find an appropriate potential participant who is interested in the resources we have to offer. We are often uncertain whether another could provide the same level of resources as the current partner. We are uncertain about the contributions the potential others will demand from us to fulfill their needs. Also, we often incur costs in other relationships with people who have a stake in the continuation of the relationship in question.

Thibaut and Kelley (1959) introduced the concept of the comparison level of the alternative. They hypothesized that the availability of alternative relationships limits the level of dissatisfaction people will tolerate before they abandon a relationship. The more access we have to alternative relationships (the less the costs of forming a new relationship), the less dissatisfaction we tolerate in a current relationship. Thus, the availability of alternative relationships limits the extent to which our needs for the resources the other controls incline us to give resources and conform to the other's wishes to secure the other's continued participation in the relationship. On the other hand, the availability of alternative relationships likewise constrains the other's behavior. The less access the other has to alternative relationships, the more we can demand adjustment in resource exchange to suit our wishes in the security that the other's lack of alternatives encourages him or her to conform to our wishes in order to secure our continued participation in the relationship.

In the research laboratory, the subject's relationship with the experimenter often constrains the subject's access to alternative relationships. When the experiment requires multiple contacts with another subject, the subject's dependence on the relationship with the other subject is increased. Subjects respond with increased ingratiation and supplication. For example, subjects conform more to the opinions of others whom they do not like when they believe they must continue working with them than when they do not (Kiesler, Zanna, & DeSalvo, 1966; Pallak & Heller, 1971). Subjects self-efface more in communications to moderately self-effacing others when they anticipate interacting with them than when they do not (Gergen & Wishnov, 1965). Subjects moderate the self-serving bias in their accounts of responsibility for group outcomes when they anticipate meeting with the others again and know that the others will see their accounts (Forsyth, Berger, & Mitchell, 1981; Norvell & Forsyth, 1984).

In their study of committed couples described earlier, Howard, Blumstein, and Schwartz (1986) found that spouses who reported higher commitment to the relationship than did their partners were perceived to use more manipulation (hints, flattery, seductiveness, reminding of past favors) and less bullying (threats, insults, violence, ridicule) than were their less committed partners. The presence of children in a relationship should intensify relationship dependence because of the costs to the children of severing the relationship. Consistent with this hypothesis, Howard, Blumstein, and Schwartz (1986) found that women with children were reported to use autocracy less frequently (insisting, claiming greater knowledge, asserting authority) than were women who had no children.

The other side of the effect of availability of alternative relationships on interpersonal behavior is reliance on the other's dependence on a relationship to make him or her responsive to demands for change. The caustic interpersonal behaviors dissatisfied spouses exchange demonstrates this effect (Billings, 1979; Gaelick, Bodenhausen, & Wyer, 1985; Nutall, 1987; Rusbult, Johnson, & Morrow, 1986). For example, Nutall asked satisfied and dissatisfied couples to exchange views about several standard scenarios of couple problems and reach consensus about who in the scenario was responsible for the problem. Husbands and wives were given slightly different information to ensure that they would have different opinions initially. The 15-minute interactions were videotaped and the members' behaviors were rated using the *Interpersonal Communication Rating Scale*. Nutall found that dissatisfied spouses used more critical and fewer cooperative behaviors than did satisfied spouses. They responded to their partners' docile and cooperative stimuli with more critical and less leading and cooperative behaviors than did satisfied spouses. The interactions of dissatisfied spouses were also marked with frequent exchanges of critical behaviors and nurturant behaviors. The exchange of critical behaviors seldom occurred between satisfied spouses, and the exchange of nurturant behaviors never occurred.

The high frequency of critical behaviors were caustic efforts to influence the other, efforts allowed by the other's determination to remain in the relationship. The exchange of nurturant behaviors is puzzling. Perhaps it represented the dissatisfied spouses' desperate efforts to maintain their troubled relationships. Perhaps it represented the spouses' efforts to appear caring, magnanimous, and blameless for conflict to themselves and their partners and to the experimenter. Whatever the meaning of the exchange of nurturant behaviors, Nutall's results are consistent with the notion that low availability of alternative relationships to the other encourages the person to engage in caustic efforts to stimulate change in the face of dissatisfaction.

Accountability and Responsibility   Seldom are the members of a relationship the only ones who have a stake in the process and outcome of their relationship. Parents want to know who their children form relationships with and what they do in the relationships. Spouses have the same concerns with each other. Children are concerned about how their parents relate to each other. Middle managers focus much of their attention on first-line supervisors' relationships with workers. Deans have much at stake in professors' relationships with students. Law enforcement officers and judges take special interest in certain relationships among citizens. Experimenters are deeply interested in subjects' relationships with each other. It is difficult to imagine a relationship in which someone outside the relationship is not interested in and affected by the process and outcome of the relationship.

People (the outsiders) who are interested in other people's (the members) relationships make the members accountable and responsible to them through their relationships with the members. Outsiders monitor the process and outcome of the members' relationships and make the availability of their resources to the members contingent on their satisfaction with what they see. Thus, the members' behavior is constrained by their interdependence with the outside person. The amount and nature of constraint is a function not only of the nature of the members' interdependence with the outsider but also the degree to which the outsider can observe the process and outcome of the members' relationship. At any given level of interdependence with the outsider, constant observation of the members' interaction maximizes its constraining effects on their behavior, whereas zero ability to monitor vitiates its effects. Members of a relationship manage the outsider's impressions of their performance through whatever means at their disposal—through their behavior toward each other if they are being observed, through self-reports to the outsider if that is the outsider's only source of information. Experiments on equity theory show the shaping effect of the form of monitoring on members' behavior (Adams & Jacobsen, 1964; Lawler, 1968).

The effect of interdependence with an outsider on behavior in a relationship depends on the nature of the outsider's interest in the relationship (putting monitoring aside). If the outsider holds one member accountable for producing a desired outcome through the relationship, and if the member is constrained to do so with a specific partner, the member is rendered highly dependent on the partner. The partner's actions control the member's ability to fulfill the outsider's expectations. If the member is not constrained to work with and can easily replace the specific partner, the member is much less dependent on the partner. In either case, the partner may be highly or less dependent on the member as a function of the member's constraints and needs. If the outsider holds both members responsible for the outcome, then they are rendered highly interdependent.

Outsiders often specify the nature of contributions members of a relationship are to make to one another and thus constrain the process of the members' relationship. For example, upper management determines who will lead and who will follow in work groups in business, military, educational, and most other organizations. Men have traditionally been expected to take the leadership role in families. In the laboratory, experimenters may designate who will lead and who will follow in groups of subjects. Assignment to a specific role constrains the behaviors the member can appear to employ in the relationship and still fulfill the outsider's expectations. When assigned to lead, the member is reluctant to appear to be obedient to the partner's demands. When assigned to follow, the member is reluctant to appear to lead.

Subjects' dependence on relationships with each other in the laboratory is largely a function of their desire to ingratiate and impress the experimenter. When the experimenter holds one member of an interaction responsible for a desired outcome that requires contributions from the member's partner, the member's dependence on the partner is enhanced. The member is constrained to behave in whatever ways are required to encourage the partner to behave in ways that allow the member to deliver the desired outcome to the experimenter. When both members are held responsible to achieve a particular outcome, the behaviors of both are constrained. When they are instructed to interact, but no particular outcome is specified, their dependence on each other is lower.

These features of experiments account for the differences Strong et al. (1988) and Shannon and Guerney (1973) reported in subjects' responses to a self-enhancing other. In the Strong et al. study, subjects were instructed to work together and achieve consensus. In keeping with the high level of relationship dependence these instructions imparted, subjects responded to their partners' (a confederate) self-enhancing with cooperation. Shannon and Guerney (1973) had college women in groups of six exchange views on a number of issues. Although their interaction was in compliance to the experimenter's instructions, they were not constrained to achieve a particular outcome. In keeping with the lower level of relationship dependence these instructions imparted, they responded to each other's self-enhancing statements with self-enhancing and critical statements of their own.

Gruszkos (1986) demonstrated the constraining effect of an outsider's specification of responsibilities in a relationship. In an experimental situation similar to that described earlier for Strong et al. (1988), Gruszkos appointed either the subject or the confederate to lead the interaction and select the best stories for the pictures. The other member was appointed to assist the leader as best she could. When working with a self-effacing partner (confederate), subject leaders employed high frequencies of self-effacing; subject assistants employed high frequencies of nurturant behaviors. Strong et al. found that subjects instructed to reach consensus used high frequencies of both self-effacing and nurturant behaviors in response to self-effacing confederates.

Making the leader subjects responsible for the outcome of the interaction intensified the subjects' dependence on the others' effective contribution to their work. Their self-effacing was probably intended to dispel the others' apparent perception that they had sufficient resources to carry out the assignment alone. They were attempting to generate greater contribution from the others by denying the resource advantage the others' behavior implied. On the other hand, subjects restrained from assisting resisted assuming leadership in the face of the leadership vacuum the leader's abdication into helplessness created. Instead, they focused on attempting to reassure and encourage the other to be more confident of her abilities through nurturant ingratiation. Gergen and Taylor's (1969) results are consistent with this interpretation of Gruszkos' leaders. Gergen and Taylor found that when the leaders in pairs of ROTC men were instructed to seek cooperation (solidarity) with their partners, they employed high levels of self-effacing. When they were instructed to focus on productivity, they employed high levels of self-promotion.

In a field setting, McGillicuddy, Welton, and Pruitt (1987) found that disputing parties cooperated more and conflicted less while working out their dispute when they were in the presence of a mediator who would reach the final decision than when the mediator was not present. These results suggest that the disputants' dependence on the arbitrator increased their dependence on each other and thus encouraged efforts to ingratiate each other and the arbitrator.

Individual Differences

The characteristics of the person that define features of relationships as opportunities or dangers are needs and beliefs about how features of relationships relate to need fulfillment. Interpersonal behavior is at base a function of the needs people seek to fulfill through relationships with others. Beliefs about how features of relationships relate to need fulfillment result from how other people's actions have impacted on needs in past and current relationships. Beliefs are the basis of evaluating whether features of a relationship pose opportunities or dangers. The resulting perceptions of opportunities and dangers are the immediate determinants of interpersonal behavior.

Differences in beliefs about how relationship features relate to needs is the source of individual differences in interpersonal behavior. People with different beliefs respond differently because they perceive different opportunities and dangers in the features of relationships. These belief differences can be assessed only indirectly. People are not aware of the beliefs that guide their behavior unless their attention has been directed to their behavior and its significance. Assessing people's beliefs directly by asking them what they are is ineffective. At best, people are unevenly aware of their beliefs. Assessing beliefs indirectly by asking people to describe how they behave in certain situations is more profitable, but people can only report the behaviors they have noticed. The behaviors they have noticed have been significant enough for others to have directed their attention to them. In any case, self-reports are interpersonal behaviors. They reflect the reporter's efforts to manage others' impressions of the reporter's characteristics in terms of the opportunities and dangers the reporter perceives in the situation.

The only reliable way to detect individual differences in interpersonal behavior is to observe how people behave in standardized situations. Differences among their behaviors reflect differences in their perceptions of the opportunities and dangers in the standardized situation and thus differences in their beliefs about how its features relate to their needs. Self-reports obtained under standardized conditions are not accurate accounts of feelings, thoughts, and actions but are presentations of self that reveal aspects of self of which the person is aware. Self-reports in standardized situations are intended to affect others' impressions in ways that benefit the person in that situation. Differences in self-reports reveal differences in awareness and beliefs. Differences in self-reports in standardized situations reveal differences among people that may be manifest in other interpersonal situations. However, the relationship between self-reports and behavior in other situations is by no means straightforward. Interpersonal behavior in all situations reflects the person's efforts to manage others' impressions and is sensitively attuned to the person's perception of the dangers and opportunities the situations present.

Several studies of relationships between personality and interpersonal behavior have used self-reports or partners' reports to assess interpersonal behaviors in relationships. Although these studies inform us about the behaviors people are aware of and are inclined to report, they yield a stilted picture of interpersonal behavior. For example, Buss, Gomes, Higgins, and Lauterbach (1987) gathered personality data and self-reports and partners' reports of the "manipulation tactics" members of dating couples used in their relationships. The tactics subjects reported were highly notable behaviors heavily loaded with hostility. Total scores on the *Tactics of Manipulation* questionnaire correlated negatively with six of the eight friendly scales and positively with six of the eight hostile scales of the *Interpersonal Adjective Scale*. Four of the six tactics and total scores had significant positive correlations with the Neuroticism scale of the *Eysenck Personality Questionnaire*. The pioneering work of Falbo and Peplau (1980) and those who have followed their lead (Cowan, Drinkard, & MacGavin, 1984; Howard, Blumstein, & Schwartz, 1986) suffer from the same biases. These studies suggest the conditions that make people aware of their attempts to influence others and reflect the impression management pressures on self-reports (Hastie, 1984; Holtzworth-Munroe, & Jacobson, 1985; Johnson, 1981).

The relationships between individual differences in self-reports and in interpersonal behavior are explored below in terms of the following characteristics: (a) dominance, (b) sex, (c) affiliation, and (d) relationship dissatisfaction and psychopathology.

Dominance   Strong et al. (1988) had subjects complete the *Interpersonal Check List* (ICL; LaForge & Suczek, 1955) after their interactions with confederates. Inasmuch as the experimental conditions had no differential effects on the students' scores on the ICL, we can examine the relationship of the subjects' scores to their responses to confederates. Subjects in two conditions—self-enhancing and self-effacing—were given different instructions for the ICL than those in the other six conditions. Therefore, the analysis includes only 60 women subjects, 10 in each of the six consistent conditions. For each subject, the eight ICL scale scores were combined using the procedure Leary (1957) suggested to generate Dominance and Affiliation dimension scores. Subjects in each experimental condition were divided into equal higher and lower groups ($N = 5$ in each group) by their scores on the Dominance and Affiliation dimensions. Because subjects were not assigned to experimental conditions on the basis of the scores, the cut scores varied from condition to condition. The significance of differences among subjects' percentages of responses (transformed) as a function of their Dominance and Affiliation scores (high or low) were assessed in eight two-way analyses of variance with repeated measures (time), one for each response behavior. Inasmuch as the analysis was exploratory rather than hypothesis testing, the same analyses were carried out within each condition. The small Ns and multiple analyses (56) certainly capitalized on type I error.

Table 1 shows the F ratios and mean percentages of response behaviors that were significantly different between high and low groups on the Dominance dimension and on the Affiliation dimension. Subjects higher on the Dominance dimension employed more nurturant behaviors overall, especially in response to critical and nurturant confederate stimuli. They also employed more critical responses to cooperative confederate stimulus behaviors and they increased self-effacing in time to persistent confederate leading stimulus behaviors.

What is striking about these results is that they present the same pattern Nutall (1987) found to distinguish the behaviors of dissatisfied spouses from satisfied spouses (see earlier discussion). This implies that more dominant women were more dissatisfied with confederate dominant behaviors (critical, nurturant, and leading) than were less dominant women. Like dissatisfied spouses, they contested with the confederates using nurturant counters to critical and nurturant stimuli. Perhaps they were expressing their greater command of the situation by being magnanimous in the face of a rigid and domineering other.

The more dominant women's increase in self-effacing behavior over time is also striking in light of the overall reduction of self-effacing behavior over time in the experiment. Self-effacing behavior communicates the impression that the other appears not to need one's resources. More dominant women's increasing use of self-effacing behavior in time may have been attempts to encourage the other to be less leading by accenting the status differential that the leading created. Gergen and Taylor (1969) and Gruszkos (1986) found that when leaders were constrained to cooperate, they self-effaced to diminish status differences. Perhaps the more dominant women were using this principle to encourage the persistently leading confederates to become

Table 1　*F* Value and Mean Percentages of Behaviors for Subjects High and Low on Dominance and Affiliation

Overall Response Behaviors and (Stimulus Response)	Dimension			Dimension Over Time				
	F	*M* High	*M* Low	*F*	*M* High		*M* Low	
					T1	T2	T1	T2
Dominance								
Nurturant	6.31	21.0	12.1					
(to critical)	17.41*	17.7	4.8					
(to nurturant)	6.79	21.1	7.1					
Critical								
(to cooperative)	12.37	6.0	1.8					
(to nurturant)	11.72	0.0	3.9					
Self-effecting								
(to leading)				8.19	2.5	11.1	3.2	3.6
Affiliation								
Self-enhancing	9.78*	3.5	9.4	5.00	3.3	2.9	5.7	13.1
(to leading)	6.36	0.0	8.0					
(to docile)	6.44	0.0	13.8					
(to distrustful)				15.27*	12.5	6.7	7.3	32.0
(to nurturant)				8.36	1.8	4.2	10.2	2.2
Cooperative								
(to distrustful)	6.45	6.7	14.5					
Docile								
(to cooperative)				6.65	7.7	3.6	1.7	6.5
Critical	8.26*	12.0	4.5					
(to cooperative)	16.83*	6.9	0.9					
Leading								
(to critical)				7.74	23.0	5.4	24.0	20.1

Note. All *p*s < .05; *p < .01.

aware of their inappropriate response to the instruction to cooperate. In all, these results suggest that high dominant women were more dissatisfied than low dominant women with the confederates' unyielding dominant behaviors and expressed their dissatisfaction in the same ways others do in highly interdependent but dissatisfying relationships.

Other studies have found that the member of a group who has the highest dominance score on the *California Psychological Inventory* (CPI) is the most likely one to be chosen by other members to lead the group (Fleischer & Chertkoff, 1986; Megargee, 1969; Nyquist & Spence, 1986). Nyquist and Spence (1986) found that women with high dominance scores who were not chosen to lead mixed-sex groups were less satisfied with the interactions than were women with low dominance scores. Self-reported dominance correlates with dominating behaviors in groups, behaviors that encourage others to employ submissive behaviors.

Sex When men and women interact, the men are likely to be chosen as the group leaders regardless of their relative dominance scores on the CPI (Fleischer & Chertkoff, 1986; Megargee, 1969; Nyquist & Spence, 1986). Numerous studies of mixed-sex groups have found that men are perceived to be and tend to act more dominant and competent in task management, whereas women are perceived to be and tend to act more conforming and affiliative (Buss, 1981; Eagly & Wood, 1982; Instone, Major, & Bunker, 1983; Wood & Karten, 1986; Wood, Polek, & Aiken, 1985). However, with information indicating status relationships or competency in task relevant areas, perceptions, leader nominations, and behavior become consistent with the information and do not reflect sex (Eagly & Wood, 1982; Fleischer & Chertkoff, 1986; Wood & Karten, 1986). These results suggest that sex differences in interpersonal behavior reflect perceived competence and status differences between men and women that arise from the positions of men and women in traditional social structure rather than differences directly associated with having an X or a Y chromosome.

Recent experiments by Nutall (1987) and Hawks (1987) are relevant to this issue. Nutall (described earlier) compared the interpersonal behaviors and response contingencies of husbands and wives (N = 40 couples) in 15-minute standardized interactions with one another. She found that husbands employed more leading behavior than did their wives, whereas the wives employed more nurturant and docile behaviors than did their husbands. Husbands responded with leading behavior to their wives' self-effacing behavior much more often than wives did to husbands' similar behavior. Compared with husbands, wives responded more with critical behavior to their husbands' docile behavior, more docile to leading behavior, and more nurturant to critical behavior. These differences in interpersonal behavior between husbands and wives reflect the historically traditional structure of marriages, with husbands more dominant and wives more submissive and ingratiating. The contingency patterns that differentiated wives suggest that they actively encouraged their husbands dominance by punishing docility and responding submissively to leading. Their use of nurturant behavior to husbands' critical behavior is the now familiar pattern of disagreement constrained by high interdependence.

Hawks (1987) observed the interpersonal behaviors of men and women in same-sex pairs in an experiment procedurally identical to Strong et al. (1988). The subjects responded to same-sex confederates who employed high frequencies of either self-enhancing or self-effacing behaviors. She had subjects describe their partners' characteristics on the *Impact Message Inventory* after the interactions and coded the interactants' behaviors using the *Interpersonal Communication Rating Scale*. She found no significant differences between male and female subjects in their perceptions of the characteristics of their same-sex interactants or in their interpersonal responses to the confederates. There were, however, highly significant differences in subjects' perceptions and interpersonal responses to the self-enhancing and self-effacing others, the same differences Strong et al. (1988) found (self-enhancing generated more docile and cooperative responses; self-effacing generated more leading, nurturant, and self-effacing responses). Hawks' and Nutall's findings, and those reviewed earlier from other experiments, support the conclusion that sex differences in interpersonal behavior reflect the different status positions of men and women in the social order rather than genetic predispositions to respond differently to others.

Hawks (1987) and Hills (1986) examined the relationship between interpersonal behavior and traditional and androgynous types based on the *Bem Sex-Role Inventory*. Hawks studied both men and women, whereas Hills examined only women. They both coded interpersonal responses to self-enhancing and self-effacing confederates in standardized situations similar to that described for Strong et al. (1988). Neither found differences between traditional and androgynous subjects in interpersonal perception or interpersonal behavior.

Affiliation   Subject behaviors that were significantly related to scores on the *Interpersonal Check List* affiliation dimension in the Strong et al. (1987) study are shown in Table 1. Compared with women who reported themselves to be highly affiliative, low affiliation women employed self-enhancing behavior more overall, and did so increasingly over time. They self-enhanced to leading and docile confederates. High affiliation women did not do so at all. They dramatically increased their self-enhancing behavior over time and employed more cooperative responses in the face of persistently distrustful others. High affiliation women decreased self-enhancing behavior over time to distrustful others. Low affiliation women initially self-enhanced in response to confederate nurturant stimuli, but dramatically decreased doing so as the interaction progressed. High affiliation women employed hardly any self-enhancing behavior with nurturant others. On the other hand, high affiliation women, compared with low affiliation women, used more critical responses overall, especially with cooperative partners. Their use of leading behavior in the face of criticism (critical behavior) deteriorated rapidly in time. Criticism did not affect low affiliation women's leading behavior.

Strong et al. (1988) reported that their subjects' use of self-enhancing responses increased in time overall. This finding was entirely a function of women low in affiliation. High affiliation women used little self-enhancing behavior and indeed slightly decreased its use over time. Self-enhancing behaviors communicate that one has more than sufficient resources to do the job. They strongly distance or separate from the other and assert self-sufficiency and superiority. They claim low dependence on the other's material resources. In a highly interdependent setting, a highly dependent other is inclined to attempt to ingratiate the superior other in an effort to maintain the relationship. High dependence on another restrains the use of self-enhancing. Apparently, high affiliation subjects perceived themselves to be more dependent on the relationship than low affiliation subjects and thus did not employ self-enhancing behavior. Low affiliation subjects perceived themselves to be less dependent on the other and were thus more free to assert their abilities, especially when the other implicitly impugned them (distrustful behavior).

The rapid retreat from leading behavior in the face of criticism for high affiliation women supports the notion that they perceived themselves to be more dependent on the other than did the low affiliation women. Their higher overall level of critical responses seems to contradict this, until we note that they were more critical when the other was behaving as if she was more highly dependent (cooperative behavior). In the safety of the others' apparent high dependence on the relationship, high affiliation women were free to express their unease with the confederates' inflexible behaviors. High self-reported affiliation appears to be associated with perceiving high dependence in relationships. High dependence restrains the person from behaving in ways that seriously threaten the continuance of the relationship. Lower self-reported affiliation appears to be associated with perceiving lower dependence in relationships. Less dependent persons in highly interdependent relationships are more likely to assert their superiority and claim dominance in the relationships. Self-reported affiliation correlates with avoidance of behaviors that generate emotional distance in, and threaten the existence of, relationships.

Relationship Dissatisfaction and Psychopathology

The interpersonal behavior correlates of self-reported dissatisfaction were presented earlier in terms of the relationship of marital dissatisfaction with the interpersonal behaviors dissatisfied spouses exchange. Dissatisfaction reflects the cost of maintaining a current relationship. The cost of maintaining a current relationship diminishes the cost of seeking an alternative relationship: There is less to be lost. If the dissatisfied person in a relationship perceives the other to be highly dependent on the relationship and the self to be less dependent, efforts to lever the partner into a more agreeable exchange will be launched with hostile dominant behaviors (self-enhancing and critical behaviors). If the person perceives the other to be highly dependent on the relationship but less dependent than the self, efforts to lever the other into a more agreeable exchange will be launched with hostile submissive behaviors (self-effacing and distrustful behaviors).

Hostile dominant behaviors deny the need for the other's resources and denigrate their value. They attempt to stimulate the other into submissive and ingratiating efforts to increase one's value to the dominant intimidator. Submissive hostile behaviors inform the other that the other's failure to provide needed resources is damaging the person, and thus imply that the other is uncaring, selfish, and personally and socially irresponsible. If these charges are not dispelled, the person's value, not only to the other but to others as well, is diminished. The danger the submissive intimidator poses is experienced as guilt. The objective is to stimulate the other into ingratiating dominance, which places the other's resources at the ready disposal of the person. The behaviors are also intended to intensify the other's dependence on the relationship. The other's value as an interactant is impugned. Lack of consideration for others implied by the charges suggest that she or he is not an attractive candidate for alternative relationships.

When a person launches a hostile campaign to stimulate change, the partner's costs in the relationship are increased. If the partner perceives the person to be highly dependent, dissatisfaction resulting from the increased costs will stimulate the partner to launch a counter campaign to encourage the person to change. The form of the campaign reflects the partner's perception of the interdependence balance in the relationship as described earlier. If both partners are highly dependent on the relationship, the result is a hostile and caustic relationship that will profoundly affect both members.

Beyond providing the members abundant practice and highly developed skills in making others miserable, prolonged struggles profoundly affect the members' beliefs about how others' behaviors affect need fulfillment. Holtzworth-Munroe and Jacobson (1985) and Fincham, Beach, and Baucom (1987) have shown that distressed spouses develop self-serving attributional patterns in which they see their partner as perniciously intending to harm and see themselves as blameless for their own negative behaviors. Whereas spouses may or may not contain their attributions to their relationship with each other, children are often triangulated into the conflict. They enter into their parents' conflict and use intimidation behaviors of their own to influence their parents for their own benefit. Because interdependence between children and parents is profound, the effects on the children's beliefs about the meaning of others' behaviors to their needs are profound.

Raush and his colleagues (Raush, 1965; Raush, Dittmann, & Taylor, 1959a, 1959b; Raush, Farbman, & Llewellyn, 1960) studied the interpersonal behaviors of six boys placed in a residential treatment center due to intolerable behaviors. The boys' interpersonal behaviors were marked by hostile behaviors, especially dominant hostile behaviors. They responded to others' behaviors, whether friendly or hostile, with hostile behaviors. Clearly, they perceived many of the interpersonal behaviors of others to pose dangers to need fulfillment and responded in ways intended to intimidate others into ingratiation and conformity. A striking characteristic of their behavior was that it was not situationally differentiated. They tended to respond with hostility in all situations, and thus their behavior was inappropriate much of the time. After several years of treatment, Raush and his colleagues found that the boys' behaviors more nearly approximated that of "normal" boys in a matched sample. Not only were the boys less hostile, but their behavior also became more situationally differentiated.

Strong (1986) compiled client and therapist behaviors in psychotherapy reported by Cutler (1958) and Swensen (1967). He found that client interview behavior was marked with high percentages of self-effacing (32.1%) and distrustful (16.5%) behaviors. In an analysis of the relationships among client and therapist behaviors that Mueller (1969) reported, Strong (1986) also found that the relationships among client and therapist behaviors changed between initial and later interviews. The changes revealed that clients employed distrustful and self-effacing behaviors less and docile and leading behaviors more over a range of therapist behaviors. These results, in combination with those of Raush and his colleagues, suggest that psychopathology is not the extreme and rigid employment of just any interpersonal behavior, but the extreme and rigid employment of hostile interpersonal behaviors.

Psychopathology results from beliefs that others are pernicious and that much of their interpersonal behavior poses dangers to need fulfillment. These beliefs are generated in highly interdependent relationships in which the members employ caustic behaviors in efforts to stimulate each other to change, in which neither will give in, and in which neither will leave. Self-reported dissatisfaction correlates with hostile behaviors in relationships. Psychopathology is a result of dissatisfaction in highly interdependent relationships.

⁴.EFERENCES

Adams, J. S., & Jacobsen, P. R. (1964). Effects of wage inequities on work quality. *Journal of Abnormal and Social Psychology, 69,* 19–25.

Bailey, K. G. (1987). *Human paleopsychology.* Hillsdale, NJ: Erlbaum.

Bavalas, A., Hastorf, A. H., Gross, A. E., & Kite, W. R. (1965). Experiments on the alteration of group structures. *Journal of Experimental Social Psychology, 1,* 55–70.

Billings, A. (1979). Conflict resolution in distressed and nondistressed married couples. *Journal of Consulting and Clinical Psychology, 47,* 368–376.

Buss, D. M. (1981). Sex differences in the evaluation and performance of dominant acts. *Journal of Personality and Social Psychology, 40,* 147–154.

Buss, D. M., Gomes,, M., Higgins, D. S., & Lauterbach, K. (1987). Tactics of manipulation. *Journal of Personality and Social Psychology, 52,* 1219–1229.

Carlsmith, J. M., Lepper, M. R., & Landauer, T. K. (1974). Children's obedience to adult requests: Interactive effects of anxiety, arousal, and apparent punitiveness of the adult. *Journal of Personality and Social Psychology, 30,* 822–828.

Carson, R. C. (1969). *Interaction concepts of personality.* Chicago: Aldine.

Clark, M. S., Ouellette, R., Powell, M. C., & Milberg, S. (1986). Recipient's mood, relationship type, and helping. *Journal of Personality and Social Psychology, 53,* 94–103.

Cowan, G., Drinkard, J., & MacGavin, L. (1984). The effects of target, age, and gender on use of power strategies. *Journal of Personality and Social Psychology, 47,* 1391–1398.

Cutler, R. L. (1958). Countertransference effects in psychotherapy. *Journal of Consulting Psychology, 22,* 349–356.

Eagly, A. H., & Wood, W. (1982). Inferred sex differences in status as a determinant of gender stereotypes about social influence. *Journal of Personality and Social Psychology, 34,* 915–928.

Falbo, T., & Peplau, L. A. (1980). Power strategies in intimate relationships. *Journal of Personality and Social Psychology, 38,* 618–628.

Fincham, F. D., Beach, S. R., & Baucom, D. H. (1987). Attribution processes in distressed and nondistressed couples: 4. Self-partner attribution differences. *Journal of Personality and Social Psychology, 52,* 739–748.

Fleischer, R. A., & Chertkoff, J. M. (1986). Effects of dominance and sex on leader selection in dyadic work groups. *Journal of Personality and Social Psychology, 50,* 94–99.

Forsyth, D. R., Berger, R., & Mitchell, T. (1981). The effects of self-serving vs. other-serving claims of responsibility on attraction and attribution in groups. *Social Psychology Quarterly, 44,* 59–64.

Gaelick, L., Bodenhausen, G. V., & Wyer, R. S., Jr. (1985). Emotional communication in close relationships. *Journal of Personality and Social Psychology, 49,* 1246–1282.

Gergen, K. J., & Taylor, M. G. (1969). Social expectancy and self-presentation in a status hierarchy. *Journal of Experimental Social Psychology, 5*, 79–92.

Gergen, K. J., & Wishnov, B. (1965). Others' self-evaluations and interaction anticipation as determinants of self-presentation. *Journal of Personality and Social Psychology, 2*, 348–358.

Gintner, G., & Lindskold, S. (1975). Rate of participation and expertise as factors influencing leader choice. *Journal of Personality and Social Psychology, 32*, 1085–1089.

Gruszkos, J. (1986). *The effects of situational motivations on interpersonal behavior.* Unpublished doctoral dissertation, Virginia Commonwealth University, Richmond.

Hastie, R. (1984). Causes and effects of causal attribution. *Journal of Personality and Social Psychology, 46*, 44–56.

Hawks, B. K. (1987). *The effects of gender and sex-role orientation on interpersonal behaviors.* Unpublished doctoral dissertation, Virginia Commonwealth University, Richmond.

Hills, H. I . (1986). The *effects of self-enhancing and self-effacing behaviors revisited: Looking for the meaning of within group differences.* Unpublished doctoral dissertation, Virginia Commonwealth University, Richmond.

Holtzworth-Munroe, A., & Jacobson, N. S. (1985). Causal attributions of married couples: When do they search for causes? What do they conclude when they do? *Journal of Personality and Social Psychology, 48*, 1398–1412.

Howard, J. A., Blumstein, P., & Schwartz, P. (1986). Sex, power, and influence tactics in intimate relationships. *Journal of Personality and Social Psychology, 51*, 102–109.

Instone, D., Major, B., & Bunker, B. B. (1983). Gender, self-confidence, and social influence strategies: An organizational simulation. *Journal of Personality and Social Psychology, 44*, 322–333.

Johnson, J. A. (1981). The "self-disclosure" and "self- presentation" views of item response dynamics and personality scale validity. *Journal of Personality and Social Psychology, 40*, 761–769.

Jones, E. E., & Pittman, T. S. (1982). Towards a general theory of strategic self-presentation. In J. Suls (Ed.), *Psychological perspectives on the self* (Vol. 1, pp. 231–262). Hillsdale, NJ: Erlbaum.

Jones, R. G., & Jones, E. E. (1964). Optimum conformity as an ingratiation tactic. *Journal of Personality, 32*, 436–458.

Kiesler, C. A., Zanna, M., & DeSalvo, J. (1966). Deviation and conformity: Opinion change as a function of commitment, attraction, and the presence of a deviate. *Journal of Personality and Social Psychology, 3*, 458–467.

Kiesler, D. J. (1983). The 1982 interpersonal circle: A taxonomy for complementarity in human transactions. *Psychological Review, 90*, 185–214.

Kolditz, T. A., & Arkin, R. M. (1982). An impression management interpretation of the self-handicapping strategy. *Journal of Personality and Social Psychology, 43*, 492–502.

LaForge, R., & Suczek, R. (1955). The interpersonal dimension of personality, III. An interpersonal check list. *Journal of Personality, 24*, 94–112.

Lawler, E. E., III. (1968). Effects of hourly overpayment on productivity and work quality. *Journal of Personality and Social Psychology, 10,* 306–313.

Leary, T. (1957). *Interpersonal diagnosis of personality.* New York: Wiley.

McGillicuddy, N. B., Welton, G. L., & Pruitt, D. G. (1987). Third-party intervention: A field experiment comparing three different models. *Journal of Personality and Social Psychology, 53,* 104–112.

Megargee, E. I . (1969). Influence of sex roles on the manifestation of leadership. *Journal of Applied Psychology, 53,* 377–382.

Mueller, W. J. (1969). Patterns of behavior and their reciprocal impact in the family and in psychotherapy. *Journal of Counseling Psychology Monographs, 16* (2, Pt. 2).

Norvell, N., & Forsyth, D. R. (1984). The impact of inhibiting or facilitating causal factors on group members' reactions after success and failure. *Social Psychology Quarterly, 47,* 293–297.

Nutall, S. B. (1987). *Interpersonal communication differences between satisfied and dissatisfied black and white married couples.* Unpublished doctoral dissertation, Virginia Commonwealth University, Richmond.

Nyquist, L. V., & Spence, J. T. (1986). Effects of dispositional dominance and sex-role expectations on leader behaviors. *Journal of Personality and Social Psychology, 50,* 87–93

Orford, J. (1986). The rules of interpersonal complementarity: Does hostility beget hostility and dominance, submission? *Psychological Review, 93,* 365–377.

Pallak, M. S., & Heller, J. F. (1971). Interactive effects of commitment to future interaction and threat to attitudinal freedom. *Personality and Social Psychology, 17,* 325–331.

Perkins, M. J., Kiesler, D. J., Anchin, J. C., Chirico, B. M., Kyle, E. M., & Federman, E. J. (1979). The Impact Message Inventory: A new measure of relationship in counseling/psychotherapy and other dyads. *Journal of Counseling Psychology, 26,* 363-367.

Raush, H. L. (1965). Interaction sequences. *Journal of Personality and Social Psychology, 2,* 487–499.

Raush, H. L., Dittmann, A. T., & Taylor, T. J. (1959a). The interpersonal behavior of children in residential treatment. *Journal of Abnormal and Social Psychology, 58,* 9–27.

Raush, H. L., Dittmann, A. T., & Taylor, T. J. (1959b). Person, setting and change in social interaction. *Human Relations, 12,* (4).

Raush, H. L., Farbman, I., & Llewellyn, L. G. (1960). Person, setting and change in social interaction: II. A normal-control study. *Human Relations, 13,* 305–333.

Rusbult, C. E., Johnson, D. J., & Morrow, G. D. (1986). Impact of couple patterns of problem solving on distress and nondistress in dating relationships. *Journal of Personality and Social Psychology, 50,* 744–753.

Shannon, J., & Guerney, B., Jr. (1973). Interpersonal effects of interpersonal behavior. *Journal of Personality and Social Psychology, 26,* 142–150.

Simpson, A., & Strong, S. R. (1987). Effects of prejudice and power on influence and attribution. *Journal of Social and Clinical Psychology, 4,* 423–432.

Smith, T. W., Snyder, C. R., & Handelsman, M. M. (1982). On the self-serving function of an academic wooden leg: Test anxiety as a self-handicapping strategy. *Journal of Personality and Social Psychology, 42,* 314–321.

Strong, S. R. (1986). Interpersonal influence theory and therapeutic interactions. In F. Dorn (Ed.), *Social influence processes in counseling and psychotherapy.* Springfield, IL: Thomas.

Strong, S. R., & Hills, H. I. (1986). Interpersonal Communication Rating Scale. *Journal of Personality and Social Psychology, 54,* 798–810.

Strong, S. R., Hills, H. I., Kilmartin, C. T., DeVries, H., Lanier, K., Nelson, B. N., Strickland, D., & Meyer, C. W., III (1988). The dynamic relations among interpersonal behaviors: A test of complementarity and anticomplementarity. *Journal of Personality and Social Psychology, 54,* 798–810.

Swensen, C. H. (1967). Psychotherapy as a special case of dyadic interaction: Some suggestion for theory and research. *Psychotherapy: Theory, Research and Practice, 4,* 7–13.

Thibaut, J. W., & Kelley, H. H. (1959). *The social psychology of groups.* New York: Wiley.

Weiner, B., Amirkhan, J., Folkes, V. S., & Verette, J. A. (1987). An attributional analysis of excuse giving: Studies of a naive theory of emotion. *Journal of Personality and Social Psychology, 52,* 316–324.

Wood, W., & Karten, S. J. (1986). Sex differences in interaction style as a product of perceived sex differences in competence. *Journal of Personality and Social Psychology, 50,* 341–347.

Wood, W., Polek, D., & Aiken, C. (1985). Sex differences in group task performance. *Journal of Personality and Social Psychology, 48,* 63–71.

Chapter 11

Not Everyone Can Tell a "Rock" From a "Lock"
Assessing Individual Differences in Speech Perception

James J. Jenkins and Winifred Strange
University of South Florida

Linda Polka
McGill University, Montreal

WHAT IS THE PROBLEM?

Native speakers of any language are familiar with the fact that most people who grow up speaking a different language have what is typically called a "foreign accent." For instance, it is rare to find a person who learned English late in life (or who learned English from a nonnative speaker) whose style of speech does not reveal that English is not his or her first language. It is commonly assumed that the accent results from an articulation problem, that is, that the habits of speech or even the motor patterns of pronunciation are resistant to change. Only recently have investigators begun to ask whether nonnative English speakers "hear with an accent" as well. This chapter sketches a series of studies that explore the perception of speech in a nonnative language and then goes on to ask, If a perceptual problem exists, what are its roots and what can be done about it?

The problem that we have chosen as an example of learning a nonnative language is the well-known difficulty that native Japanese speakers experience when learning the American English /r/ and /l/. Of course, this difficulty is by no means restricted to native Japanese speakers.

Speakers of many languages—for example, Cantonese, Korean, and Vietnamese—have similar problems. The distinction between /r/ and /l/ is important in the English language because it is *phonemic,* meaning that this distinction differentiates many otherwise identical words (e.g., "rock" vs. "lock," "grass" vs. "glass," "correct" vs. "collect"). Native speakers of American English make this perceptual differentiation easily and accurately under all sorts of listening conditions. The distinction is not a phonemic contrast in Japanese, however. There is a speech sound in Japanese that is referred to as /r/ but it is a "flapped-r." To American ears, it sounds most like a "flapped /d/," such as the sound of /d/ in the word "rider." Most important, there is no contrast in Japanese between this sound and anything that resembles an /l/ sound. When Japanese speakers hear an American /r/ or /l/ at the beginning of a syllable, they may perceive the sound as the Japanese /w/, presumably because that speech sound is the only one in Japanese that is similar to either of the /r/ or /l/ sounds in American English.

As an aside, we should note that the American /r/ and /l/ may be unusually difficult speech sounds to articulate even for native speakers of American English. The mastery of these sounds, in fact, develops late in children's productions and perception (Sanders, 1972; Strange & Broen, 1980), and /r/ is one of the most commonly mispronounced sounds in adult speech. A common substitution for /r/ by young children is /w/, as in their pronunciation of "wed" for "red" or "wabbit" for "rabbit." It is possible that this class of speech sounds, called *liquid glides,* is an especially sensitive candidate for the examination of the hypothesis of "hearing with an accent."

Production and Acoustic Structure of /r/ and /l/

The first surprising feature of the two speech sounds of /r/ and /l/ is that there is no one way of articulating the sounds. Delattre and Freeman (1968) pointed out that there are four quite different ways of producing an American English /r/. These different articulations, however, yield almost indistinguishable results in terms of the speech sound that the listener hears. Common methods of producing these sounds when they occur at the beginning of a syllable are as follows. For /r/, the tongue tip turns up against the hard palate just behind the dental ridge with the lateral edges of the tongue in contact with the sides of the palate, but without the middle of the tip forming a closure. This tongue position, incidentally, is referred to as a *retroflex, palato-alveolar central* position. The syllable-initial /l/, on the other hand, is made with the tongue tip in contact with the middle of the dental ridge, but with the lateral edges of the tongue lowered and not in contact with the hard palate. This position is referred to as an *alveolar lateral* position. If the American reader will pronounce "rock" and "lock" and pay attention to the position and action of the tongue tip, these verbal descriptions may be easily associated with a proprioceptive experience.

An acoustic analysis of /r/ and /l/ shows that change in the frequency spectrum, mainly in the higher frequencies, is the chief, though not the only, difference between these two sounds. Figure 1 shows spectrograms of a male voice saying "rah" and "lah."[1] The most salient acoustic difference between "rah" and "lah" is in the third major resonance of the vocal tract, called the *third formant*. As can be seen in the figure, the third formant rises rapidly from a low frequency for the /r/ but is almost level for the /l/. This was the acoustic variable that we chose to examine in our first study of the perception of /r/ and /l/ by native Japanese speakers.

PERCEPTION OF /R/ VERSUS /L/ BY AMERICAN AND JAPANESE LISTENERS

Cross-Language Study of Adults

The first study of Japanese and American listeners was carried out as a collaboration of investigators at the University of Minnesota, Haskins Laboratories in New Haven, and the University of Tokyo (Miyawaki, Strange, Verbrugge, Liberman, Jenkins, & Fujimura, 1975). The technique employed was one that had been developed by the Haskins researchers for the study of the critical physical variables in speech perception (see Liberman, Cooper, Shankweiler, & Studdert-Kennedy, 1967). Typically, speech stimuli were synthesized on a special device that permitted control of the acoustic parameters involved in each syllable. This made it possible to create speech syllables that differed from each other in a known and precisely controlled way. A common form of the experiment used a series of syllables that interpolated between one speech syllable and another in physically equal steps. Tokens from this series were then presented to listeners, who then identified them as one speech sound or another. The listeners' responses then revealed the critical physical parameters that marked the boundary between the two speech sounds. The stimuli also permitted tests of *discriminability*, that is, the extent to which listeners could tell one token in the series from an adjacent token, or a token two steps apart, or three steps apart.

---

[1] A spectrogram displays time on the abscissa and frequency on the ordinate. Thus, like musical notation, it shows the pitch of the various components of the speech signal as they change over time. The spectrogram has proved to be one of the most informative ways of displaying the acoustics of speech.

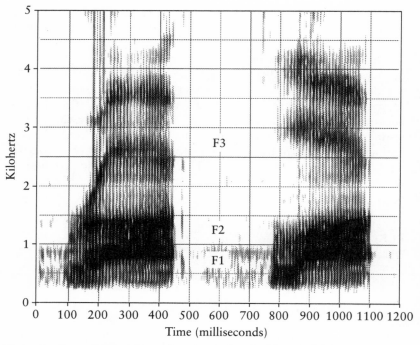

Figure 1   Spectrogram of a male voice saying "rah" and "lah"

For the experiment we are exploring here, a series of 13 synthetic speech stimuli was developed at Haskins Laboratories. The syllable at one end of the series was modeled after a good instance of an American English syllable, "rah," /ra/. The syllable at the other end of the series was modeled after an American English "lah," /la/. The stimuli at the beginning and end of the series are shown in Figure 2. For intermediate synthetic syllables, moving along the series from /ra/ to /la/, the third formant originated at a higher frequency, starting at a position about 167 Hz (cycles per second) higher for each step. All other acoustic parameters of the stimuli were held constant. Thus, the onset and frequency transition of the third formant was the only difference among the stimuli. Somewhere between the seventh and eighth stimulus, the synthetic stimuli began to sound like /la/ to the American listeners and continued to sound like /la/ to the end of the series.

The American listeners in the study performed the following three tasks:

- *Syllable Identification.* The 13 stimuli were presented 10 times each in random order for a total of 130 trials; listeners were asked to label each syllable they heard as beginning with "r" or "l."

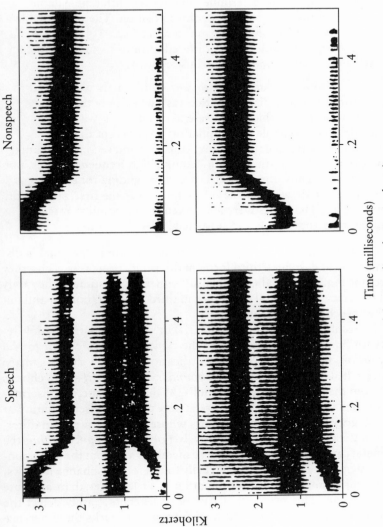

Figure 2 Spectrograms of endpoints of the speech and nonspeech series

Adapted from "An Affect of Linguistic Experience: The Discrimination of /r/ and /l/ by Native Speakers of Japanese and English," by K. Miyawaki, W. Strange, R. R. Verbrugge, A. M. Liberman, J. J. Jenkins, and O. Fujimura, 1975, *Perception & Psychophysics, 18.* Reprinted with permission. © Psychonomic Society, Inc.

- *Syllable Discrimination.* Listeners were asked to detect differences between stimuli in an oddity discrimination task. In this task, three syllables were presented in each trial. Two of the stimuli were identical and one was different (AAB, ABA, BBA). The listener's task was to determine whether the different syllable occurred in the first, second, or third position. The odd syllable always differed by three steps in the series (e.g., 1-4, 2-5, 3-6). Thus, all discrimination pairs differed in third formant frequency onset by the same amount in acoustic terms.

- *Isolated Third Formant Discrimination.* Listeners were asked to perform the oddity discrimination task when only the third formant of the syllables was presented. This task was exactly parallel to the syllable discrimination task, except that the remainder of the syllable context (the first and second formants) was removed. The stimuli sounded like high frequency glides, not like speech. Thus, the listener heard three gliding tones and was asked to decide whether the odd syllable was the first, second, or third glide. The glides were also taken from stimuli that were three steps apart along the series (e.g., 1-4, 2-5, 3-6).

The Japanese listeners were asked to perform only the syllable discrimination and isolated third formant discrimination tasks. Thus, they were not required to label or identify either set of stimuli; they only had to detect the physical difference in third formant, both in and out of the speech-syllable context.

The results are shown in Figure 3. The syllable discrimination results for American listeners show the typical findings of *categorical perception,* that is, the pooled identification function shows a sharp break, called the *phonetic category boundary,* between /r/ and /l/ choices (between the sixth and eighth stimuli). At the same time, the discrimination function shows a peak of relatively accurate discrimination at the category boundary (i.e., for pairs whose members are from different phonetic categories), but relatively poor performance *within* the phonetic categories (i.e., pairs whose members are from the same phonetic category). This finding is typically found for consonants; it shows, rather surprisingly, that discrimination is little better than absolute identification. This means that American listeners readily detect the acoustic difference in the third formant when it marks the difference *between* phonetic categories but fail to detect a difference of the same physical magnitude when it falls *within* a speech category. (See

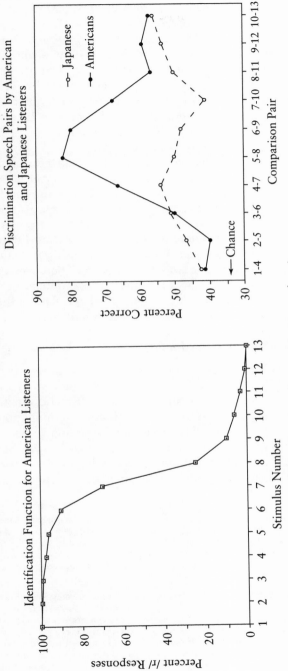

Figure 3 Identification and discrimination functions for a synthetic speech series

Adapted from "An Affect of Linguistic Experience: The Discrimination of /r/ and /l/ by Native Speakers of Japanese and English," by K. Miyawaki, W. Strange, R. R. Verbrugge, A. M. Liberman, J. J. Jenkins, and O. Fujimura, 1975, *Perception & Psychophysics*, 18. Reprinted with permission. © Psychonomic Society, Inc.

Liberman et al., 1967, Repp, 1984, and Strange & Jenkins, 1978, for discussions of categorical perception of speech.)[2]

In sharp contrast, the pooled Japanese discrimination function for these synthetic speech stimuli is relatively flat—only slightly above chance—and shows no discrimination peak in the vicinity of stimuli 6, 7, and 8. This suggests immediately that the Japanese listeners' difficulty with /r/ and /l/ is not merely a labeling or production problem. As surprising as it may seem to a speaker of American English, the Japanese listeners do not hear the difference between the /r/ and /l/ that is so readily apparent to the American ear.

When one examines the discrimination of the isolated third formant series, however, a very different outcome is found, as can be seen in Figure 4. Both the American and Japanese listeners showed highly accurate discrimination of all comparison pairs. This means that performance on the syllable discrimination test was not a result of some physical inability to discriminate the relevant acoustical differences, but, rather, that these differences did not function as meaningful cues when they were in the acoustic complex of speech. Thus, even though the Japanese listeners can readily discriminate the differences in third formant patterns when the sounds are presented in isolation, they fail to discriminate speech syllables that differ in exactly that respect.[3]

Discrimination of /r/ and /l/ by Infants

At the same time that Miyawaki et al. (1975) were conducting their study, Eimas (1975) engaged in a similar study with infants in the United States, employing the identical series of synthetic stimuli. Using a conditioning technique to test the infant's discrimination of a sound change from one stimulus to another, Eimas showed that two- and three-month-old babies growing up in an English-speaking environment could discriminate synthetic speech syllables that crossed the American English-speaking adult /r/-/l/ phonetic category boundary

---

[2]The finding that discrimination is constrained by identification is what distinguishes categorical perception from continuous perception. Continuous perception is the more typical finding in psychophysical experiments. It is characterized by the independence of identification and discrimination, that is, subjects are able to discriminate stimuli regardless of the labels they attach to them. Perception of pitch and color are examples of stimulus dimensions that are continuously perceived.

[3]It could be argued that the lower formants mask the third formant when the sounds are combined in a speech syllable and thus prevent Japanese listeners from utilizing their ability to discriminate the third formant. However, this argument seems unlikely on several grounds. For our purposes here, it is sufficient to point out that American listeners do discriminate the speech stimuli that differ in terms of the third formant only at the phonetic category boundary. Thus, physical masking of the third formant cannot be responsible for the difference in performance of the two groups of subjects.

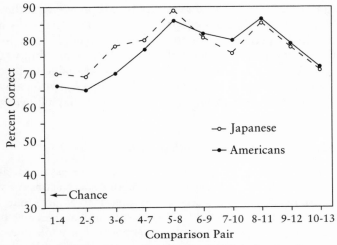

Figure 4   Discrimination of nonspeech pairs by American and Japanese listeners

Adapted from "An Affect of Linguistic Experience: The Discrimination of /r/ and /l/ by Native Speakers of Japanese and English," by K. Miyawaki, W. Strange, R. R. Verbrugge, A. M. Liberman, J. J. Jenkins, and O. Fujimura, 1975, *Perception & Psychophysics, 18.* Reprinted with permission. © Psychonomic Society, Inc.

but *did not* discriminate syllables from within a phonetic category. That is, the infants discriminated stimulus 5 and stimulus 8 but did not discriminate stimulus 1 and stimulus 4 (both of which adults labeled /r/) or stimulus 9 and stimulus 12 (both of which adults labeled /l/).

When Eimas tested infants' discrimination of the isolated third formant stimuli—the nonspeech condition—*none* of the stimulus pairs were discriminated. Although these data cannot support the notion that infants hear the speech sounds in a truly categorical manner, they do support the interpretation that there is an innate sensitivity to acoustic differences in speech patterns that are utilized in some languages to distinguish phonetic categories.[4]

If one assumes, as we do, that all normally developing human infants have essentially the same sensory equipment, it is reasonable to suppose that Japanese infants have the same innate sensory capabilities as U.S. infants. And, of course, we know that Japanese-Americans raised in this country have no difficulty acquiring unaccented

---

[4]It is important to notice that a parallel sensitivity is not found with the nonspeech stimuli, even though these stimuli contain the only acoustic component that is changing in the speech stimuli. This fact suggests that the perception is dependent on some relational properties of the acoustics of the syllable that are exploited by the speech system. It also argues against the hypothesis discussed in Footnote 2 that the third formant differences in the syllables are masked by lower frequency components.

American English. The lack of exposure to a language with the /r/-/l/ distinction, as was the case for Japanese adults, must markedly affect the individual's perception of these complex sounds later in life. Thus, the question arises: What happens to the infants' ability to discriminate these speech sounds so that it is not available to Japanese adults, like the ones that we studied in Tokyo? Is it irrevocably lost or is it a matter of reeducating the attention or reshaping perceptual habits?

The Relation of Production and Perception

At the time that these studies were conducted, we assumed, as did most investigators, that reliable production of a speech contrast was a guarantee of its perception. It seemed reasonable to assume that if one could produce a contrast reliably, one must be able to perceive it. On the other hand, it seemed reasonable to suppose that while one might be able to discriminate a nonnative speech contrast reliably when listening to the speech tokens, one still might not be able to produce the contrast accurately. A search of the literature on this topic, however, failed to confirm these beliefs. Goto (1971) performed a study of native Japanese speakers who had learned English as a second language. He evaluated both the production and perception of the American English /r/ and /l/ in natural speech. He found that some of his Japanese subjects who could produce good /r/ and /l/ tokens (as judged by a panel of native American English listeners) did not perform as well in perceptually differentiating these sounds when they were produced by American speakers. Indeed, the Japanese subjects were not highly successful in classifying their own recorded productions when they were played back to them!

Sheldon and Strange (1982) repeated and extended the research of Goto with a small sample of Japanese college students who had been in the United States for at least one year and who were reported by their professors to have good English language skills. In the first phase of the experiment, the students were asked to pronounce English words that formed minimal pairs with /r/ and /l/ (e.g., "glass"-"grass," "rock"-"lock," "correct"-"collect"). These productions were recorded and later evaluated by a panel of American listeners. The results confirmed that five of the students were in good command of English production; the American judges correctly identified 99% of the words as the speakers intended. One month later, in the second phase of the experiment, the Japanese subjects were tested on identification of recorded words spoken by the American speakers, and the words they had spoken. As expected, even these Japanese listeners with a good command of the English language made more errors identifying the Americans' productions (11% errors in contrast to 1% errors) than did the American listeners. When these Japanese listened to their own productions, the results confirmed Goto's finding. Although the American listeners made only 1% errors, the Japanese made 10% errors. And when each subject was scored only on the perception of his or her own productions, the error rate was 7%.

The Sheldon and Strange study also examined error rates in terms of the position of the /r/ or /l/ in the syllable. The error rates were highest in prevocalic consonant clusters (e.g. "grass"-"glass"), intervocalic positions (e.g., "berry"-"belly"), and in syllable initial position (e.g., "rock"-"lock"). There were very few errors on /r/ and /l/ at the end of the syllable (e.g., "bar" - "ball"). Thus, their study made several things clear. First, accurate production of nonnative phonemes does not ensure that perceptual differentiation has been mastered. Second, not all syllabic locations of /r/ and /l/ are equally difficult perceptually.

The finding with respect to the differential errors in different syllabic positions was verified in Goto's (1971) data and has been confirmed in further studies of Japanese speakers in the United States by Mochizuki (1981) and by Pisoni and his colleagues (Pisoni, Lively, & Logan, 1994; Logan, Lively, & Pisoni, 1991). This suggests, of course, that the accurate perceptual classification of /r/ and /l/ is not a matter of detecting and classifying a simple acoustic constant of some sort but, rather, is a matter of attending to a complex of acoustic variables that differentiate the phonemes in a variety of context-sensitive ways.

HOW DO PERCEPTUAL CATEGORIES CHANGE?

The Role of Experience and Training

Both common sense and data suggest that at least some adults can learn to perceive and produce the phonemes of a second language as a function of practice and exposure to speaker-listener interactions in the language. In the case of the Japanese perception of /r/ and /l/, MacKain, Best, and Strange (1981) have provided relevant experimental data. Their study, conducted wholly in the United States, examined identification and discrimination abilities of Japanese adults with different amounts of experience with American English.

To prepare for their study, the investigators developed a new /r/-/l/ series at Haskins Laboratories, using the spoken words "rock" and "lock" as the endpoints of the series. This 10-step series sounded more natural than the series used in the earlier studies and varied on more parameters: onset and transition of the third formant (as before), onset and transition of the second formant, and the rate of change of the first formant transition. All these acoustic parameters vary systematically in natural speech, although they may not all be *necessary* for native American English speakers to perceive the difference.

MacKain et al. (1981) divided their Japanese subjects into two groups on the basis of three criteria: length of time they had lived in the United States, amount of intensive conversational English training, and amount of interaction with native speakers of American English. They also tested a group of native speakers of American English for comparative purposes. All subjects were presented with three tasks:

- *Identification.* This consisted of identification of each stimulus in the synthetic series as "rock" or "lock"; as before, the stimuli were presented repeatedly in random orders.

- *Oddity Discrimination.* As in Miyawaki et al. (1975), three stimuli were presented (two identical and one different) and the listener had to determine which one of the three was different. All comparison pairs differed by three steps along the series.

- *AXB Discrimination.* The listener's task was to determine whether the second of three stimuli was identical to the first one or to the third one. As in the oddity task, all pairs differed by three steps. (The AXB task is presumed to be easier than the oddity task because both stimulus uncertainty and memory load are reduced in such a task.)

Figure 5 summarizes the results of the study. The findings for the American subjects are again typical of those showing categorical perception. The pooled identification function shows an abrupt crossover at the phonetic category boundary, and the discrimination functions show marked peaks of relatively accurate discrimination in the neighborhood of that boundary.

In sharp contrast, the group of Japanese who had little experience with and instruction in spoken English showed identification functions that were nearly flat; that is, they responded little better than chance when they were trying to identify the synthetic stimuli as "rock" or "lock." Further, these subjects showed little ability to discriminate syllables at *any* point along the series. Even on the easier of the two discrimination tasks (AXB), they had great difficulty. Performance was not above chance in either discrimination test.

On the other hand, the Japanese with intensive conversational training and more exposure to and interaction with native speakers of American English produced fairly clear boundaries on their identification functions. Their ability to identify these synthetic syllables was

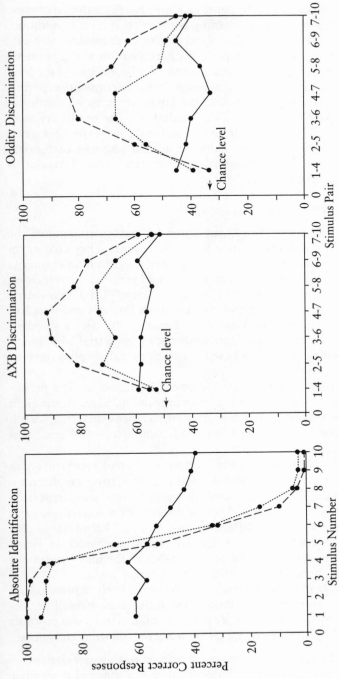

Figure 5 Identification and discrimination functions for three groups

--●-- Americans (10)
⋯●⋯ Japanese—experienced (5)
—●— Japanese—not experienced (7)

Adapted from "Categorical Perception of English /r/ and /l/ by Japanese and Bilinguals," by K. S. MacKain, C. T. Best, and W. Strange, 1981, *Applied Psycholinguistics*, 2. Reprinted with the permission of Cambridge University Press.

little different from that of the American listeners, suggesting that these Japanese were, so to speak, listening without an accent. In addition, these subjects showed considerable ability to discriminate cross-category stimuli and displayed a peak in discrimination at the phonetic category boundary. Although these listeners had not achieved the level of performance of the American speakers, their discrimination performance was significantly better than the Japanese group with little experience. As MacKain et al. (1981) concluded, "The results are most encouraging, for they demonstrate that native Japanese speakers learning to converse in English as adults can achieve phonetic categorization of /r/ and /l/ that approximates the categorization behavior of native English speakers" (p. 387).

Perceptual Training in the Laboratory

Strange and Dittmann (1984) attempted laboratory training of the /r/-/l/ distinction with eight native Japanese speakers. They used a synthetic stimulus series in an extensive course of discrimination training. The stimulus series simulated a male voice and varied concurrently on several acoustic parameters from "rock" to "lock." Training involved a same-different discrimination task in which listeners attempted to discriminate series members against a standard "r" and a standard "l." Listeners received immediate feedback on each trial over an extensive training period (14 to 18 sessions with a total of approximately 2,500 training trials).

Gradual, but substantial, improvement in discrimination performance was observed during the course of training. Seven of the eight subjects showed generalization of training to more demanding identification and oddity discrimination tasks, although performance was still not nativelike.

Pre- and posttraining performance on a different synthetic series was also studied. These tests examined the identification and discrimination of a "rake"-"lake" series, which was acoustically different from the "rock"-"lock" series, both because it simulated a female voice and also because it involved a different vowel context. Performance also improved (but to a lesser extent) for five out of seven subjects. However, the effects of training did not generalize to the identification of natural productions of words containing initial /r/ and /l/.

Considerable individual variability was noted both at pretests and in response to training. To capture these differences, overall performance on identification and oddity discrimination pretests and posttests was described by Strange and Dittmann using the following categories:

- *Chance.* The subject's responses conformed to a chance pattern, and the subject could not reliably identify any stimulus more than

80% of the time or discriminate any pair of items more than 58% of the time.

- *Inconsistent.* The subject's responses showed irregular or nonmonotonic functions, but performance was above chance in labeling stimuli at some points along the series. Discrimination results were not predictable from identification boundaries.

- *Continuous.* The subject's identification functions showed a steady change in labeling probabilities across the series with at least three of the four endpoint stimuli correctly identified more than 80% of the time. Discrimination was above chance for some of the stimulus pairings.

- *Categorical.* The subject's responses showed a pattern of identification and discrimination much like that of a native speaker.

Of the seven subjects who completed all of their testing, one subject changed from continuous to categorical perception on both the "rock"-"lock" and "rake"-"lake" series as a function of training. Three subjects changed from inconsistent or continuous perception to categorical perception on the "rock"-"lock" trained series and continuous perception on the "rake"-"lake" transfer series. Two subjects changed from chance or inconsistent to continuous perception on both series. Finally, one subject's inconsistent perception at pretest did not change. Considering the extensive training involved in this study, Strange and Dittmann (1984) concluded that modification of perception of the /r/-/l/ contrast in adults appears in general to be "slow and effortful." They further recommended that future studies be designed in such a way that subjects

> learn to abstract the relevant parameters which differentiate the phonemes while ignoring the acoustic and phonetic contextual variations that are not distinctive with respect to the contrast. This would include training of the contrast with more than one set of stimuli and in more than one phonetic context. (p. 141)

In a dissertation by Underbakke (1987) and in subsequent work by Miranda, Underbakke, Strange, and Micceri (1989), several strategies of training the perception of /r/ and /l/ were employed in a factorial design. One factor investigated differential effects of the training task: *identification* ("Label this as rock or lock") or *discrimination* ("Are these two syllables the same or different?"). A second factor compared *gradient* training, in which stimuli closer to the phonetic boundary were presented on successive training days, versus *prototype* training, in which the series endpoints or "clear cases" were used throughout training. A third factor compared training on only *one stimulus context* at a time ("rook"-"look" training, then "rake"-"lake" training, and, finally, "rock"-"lock" training) versus training on *mixed contexts,* where all three series were presented in each training session.

Native Japanese speakers who had little experience with American English were again the trainees. Several pre- and posttraining production and perception tests were administered, and every training session was followed by a brief identification test to chart the progress of learning. Thirty-minute training sessions were given each day for a total of nine training days.

The training resulted in improvement in the identification of the clearest instances of /r/ and /l/ for all training subjects. However, the observed improvements showed no overall differences based on types of training used. Furthermore, *production* of /r/ and /l/ by the subjects in the training groups improved significantly, whereas it did not for control subjects, who received no training. Again, there were no differences between groups of subjects experiencing the different types of training. However, for subjects with the poorest pretraining perception, training on prototypes appeared to lead to the greatest improvement in production. Finally, there was slight improvement for all training groups in the identification of /r/ and /l/ in samples of natural speech, but the differences were not statistically different from the control group. Overall, it seems clear that small gains in perception and production can be obtained from intensive perceptual training, but that no particular type of training seems to be favored, and the transfer from synthetic training materials to the perception of natural speech appears to be limited.

Studies of the training of /r/ and /l/ are currently being conducted in several laboratories. Logan, Lively, and Pisoni (1991), for example, reported the work of the Speech Research Laboratory at Indiana University on this very issue. To summarize the work briefly, these investigators have trained native Japanese speakers on the perception of /r/ and /l/ with identification procedures rather than discrimination procedures. In addition, their training materials were real words spoken by several different speakers (instead of synthetic stimuli) and included words with /r/ and /l/ in several different contexts. Overall, they found an improvement of about 8% (from about 78% correct to about 86% correct) as a result of three weeks of training. Interestingly, they found no improvement in the perception of initial /r/ and /l/ (e.g., "rock"-"lock"), which remained at about 80% correct. The largest improvement (from about 59% correct to about 79% correct) was in the identification of /r/ and /l/ in the context of a word-initial consonant cluster (e.g., "glass"-"grass"), where identification was poorest in the pretests.

In general, it appears that the results of training experiments directed at improving the perception of /r/ and /l/ seem to be modest. Changes in perception tend to be specific to the materials used in the training setting, and overall improvements in accuracy of identification seem to hover in the neighborhood of about 10%. At this point, we must ask whether these findings are specific to this particular contrast or whether they serve as a demonstration of a more general state of affairs. A brief review of the role of experience in shaping the perception of speech categories therefore is in order.

REORGANIZATION OF PERCEPTUAL CATEGORIES BY LINGUISTIC EXPERIENCE

Infant Studies

Developmental research supports the idea that very young infants start life with the ability to discriminate almost all phonetically relevant acoustic differences. Numerous studies using synthetic speech series have shown that infants differentiate stimuli that constitute different phonetic categories in some language, but infants generally fail to differentiate stimuli that are not differentiated in any language (see reviews by Aslin, Pisoni, & Jusczyk, 1983; Eimas, 1975; Kuhl, 1978; Werker & LaLonde, 1988). Unlike adults, infants can discriminate phonetically relevant contrasts regardless of whether they are phonemic in the language they are being exposed to (Laskey, Syrdal-Laskey, & Klein, 1975; Streeter, 1976; Werker & Lalonde, 1988; Werker & Tees, 1983). Thus, infant speech perception appears to be phonetically relevant, but language universal (Werker, 1989).

A critical question, then, is when does this universal pattern of perception change to the language-specific pattern of perception shown by adults? In a recent series of studies using natural speech stimuli, Werker and her colleagues have gathered data on speech perception from different age and language groups (Werker, Gilbert, Humphrey, & Tees, 1981; Werker & Tees, 1983, 1984a, 1984b). This research provides strong evidence that this "reorganization" of speech perception occurs around the infant's first birthday.

The research tested speech contrasts from English, Hindi, and Salish, a Canadian-Indian language. (None of the Hindi or Salish contrasts used in the study are phonemic in English.) In both cross-sectional and longitudinal studies involving subjects six to 12 months old, Werker and her colleagues showed that the ability to differentiate non-English consonant contrasts among infants growing up in English-speaking homes declined; by age 11 to 12 months, the English-learning infants no longer differentiated the Hindi and Salish contrasts, although they continued to perform well on the English contrast. Additionally, they found that 12-month-olds from Hindi- and Salish-speaking environments continued to discriminate the Hindi and Salish contrasts, respectively.

In another study, Tees and Werker (1984) showed that English-speaking children aged 4, 8, and 12 were also unable to differentiate the nonnative contrasts under the same testing conditions. Werker concluded that perceptual reorganization takes place as children learn the phonological structure of their first language. This reorganization appears to occur by the end of the first year, about the same time that children typically begin to produce their first words.

Second-Language Learning

Investigators have also studied changes in speech perception during the course of second-language learning (e.g., MacKain et al., 1981). Williams (1980) examined perception of stimuli varying in voice onset time (e.g., the difference in English between /b/ and /p/) by children who were native speakers of Puerto Rican Spanish learning English as a second language. (Spanish and English differ in the timing of the voicing boundary.) The children varied in both age (8- to 10- vs. 14- to 16-year-olds) and in their amount of exposure to English (0 to 6 months, 1.5 to 2 years, 3 to 3.5 years). The six groups of children were tested on both identification and discrimination of a /b/-to-/p/ series in the categorical perception paradigm.

The boundaries in identification functions for all the children fell between the boundaries observed for monolingual English speakers and monolingual Spanish speakers. The boundaries for Spanish children with more exposure to English were shifted more toward the English monolingual crossover. Also, within groups with equal amount of exposure to English, the shifts toward English boundary values were greater in the younger children than in the older children, although this trend was not statistically reliable. Thus, as in the study by MacKain et al., the amount of language experience appeared to be an important factor influencing the modification of speech perception during the course of second-language learning.

Whether the age at which children are exposed to this experience is a factor is unclear. Tees and Werker (1984) found that exposure to Hindi in the first two years of life (with no subsequent exposure) enabled college students taking beginning Hindi to perceive Hindi contrasts after only two weeks of study, whereas students without such early exposure who had a full year of Hindi instruction were not able to perceive the most difficult Hindi contrast. Flege and Eefting (1987) reported that 9- to 10-year-old Spanish-speaking children who began learning English at 5 to 6 years of age were able to identify a /d/-to-/t/ synthetic series, just as monolingual English-speaking children could. They also produced the English /d/ and /t/ without a noticeable accent. Thus, it appears that exposure to a second language in the preschool years leads to more nativelike patterns of perception and production of a second language than exposure later in childhood.

CURRENT VIEWS ON
CROSS-LANGUAGE PERCEPTION

When we attempt to assess the current state of our knowledge and plan for future experimentation, it is useful to employ the tetrahedral model advanced by Jenkins (1979) to describe the factors influencing the perception of nonnative speech sounds. Jenkins' model reminds us that in order to determine the outcome of any particular experimental study, experimentation in any cognitive domain must consider four interacting factors: (a) stimulus materials (e.g., natural vs. synthetic speech), (b) criterial tasks (e.g., identification, discrimination), (c) orienting tasks (e.g., instructions, cognitive strategies, training regimes), and (d) differential characteristics of the subjects (e.g., particular native language, age, degree of experience with the nonnative language). Next, we briefly consider some issues raised in specific areas and suggest some of the possible interactions among these variables.

Stimulus Materials

The research reviewed earlier has drawn attention to the question of whether we should train with natural or synthetic materials. In part, the answer to that question depends on the nature of our overall objective. If we are pursuing a particular hypothesis about the process of perceptual learning (e.g., whether particular cues should be made salient in training and then faded as training proceeds), then we must choose synthesized or electronically altered materials (Jamieson & Morosan, 1989). If, on the other hand, we are largely concerned with achieving a perceptual skill that will be useful in day-to-day discourse, the choice may well be to use natural stimuli and multiple talkers (several different speakers of the language to be learned).

There is, however, a more subtle interest in a different aspect of the stimuli, namely, how the phonemes in the second language relate to the phonemes in the first language. The research to date, of which only a little has been reviewed here, strongly suggests that some speech sound contrasts are relatively easy to learn for some people, while other contrasts are especially difficult. Best (1994; Best, McRoberts, & Sithole, 1988) has recently proposed a systematic description of the role of phonemic status and phonetic similarity in the perception of nonnative contrasts. Best argues that attention is focused on the phonemic (functional) level during ordinary speech perception and that listeners perceptually assimilate nonnative speech sounds to their native phonemic categories whenever possible. Four types of perceptual assimilation patterns have been suggested:

- *Type 1, Single-Category Assimilation,* in which both phones of the nonnative contrast are assimilated as (i.e., heard as) variants of a single native phoneme category

- *Type 2, Two-Category Assimilation,* in which the contrasting phones are assimilated into different native phoneme categories

- *Type 3, Category Goodness Difference Assimilation,* in which one phone is better assimilated to a native category than the other, that is, one is heard as a good native speech sound and the other is heard as a poor version of the same sound

- *Type 4, Nonassimilation,* in which both phones are phonetically dissimilar to any native category and therefore are not processed as phonologically relevant speech sounds at all; in this case, the sounds are heard as being outside of speech

Using this classification scheme, Best predicts that when nonnative contrasting phones are both assimilated to a single native category (Type 1), it will be difficult to learn to differentiate the phones. Further, she predicts that the ability to discriminate this contrast will decline early in infancy, if the contrast is not phonemic in the language being learned. Differentiation of nonnative phones that are assimilated in the other three ways is predicted to be less difficult. Perceptual differentiation should be observed in adults after a limited amount of training, and the ability to discriminate the contrasting phones should not decline markedly during infancy. These predictions assume that the second and third patterns of assimilation exploit phonetically relevant information that the listeners use to differentiate the nonnative phones. For Type 2, nonnative phones that are assimilated as opposing category contrasts will be perceived as analogous to a native phonemic contrast. Phones assimilated according to their goodness of fit (Type 3) will be differentiated on the basis of the degree of their perceived similarity to a single native phoneme category. Finally, phone pairs that are nonassimilated are predicted to be differentiated readily by adults if they can be discriminated in terms of acoustic properties without reference to native phonemic categories. Whether they would be integrated in ordinary speech perception, however, is not clear.

Returning to the chief example in this chapter, we would argue that perception of the /r/-versus-/l/ contrast by Japanese listeners represents a single-category type of assimilation. Because /l/ does not occur in Japanese and the Japanese /r/ is not phonetically similar to the American English /r/, Japanese listeners probably perceive both the English /r/ and /l/ as instances of the single category in Japanese—perhaps the glide sound /w/. Whether perception of /r/ and /l/ by Japanese infants declines during infancy has not yet been determined.

Best and Strange (1992) found a considerable difference between perception of an American English /r/-/l/ series and an American English /w/-/r/ series by Japanese listeners. Perception of the /w/-/r/ series by Japanese listeners was more categorical than perception of the /r/-/l/ series. The difference can be accounted for within Best's framework. Best and Strange predicted that the /w/-/r/ series was an example of category goodness assimilation, that is, Japanese listeners would recognize the American English /w/ as quite similar to the unrounded Japanese /w/ and would recognize the /r/ as a poorer instance of the same /w/ category.

Another reason for paying particular attention to the stimuli employed in our studies is that certain classes of speech sounds may simply be more difficult than others for adults to learn to perceive. In part, this may be the result of intrinsic differences in salience of acoustic-phonetic and articulatory-phonetic properties. The perceptual difficulties experienced by Japanese listeners in perceiving /r/ and /l/, even after extensive laboratory training, suggest that nonnative *place* contrasts are particularly difficult. (Such contrasts are discriminated primarily by differences in the frequency spectrum that are associated with differences in articulatory position and gesture, cf. Strange & Dittmann, 1984.) Conversely, training studies involving *voicing* contrasts have shown that perception of nonnative voice onset time categories can be improved relatively easily with laboratory training, at least for selected subjects (Pisoni, Aslin, Perey, & Hennessy, 1982; McClaskey, Pisoni, & Carroll, 1983). (Voice onset time is a temporal cue for voicing of stop consonants associated with the timing of the laryngeal gesture.) It is notable that the only study that reported transfer to natural speech of training with synthetic speech involved a voicing contrast (Jamieson & Morosan, 1986).

The suggestion that *place* and *voicing* contrasts differ in intrinsic difficulty is further supported by Tees and Werker (1984). These investigators used naturally produced stimulus materials to train English speakers to differentiate natural (unedited) consonant-vowel productions of two Hindi contrasts. To train the subjects, they used a category change procedure; they allowed the subjects to switch back and forth between samples of the contrasting categories whenever they wished. After every 50 subject-determined change trials, the subjects were tested on their ability to detect experimenter-determined category changes. One group of subjects was trained on a Hindi place contrast; another group was tested on a Hindi voicing contrast. Fourteen of 15 subjects reached criterion performance on the voicing contrast by the end of 300 training trials, and 11 of these subjects demonstrated retention of this ability when tested 30 to 40 days later. The Hindi place contrast was more difficult. Only 7 out of 15 subjects reached criterion by the end of 300 training trials, and only three retained the ability to differentiate the contrast when retested at the later date.

It is apparent that training perception of nonnative contrasts in a linguistically relevant manner is not equally difficult for all kinds of speech contrasts. Some contrasts are harder to acquire than others. (For further discussion, see Burnham, 1986.)

Criterial Tasks

In many training experiments, the focus is on improvement in the experimental task and the specific material on which the subject is being trained. It is obvious, however, that a more general goal is appropriate if we are concerned with learning to perceive the sounds of a second language in a natural context. The real goal is the ability to identify the relevant classes of speech sounds that make a difference in that language. Ideally, one should strive for rapid and effortless categorization of the speech sounds so that the lexical, syntactic, and semantic levels of language processing may proceed unhindered. Thus, one may argue that the most appropriate criterial task is speedy identification of phonemic categories in the varied contexts of natural speech. Of course, as we strive to perfect training techniques, other partial goals may be appropriate to evaluate the progress of the work and the particular virtues of one training approach or another. In the long run, however, we take it that the perception of natural speech is our most common goal.

Orienting Tasks

An important question of current concern in cross-language speech perception studies is, What types of training tasks can provide the kind of perceptual experience that will generalize to those criterial tasks that are akin to natural language processing? That is, What types of instructions, displays, activity, feedback, rewards, and the like lead to optimal learning? Current attempts to train subjects to differentiate nonnative speech contrasts reveal the limits of our understanding of this aspect of speech perception.

Consider, for example, the effect of feedback, which, by tradition, one would suppose has an important role in training. Surprisingly, research that directly examines the role of feedback in this area of perceptual learning is sparse. Werker and Tees (1984b) compared performance of two groups of English subjects in differentiating the Hindi retroflex/dental contrast in an AX ("same" or "different") discrimination task with a short (250 ms) interstimulus interval. One group received feedback during the first block of trials, while the other group did not. Although there was a nonsignificant trend in favor of the group that received feedback, both groups improved during the course of the AX task. Werker and Tees concluded that while providing feedback may have facilitated performance, it was not the operative variable in the subjects' improvement. Since the effect of feedback may well be different in particular training tasks, the role of feedback in other orienting tasks (e.g., in identification or categorization tasks) should also be examined.

Jamieson and Morosan (1986) discussed possible reasons why most cross-language training studies done prior to 1986 may have failed to show positive results (see also Pisoni, Lively, & Logan, 1994). These critiques emphasized the selection of an appropriate task for training. They maintained that training should involve *identification tasks* rather than discrimination tasks. Jamieson and Morosan point out that although previous research indicated that subjects show substantial improvement in accuracy during discrimination training, this improvement rarely transfers to the categorization of nonnative speech contrasts. They maintain that the discrimination training tasks that have been used in most training studies have the undesirable effect of enhancing sensitivity to within-category differences. Such sensitivity to intraphonemic differences is not relevant in the perception of categories and may interfere with category formation by focusing the subject's attention on the very information that should be ignored. Jamieson and Morosan recommend identification tasks because such tasks focus the subject on *categorization* of a stimulus set, which requires both accurate discrimination of relevant between-category differences *and* recognition of within-category similarities.

Even here, however, it is not clear that one recommendation will suffice. Neither Jamieson and Morosan nor Pisoni et al. directly compared identification and discrimination. There is a possibility, suggested by Underbakke (1987) and Strange (1992), that beginning learners might profit most from discrimination training, whereas advanced learners might be best served by identification training. That is, for beginning learners, discrimination tasks that emphasize differentiation of types are needed. After subjects can differentiate clear cases of each type, then identification tasks that emphasize the elaboration of categories (the abstraction of similarities among tokens of a type) may be optimal. If this is indeed the case, the hypothesized two-way inter-action, 2 (beginning vs. advanced learners) × 2 (discrimination vs. iden-tification training), constitutes the type of interaction that Cronbach (1957, 1975) has encouraged researchers to identify and respect.

Individual Subject Variability

Substantial individual differences in cross-language speech perception have been noted by researchers in this area, yet the role of individual differences has not been explicitly addressed and the bases for indi-vidual differences in speech perception are not well understood. Indi-vidual differences have received some attention in the second-language learning literature as part of the general interest in assessing language aptitude. However, measures of language aptitude often assess pho-netic ability by using imitation tasks that fail to distinguish between perceptual and production skills (Flege, 1988). Thus, they do not explain the underlying variables that may be involved.

Tees and Werker (1984), as mentioned earlier, found that individu-als who were exposed to Hindi up to the age of two (and not thereaf-ter until they took courses in Hindi in college) were able to learn to perceive the Hindi retroflex-dental contrast after brief exposure, whereas subjects without such early experience could not perceive the contrast even after a year of Hindi language instruction. Such findings have important implications for understanding differences in cross-language perception and strongly suggest that we should look to early experience as one important source of individual differences.

It is also important to notice that in almost every study reported above, there have been impressive unexplained individual differences. In the original study by Miyawaki et al. (1975), three Japanese sub-jects (out of a sample of 22) had peaks of high accuracy in their dis-crimination of /r/ and /l/ stimuli. Two of the subjects were female, each of whom had spent four years of her adolescence in countries where either English or German was spoken. Each was considered fluent in her second-language. It is presumed that this extensive exposure and second-language learning accounted for their performance. The re-maining subject, however, was a 43-year-old male whose English train-ing had taken place entirely in Japan, where emphasis was placed on reading and writing. No explanation was given for his superior dis-crimination performance. Similarly, in the study by MacKain et al. (1981), one subject in the inexperienced group showed high peaks of discrimination for which no explanation was given. Strange and Dittmann (1984) also found highly variable perceptual performance and widely different results of training among their subjects. Although these cases again implicate the role of experience, it appears that there must be other variables that contribute to perceptual performance in identification and discrimination of foreign speech sounds.

In current work in our laboratories, we have begun studies aimed at teaching U.S. subjects to discriminate and categorize the Hindi retroflex-dental contrast (see Polka, 1989, 1991, 1992; Pruitt, Strange, Polka, & Aguilar, 1990; Strange, 1992). In the studies thus far, we have found a small number of subjects who seem to grasp the contrast. In the course of their first two training trials, their errors dropped to less than 10%. The majority of subjects showed gradual improvement over the course of training. Finally, another group showed no evidence of learning at all, making the same scores at the end of training as they did in the beginning. At present, neither gender nor age seem to be implicated. We cannot identify the source of these differences.

FUTURE RESEARCH

This chapter began by asking whether people learning a second language "listened with an accent." The answer to that question appears to be a resounding affirmative. It appears to be generally the case that some phonemic contrasts may be exceedingly difficult for speakers of another language to master. In spite of high motivation and great effort on the part of the second-language learners, some new contrasts are extraordinarily hard to perceive with the same effortless skill of a native speaker of the language.

Experimental procedures aimed at training listeners to achieve the relevant perception have had modest degrees of success. Skill in pronunciation is no guarantee that the perceptual skill has been mastered. High degrees of practice on training materials lead to improvement, but gains tend to be quite specific to the training material itself and resist generalization to the variety of contexts present in daily life. Nevertheless, it is clear that over a long period of time, experience with the second language leads to increasingly nativelike perception of the new language contrast.

The evidence from developmental perception studies shows that prelinguistic infants are sensitive to all or most of the differences in speech sounds that function to define phonetic classes in the languages of the world, implying that they are universal perceivers. By the time they are one year of age, however, it appears that infants are able to discriminate easily only the speech sounds that are important in the language that they are learning naturally, the language that surrounds their lives. Important questions, then, are, What kinds of reorganization take place in the perceptual system? How does this reorganization take place? What is the mechanism of reorganization? And how may the organization be altered by further manipulation of experience and circumstances?

In this chapter, it has been suggested that learning to perceive foreign speech sounds involves complex phenomena that have many different sources and many manifestations. We cannot expect a simple answer to the questions raised here; therefore, we must conduct our research in a way that enables us to investigate several variables and their interactions systematically. In particular, it is suggested that we employ the tetrahedral model of training studies to guide our experimental investigations. If we want generalization, then we must examine a variety of stimulus materials produced by a variety of speakers using a variety of contexts. We must be sensitive to the fact that not all contrasts behave in the same way. If Best's assimilation model (Best, 1994) is correct, for example, there may be several different relationships to consider, depending on the characteristics of the particular native language and second language that are involved. In addition, there may be classes of contrasts or sounds that are especially easy or difficult to perceive because of their acoustic or gestural nature.

We will surely want to try out new training tasks as our knowledge of perceptual learning matures. The debate about the relative goodness of discrimination tasks versus identification tasks is not yet settled, and the possibility exists that different tasks may be most suitable for learners of different skill levels.

Finally, we need more informed and detailed study of the individual differences that learners bring to a given situation. It appears that all normally developed children learn their native language with no obvious effort, assimilating the language or languages around them. Learning a second-language, however, seems to be a very different matter. We are typically ill informed about second-language learners' perceptual problems because perceptual competencies are rarely tested (although production competencies are usually painfully obvious). We need to launch a thorough campaign of study that examines background variables, the ability variables, and the cognitive variables that underlie the ability to acquire the phonological system of a nonnative language.

Preparation of this chapter was supported in part by a grant from the National Institute of Deafness and Communicative Disorders, DC-00323, with Winifred Strange and James Jenkins as coprincipal investigators. Much of the work discussed herein also owes a debt to Haskins Laboratories and to the support given to Haskins Laboratories by the National Institute of Child Health and Human Development.

REFERENCES

Aslin, R. N., Pisoni, D. B., & Jusczyk, P. W. (1983). Auditory development and speech development in infancy. In M. M. Haith & J. Campos (Eds.), *Carmichael's manual of child psychology, Vol. II, Infancy and the biology of development* (4th ed., pp. 573–687). New York: Wiley.

Best, C. T. (1994). The emergence of native-language phonological influences in infants: A perceptual assimilation model. In J. C. Goodman & H. C. Nussbaum (Eds.), *The development of speech perception* (pp. 167–224). Cambridge, MA: MIT Press.

Best, C. T., McRoberts, G. W., & Sithole, N. M. (1988). Examination of perceptual reorganization for non-native speech contrasts: Zulu click discrimination by English-speaking adults and infants. *Journal of Experimental Psychology: Human Perception and Performance, 14,* 345–360.

Best, C. T., & Strange, W. (1992). Effects of language-specific phonological and phonetic factors on cross-language perception of approximants. *Journal of Phonetics, 20,* 305–330.

Burnham, D. K. (1986). Developmental loss of speech perception: Exposure to and experience with a first language. *Applied Psycholinguistics, 7,* 207–240.

Cronbach, L. J. (1957). The two disciplines of scientific psychology. *American Psychologist, 12,* 671–684.

Cronbach, L. J. (1975). Beyond the two disciplines of scientific psychology. *American Psychologist, 30,* 116–127.

Delattre, P., & Freeman, D. C. (1968). A dialect study of American R's by X-ray motion picture. *Linguistics, 44,* 29–68.

Eimas, P. (1975). Speech perception in early infancy. In L. B. Cohen & P. Salapatek (Eds.), *Infant perception: From sensation to cognition* (Vol. 2). New York: Academic Press.

Flege, J. E. (1988). The production and perception of foreign speech sounds. In H. Winitz (Ed.), *Human communication and its disorders: A review* (pp. 224–401). Norwood, NJ: Ablex.

Flege, J. E., & Eefting, W. (1987). Production and perception of English stops by native Spanish speakers. *Journal of Phonology, 15,* 67–83.

Goto, H. (1971). Auditory perception by normal Japanese adults of the sounds "L" and "R." *Neuropsychologia, 9,* 317–323.

Jamieson, D. G., & Morosan, D. E. (1986). Training non-native speech contrasts in adults: Acquisition of the English /ð/-/θ/ contrast by francophones. *Perception & Psychophysics, 40,* 205–215.

Jamieson, D. G., & Morosan, D. E. (1989). Training new, nonnative speech contrasts: A comparison of the prototype and perceptual fading techniques. *Canadian Journal of Psychology, 43,* 88–96.

Jenkins, J. J. (1979). Four points to remember: A tetrahedral model of memory experiments. In L. S. Cermak & F. I. M. Craik (Eds.), *Levels of processing in human memory* (pp. 429–446). Hillsdale, NJ: Erlbaum.

Kuhl, P. (1978). Predispositions for the perception of speech-sound categories: A species-specific phenomenon? In F. D. Minifie & L. L. Lloyd (Eds.), *Communicative and cognitive abilities: Early behavioral assessment.* Baltimore: University Park Press.

Laskey, R. E., Syrdal-Laskey, A., & Klein, R. E. (1975). VOT discrimination by four- to six-and-a-half-month-old infants from Spanish environments. *Journal of Experimental Child Psychology, 20,* 215–225.

Liberman, A. M., Cooper, F. S., Shankweiler, D. P., & Studdert-Kennedy, M. (1967). Perception of the speech code. *Psychological Review, 74,* 431–461.

Logan, J., Lively, S., & Pisoni, D. (1991). Training Japanese listeners to identify English /r/ and /l/: A first report. *Journal of the Acoustical Society of America, 89,* 874–886.

MacKain, K. S., Best, C. T., & Strange, W. (1981). Categorical perception of English /r/ and /l/ by Japanese bilinguals. *Applied Psycholinguistics, 2,* 369–390.

McClaskey, C. L., Pisoni, D. B., & Carroll, T. D. (1983). Transfer of training of a new linguistic contrast in voicing. *Perception and Psychophysics, 34,* 323–330.

Miranda, S., Underbakke, M., Strange, W., & Micceri, T. (1989). Training methods for the facilitation of Japanese students' perception of American English /r/ and /l/. *Journal of the Acoustical Society of America, 86,* (S1), S102 (A).

Miyawaki, K., Strange, W., Verbrugge, R. R., Liberman, A. M., Jenkins, J. J., & Fujimura, O. (1975). An effect of linguistic experience: The discrimination of /r/ and /l/ by native speakers of Japanese and English. *Perception & Psychophysics, 18,* 331–340.

Mochizuki, M. (1981). The identification of /r/ and /l/ in natural and synthesized speech. *Journal of Phonetics, 9,* 283–303.

Pisoni, D. B., Aslin, R. N., Perey, A. J., & Hennessy, B. L. (1982). Some effects of laboratory training on identification and discrimination of voicing contrasts in stop consonants. *Journal of Experimental Psychology: Human Perception and Performance, 8,* 297–314.

Pisoni, D. B., Lively, S. E., & Logan, J. S. (1994). Perceptual learning of non-native speech contrasts: Implications for theories of speech perception. In J. C. Goodman & H. C. Nussbaum (Eds.), *The development of speech perception* (pp. 121–166). Cambridge, MA: MIT Press.

Polka, L. (1989). *The role of experience in speech perception: Evidence from cross-language studies with adults.* Unpublished doctoral dissertation, University of South Florida, Tampa.

Polka, L. (1991). Cross-language speech perception in adults: Phonemic, phonetic, and acoustic contributions. *Journal of the Acoustical Society of America, 89,* 2961–2977.

Polka, L. (1992). Characterizing the influence of native language experience on adult speech perception. *Perception & Psychophysics, 52,* 37–52.

Pruitt, J., Strange, W., Polka, L., & Aguilar, M. C. (1990). Effects of category knowledge and syllable truncation during auditory training on American's discrimination of Hindi retroflex-dental contrasts. *Journal of the Acoustical Society of America, 87* (Suppl. 1), S72.

Repp, B. (1984). Categorical perception: Issues, methods, findings. In N. J. Lass (Ed.), *Speech and language: Advances in basic research and practice* (Vol. 10, pp. 243–335). New York: Academic Press.

Sanders, E. K. (1972). When are speech sounds learned? *Journal of Speech and Hearing Disorders, 37,* 55–63.

Sheldon, A., & Strange, W. (1982). The acquisition of /r/ and /l/ by Japanese learners of English: Evidence that speech production can precede speech perception. *Applied Psycholinguistics, 3,* 243–261.

Strange, W. (1992). Learning non-native phoneme contrasts: Interactions among subject, stimulus, and task variables. In Y. Tohkura, E. Vatikiotis-Bateson, & Y. Sagisaka (Eds.), *Speech perception, production and linguistic structure* (pp. 197–219). Tokyo: OHM Publishing.

Strange, W., & Broen, P. A. (1980). Perception and production of approximate consonants by three-year-olds: A first study. In G. H. Yeni-Komshian, J. F. Kavanagh, & C.A. Ferguson (Eds.), *Child phonology: Vol. 2 perception* (pp. 117–154). New York: Academic Press.

Strange, W., & Dittmann, S. (1984). Effects of discrimination training on the perception of /r-l/ by Japanese adults learning English. *Perception & Psychophysics, 36*, 131–145.

Strange, W., & Jenkins, J. J. (1978). The role of linguistic experience in the perception of speech. In R. D. Walk & H. L. Pick, Jr. (Eds.), *Perception and experience* (pp. 125–169). New York: Plenum Publishing.

Streeter, L. A. (1976). Language perception of two-month-old infants shows effects of both innate mechanisms and experience. *Nature, 259*, 39–41.

Tees, R. C., & Werker, J. F. (1984). Perceptual flexibility: Maintenance or recovery of ability to discriminate non-native speech sounds. *Canadian Journal of Psychology, 38*, 579–590.

Trehub, S. E. (1976). The discrimination of foreign speech contrasts by infants and adults. *Child Development, 47*, 466–472.

Underbakke, M. (1987). *Training Japanese students of English to perceive American English /r/ and /l/ categorically.* Unpublished doctoral dissertation, University of South Florida, Tampa.

Werker, J. F. (1989, January/February). Becoming a native listener. *American Scientist, 77*, 54–59.

Werker, J. F., Gilbert, J. H. V., Humphrey, K., & Tees, R. C. (1981). Developmental aspects of cross-language speech perception. *Child Development, 52*, 349–355.

Werker, J. F., & LaLonde, C. E. (1988). Cross-language speech perception: Initial capabilities and developmental change. *Developmental Psychology, 24*, 672–683.

Werker, J. F., & Tees, R. C. (1983). Developmental changes across childhood in the perception of non-native speech sounds. *Canadian Journal of Psychology, 37*, 278–286.

Werker, J. F., & Tees, R. C. (1984a). Cross-language speech perception: Evidence for perceptual reorganization during the first year of life. *Infant Behavior and Development, 7*, 49–63.

Werker, J. F., & Tees, R. C. (1984b). Phonemic and phonetic factors in adult cross-language speech perception. *Journal of the Acoustical Society of America, 75*, 1866–1878.

Williams, L. (1980). Phonetic variation as a function of second-language learning. In G. H. Yeni-Komshian, J. F. Kavanagh, & C. A. Ferguson (Eds.), *Child Phonology: Vol 2. perception* (pp. 185–216). New York: Academic Press.

Part Five

Commentaries

We end this volume with three provocative pieces. In Chapter 12, David Premack proposes the surprising thesis that individual differences would have caused the human race to fragment were it not for three countervailing forces: (a) *pedagogy*—the ability of humans to teach one another, which promoted conformity (not just among people, but also between generations) and enabled human innovation to survive; (b) the predisposition to "share experience," which allowed language and pedagogy to evolve; and (c) the relative lack of creativity in the human race, which slowed the rate of fragmentation.

In Chapter 13, Howard Tinsley casts a critical yet sympathetic eye on Minnesota psychology. To Tinsley, the distinctive hallmarks of Minnesota psychology are an individual differences/developmental viewpoint, methodology, integration, and application. He illustrates these hallmarks by drawing on the chapters by Betz, Campbell, Rounds, and Waller, Lykken, and Tellegen in this volume, and his work with Diane Tinsley on leisure. Tinsley points out that individual differences psychology is interested in more than just status, that it examines origins and causes as well as implications. But Tinsley also does not hesitate to point out that preoccupation with methodology and multivariate data-analytic procedures can easily obscure the goal and lead to a form of fixation or addiction; that quantity of research cannot substitute for integration and can result in the kind of intellectual dead end that Betz describes in the case of masculinity-femininity in her chapter; and that the application of science to the amelioration of human and societal problems is of the utmost importance.

In Chapter 14, John Holland provides a vigorous defense of the neobehaviorist, evidence-oriented view of science, that is, Minnesota "dust-bowl empiricism." He attacks the current establishment that seems to favor complexity over simplicity, explanation over description, theory over data; an establishment that is ruled by

327

interlocking editorships and editorial boards, which prizes respectability and correctness, and avoids controversy; an establishment that unduly depends on grants, fosters "grantsmanship," and thwarts unconventional and creative initiative. Holland's piece was the featured address at the 40th anniversary celebration of counseling psychology at Minnesota—a fitting conclusion to this Festschrift for the founder of the Counseling Psychology Program at the University of Minnesota's Department of Psychology—Lloyd H. Lofquist.

Chapter 12

On the Control of Human Individual Differences

David Premack
University of Pennsylvania and
Laboratoire de Psycho-biologie de l'Enfant, Paris

Let me begin by observing that the University of Minnesota was a highly appropriate place for the study of individual differences. Unlike a certain school in a neighboring state, where a party line summoned everyone to the same truth, at Minnesota in the early 1950s there was no established truth—only the pursuit of truth by widely different paths, with no guarantee of safe arrival. In many respects, there were not even guides; one was supposed to take the trip alone. To be sure, some of the liberty resulted more from neglect than an explicit policy—clearly the case with the experimental curriculum—yet even the better-defined clinical curriculum did not impose a unitary view. Although I have found many campuses over the years where I preferred the weather (not to mention the architecture), I have found few where I preferred the intellectual climate.

The Minnesota policy was not an idealistic one, however; it was, for reasons that I will make clear in this chapter, quite realistic, though, at the same time, somewhat dangerous. Realistic because, in fact, individual differences among human species are enormous—greater than in any other species. Humans are not only more intelligent than other species, more talkative, more this, that, and the other, but also more different from one another than are members of any other species—a difference that is far less observed. A comparative atlas of brains would, I believe, show clearly that human brains differ from one another more than do brains of any other species. Hence, an educational policy that fostered disparate views is well suited to the human species; whereas one that promulgated a monolithic view is less well suited and would fit other species better.

THE THREAT OF HUMAN
INDIVIDUAL DIFFERENCES

But I have made two claims about Minnesota policy: not only that it was realistic, but also that it was dangerous. Before dealing with the latter claim, let me digress to say I regret the lack of data that prevents demonstrating the uniqueness of human individual differences in a more quantitative manner. While I am convinced that human minds differ in far greater degree than do the minds of other species, this is still a clinical impression based on 40 years of comparing different species. The only data that comes to mind is Tyrell's celebrated failure to breed intelligence in rats. Has it since been discovered that he proceeded incorrectly, or is it rather that, as I suspect, the variability in rat intelligence is too small for breeding to produce significantly different strains?

In lieu of data, one can also argue that individual differences must be proportional to complexity and that the complexity of human mental machinery certainly exceeds that of all other species; therefore, human individual differences must exceed that of other species. But this, too, is only argument.

The absence of data also keeps us from appreciating some of the problems that would arise in attempting to make the comparisons. What measures should be used in comparing the individual differences of rats and people? Perhaps we should test both species on the same (size-adjusted) maze, and then compare the variance of their scores? But if we did, humans might show less variance than rats, proving only perhaps that the maze is too simple and does not bring into play those human resources for which individual differences are large. Simply comparing the two species on a common apparatus is not sufficient; we must compare them on a set of problems covering a broad range of difficulty. As problem difficulty increases so should the variance of the scores of each species, but at a markedly greater rate for humans than for rats. Notice that this approach presupposes theories of both rat and human competence, theories sound enough to permit judiciously choosing the problems on which to test each species. This may largely explain why the data are missing.

Why is the Minnesota policy, though realistic, nonetheless dangerous? Because, it seems to me, a society composed of individuals whose brains are as different as are those of a group of humans is in danger of coming apart. The centrifugal force arising from the combined differences of that magnitude must be enormous! (Or do some differences annul others?) In any case, something must be done to hold such a group together. Therefore, an educational policy that not only tolerates but also even encourages different views must be something of a danger.

To get a sense of the human potential for disunity, we need not look at pictures of human brains or read theories about their development (e.g., Edelman, 1987)—theories that in emphasizing developmental rather than genetic factors help explain some of the individual differences—instead, we can test young children. Even the simplest of tests will reveal the diversity of children.

For example, sit on the floor with a child, draw a chalk oval on the floor, and then lay out parts of a face before the child—cardboard eye, nose, and mouth shapes—implicitly inviting the child to assemble the face inside the oval. Many children eagerly seize the pieces, forming them into a face, attacking and solving the problem immediately. Others turn the pieces over, discovering the blank undersides, and then play with the unindividuated pieces to form "towers." Still others, whom I will turn to in a moment, make a face and then modify it. A few become pale, glance about nervously, and never touch the pieces. The problem is too unstructured for them because they have not been told what to do—thus, they panic, glancing about for a way to escape. And yet still others respond in different ways. The individual differences brought out by even this simple experiment are striking!

INDIVIDUAL DIFFERENCES
AND THE ABUSE OF POWER

Immorality has many sources, individual differences, as we shall see in this section, among them. But consider first two other basic factors that contribute to immorality: We live in a world of limited resources and we strongly prefer some resources over others. This combination already makes it likely that some individuals will be susceptible to control by others, for reasons that I will clarify shortly, though it does not by itself make immorality inevitable. We could share the limited resources equitably. Indeed, there is some suggestion that during the Pleistocene, our ancestors approximated this benign condition, not with everyone, of course, but at least among other group members. Contemporary hunter-gatherers have been observed to share in this manner; moreover, the distribution of power between the sexes in some of these groups is remarkably equitable (Lee & Devore, 1976). However, with the event of pastoralism and, especially agriculture, possession and power became concentrated in the hands of a few. The inequity did not come from the practice of agriculture per se but from the large populations that it made possible. Sharing is more likely to occur among members of a band than of a large group.

Those having power gained control of access to preferred items, putting them in a position to force others to "work" to obtain these items. That people will work—that is, do more of a nonpreferred act than they would normally—to obtain access to preferred items is nothing more than applied reinforcement theory. A preferred item made contingent upon responding to a less preferred item leads inevitably to an increase in responding to the less preferred item (Premack, 1959, 1965). Work is reinforcement theory in action.

Interestingly, we are the only species that works, that is, the only species in which some control others by work, that is, by gaining access to preferred items and requiring others to carry out less preferred acts to gain access to more preferred ones. Why is this so? What principles apply to humans that do not apply to nonhumans? It cannot be reinforcement—all vertebrates are subject to the control by reinforcement. Nor can it be preference, or the fact that nonhumans do not live in worlds of limited resources.

Of course, pastoralism and agriculture are not found widely. Except for social insects (Wilson, 1975), they are found only in humans. To engage in agriculture, one must have either the right instincts (ants) or knowledge of biological principles, which we have reason to believe has its origins in the domain-specific knowledge of the infant or child (cf. Carey, 1995; Keil, 1995). So nonhumans do not work and do not control one another by applied reinforcement theory, in part because of cognitive factors.

But individual differences play a role in bringing about work. Limited resources and preference are a highly catalytic pair, but add massive individual differences to this pair and work—the control of one individual by another—is all but inevitable. When differences in ability are as great as they are among humans, it is virtually certain that power will come to be distributed inequitably, that some will gain access to preferred resources, and, therefore, that others will be forced to work to gain access to these captive resources. Limited resources, preference, reinforcement, massive individual differences—this combination assures "work"—the control of one individual by another and repeated opportunity for abuse of power or immorality.

A society made up of individuals so different must have a great potential for disunity. Human groups must have mechanisms that serve to reduce the differences among their members and thus protect them against disunity. Consider four mechanisms found in humans that could in principle serve to counteract individual differences and help bind humans together.

IMITATION AND PEDAGOGY

Most species rely on learning to produce uniformity across generations. Because nonhuman animals do not make fundamental changes in their environment, each generation grows up in the same world. Therefore, each generation learns largely the same things. Humans, however, operate vigorously on their environments, changing them continually, virtually assuring that parent and child will not grow up in the same world. Therefore, learning alone will not produce conformity across generations in humans.

Imitation

Imitation is the first of two devices that compensate for the inability of learning to assure continuity across generations in the human case. Humans imitate virtually from the time of birth (Meltzoff & Moore, 1983), but nonhuman primates do not. "Monkey see, monkey do" is a misleading adage. And monkeys are not alone in their failure to acquire new modes of problem solving by observing a model; wild chimpanzees evidently share this inability (Visalberghi & Fragaszy, 1990). Only when reared by humans do chimpanzees imitate extensively (Premack & Premack, 1994).

Pedagogy

Pedagogy, the teaching of one individual by another, is the major device by which humans achieve conformity, both within and between generations. Though one finds precursors of pedagogy in nonhuman animals (e.g., Premack, 1984, 1991), the full-fledged version is found only in humans. Only the human parent trains his or her child over and over until the child's behavior conforms with a well-defined standard. Interestingly, while the failure of most species to do this can be readily explained on cognitive grounds, the failure of the chimpanzee cannot be so explained. The chimpanzee has the major cognitive prerequisites for pedagogy, including a theory of mind, that is, the attribution of mental states to others, and yet it does not engage in pedagogy. It seems necessary to explain the chimpanzee's failure on conative or motivational grounds.

Two motivational factors are weak or lacking in the ape. One is an aesthetic factor. Strong in humans, this factor is either weak or absent in animals. For instance, humans not only train others, they also train themselves (Premack, 1984, 1991). They spend hours practicing, honing their skills, not for extrinsic reward but to bring the skill (or the artifact produced by the skill) into conformity with an aesthetic ideal. Moreover, the same standards that guide an individual's practice also guide his or her pedagogy. These standards are responsible for the compunctious character of human pedagogy and for the fact that human intervention is not desultory, as it is in the chimpanzee, which may occasionally correct an offspring once or twice, but is pursued relentlessly until the child attains the standard. Practice, the training of self, and pedagogy, the training of others, go hand in hand. One is not found without the other. By and large, in the nonhuman animal, one finds neither, not the honing of personal skills nor the training of the other (see Premack, 1991, for the occasional exception).

Pedagogy is more certain to bring about conformity between parent and child than is either learning or even learning combined with imitation. A parent does many things that a child cannot acquire through either learning or imitation. This is true not only of modern skills—reading, writing, arithmetic—but also of ancient ones—lithic tool making (in which the construction of a tool is carried out in three or four stages). To teach these skills, the expert cannot rely on the novice's observation but must also observe the novice (unlike imitation, where only the novice observes the expert) and then judge and correct the person. Therefore, there is a need for pedagogy in the human case, not only because humans continually change their environment , which greatly limits the contribution that learning can make to conformity, but also because certain human skills simply cannot be acquired without the judgment and intervention of a second party. Human conformity depends on pedagogy.

Nonhuman animals have no skills that depend upon the intervention of a second party. For instance, there is nothing an adult chimpanzee does that a young chimpanzee does not acquire on the basis of learning (and perhaps imitation, though in the wild chimpanzee, even the imitation is in doubt).

Pedagogy makes a further contribution to human conformity. It contributes to the survival of innovations by gifted members of the population. Again, the disparity of human intelligence is such that the innovation of a specialist is unlikely to be acquired by nonspecialists unless they are given pedagogic assistance. By specialist, I mean not only scientists and mathematicians but also, for example, household cooks. Some innovations may be simple enough to be acquired on an observational basis, but even a good household cook can invent procedures that only another expert could acquire without instruction.

Indeed, the very concept of expert or specialist applies only to humans. Specialized competence comes in part from the modularity of human intelligence, which is far more marked in humans than in other species and is itself a source of individual differences.

When in human or protohuman history did "exceptional" tools, tools that bore the mark of an expert and that stood out from others, first appear? Whatever the date, the occurrence was a likely harbinger of fundamental changes in human culture. For division of labor—more basic even than that which is based on sex—lay ahead. Notice that in most species, sex is the only major source of diversity—that and age. Whereas in the human, though sex and age are major sources of diversity, competence (i.e., the variation in competence) is yet another fundamental source.

In brief, human groups need pedagogy so that children will acquire adult skills, so that the innovations of gifted members will be perpetuated, and so that potentially different minds will acquire the same beliefs and conform to the same traditions. There is no surer way to produce conformity than to teach it.

THE DISPOSITION TO SHARE EXPERIENCE

A second device that can serve to keep human individual differences under control is a disposition to share experience. This disposition, which is part of the general human social competence, is detectable from early infancy. For instance, a six-month-old infant clinging to a teddy bear makes eye contact with an observer, then glances at his teddy bear, inviting the observer to share with him the presence of the bear and the child's possession of it. In the child of 11 or 12 months, who is likely to possess a few words, the evidence takes a more conspicuous form. The child points excitedly at an object, almost always calling out its name repeatedly, and at the same time avidly seeking eye contact with her observer (Bates, 1976; Premack, 1990).

The child is not requesting the object, as tests have shown (Premack, 1990), but rather is inviting the recipient to share the excitement of the object the child has encountered. No comparable behavior has been reported in chimpanzees, neither visual behavior analogous to that of the preverbal child nor combined visual-verbal behavior (in the language-trained animal) analogous to that of the older child.

The disposition to share experience is likely to have played a key role in the evolution of the human species. Language and pedagogy being independent—one does not need language to teach another— the combination of these two competencies could have resulted in four kinds of species: those with both language and pedagogy, those without either, and those with one or the other. However, we do not find "mixed" cases, that is, species having language without pedagogy or having pedagogy without language. Rather, we find species with either both competencies or neither.

This restriction on the logical possibilities can be explained by the disposition to share experience. Given this factor, both language and pedagogy are likely to evolve; without it, neither is. The common code or sharing symbols that language presupposes is unthinkable without a disposition to share experience. Such a disposition seems equally essential for the evolution of pedagogy, for pedagogy involves bringing others into conformity with the standards one applies to oneself. The absence of this disposition might well explain the absence of both language and pedagogy in the chimpanzee. A high price to pay for what on the surface would appear to be a secondary factor!

CREATIVITY

A third factor that may counter individual differences and keep humans from fragmenting is the fact that, contrary to common belief, humans are only a modestly creative species. Though humans cherish creativity—sometimes even characterizing themselves as the inventive species—they are not as inventive as they suppose, as I will show in this section. They are not, I would argue, because they cannot afford to be. Perhaps if individual differences among humans were not as great as they are, humans could then be more creative. But under the circumstances—dangerous centrifugal force of high individual difference—even the little creativity in which humans engage may pose a risk.

Three pieces of evidence point to serious limitations in human creativity. The first comes from a venerable study (for which I can no longer find the reference) showing the small percentage of professional chemists who engage in publication, that is, who have gone on to publish work after their thesis (something less than 10%). Moreover, publication itself is at best a necessary condition for creativity. What proportion of published work can honestly be called creative? Even if we estimate this in a most generous fashion, we are still left with the fact that, say, more than 95% of chemists do not engage in creative chemistry. Is this peculiar to chemistry or, as our next example suggests, more representative than peculiar?

Mathematics is a field that has an unusual relation to creativity. Because of its formal nature, stricter judgments of creativity are more possible in math than in other fields. As a consequence, a creative contribution for the Ph.D. in math is a serious requirement, not simply part of the doctoral rhetoric as it is in most fields. The result has been a chronic shortage of Ph.D.s in math—a shortage that has come to public attention because it results in a shortage of teachers. A doctorate is required to teach math at the university level, and there are too few candidates to meet university teaching needs. People have considered awarding two degrees—one requiring creativity, the other merely competence with regard to existing math—and then accepting both as qualification for university-level teaching.

For our purposes, the interest in the math example is the comment it makes about human creativity. In a field in which creativity is subject to serious judgment, the proportion of specialists who can meet the criterion is so small that a practical problem exists. We may ask the same question of mathematics that we asked earlier of chemistry. Is math peculiar? Or, suppose creativity could be judged as strictly in other fields as it can be in math. Would the teacher shortage then be confined to math? This is not, I think, the kind of pickle that a highly creative species would ever find itself in.

The third piece of evidence returns us to children and the simple test we considered earlier. In the course of reassembling the face, some percentage of children improvise. Having begun with a veridical reconstruction—placing the mouth, nose, and eyes in proper positions, which is the modal order of reassembly—they transform the face, changing it into something noncanonical. For example, they may place both eyes on the left side of the face or interchange eyes and mouth or produce a squashed face by pushing the features together. Still others abandon the face and make figures that would rarely be interpretable were it not for the child's accompanying remark, "Now it's a bug," "Now it's a snake," and so on.

When making noncanonical faces and when "changing the topic" by converting the face into a bug, children show a decided heightening of affect. Facial expression and affective tone are like those found in humor or wit. They laugh, giggle or smile, and increase eye contact, as though they were saying to the observer, We both know that I know better and that I'm now engaged in another enterprise.

The percentage of children who made such transformations, in a sample of 55 five- to seven-year-olds, was about 9% (roughly the same percentage of chemists who publish). We tried to increase this figure, but could find no way to do so (short of telling the child to make such changes). We did, however, succeed in increasing the rate of improvisation in children already identified as transformers from earlier tests by changing the stimulus material that was given to them (Premack, 1975).

Although humans regard themselves as an inventive species, and even characterize themselves in this light, the evidence noted here suggests that the level of creativity in humans is modest. A minority of chemists publish, so few mathematicians can meet strict standards of creativity that a shortage of teachers has resulted, and few children improvise, most simply reconstructing veridical figures. I did not select these cases from a larger set, leaving out others that would support the opposite conclusion. Indeed, I should like to know of other cases that could be used to estimate creativity in humans.

CONCLUDING REMARKS

Among the features that distinguish the human species are, I believe, individual differences of an unusually large magnitude. Humans differ more from one another in intelligence and other mental capacities than do other species. Although, regrettably, this claim is based on clinical impression rather than data, if data were seriously sought there are excellent reasons for supposing that they would be found. For example, attempts to breed rats differing in intelligence failed, whereas human differences in intelligence are well established. Further, human intelligence has a modularity or degree of modularity that is lacking even in the chimpanzee. There is no question that complexity and individual differences go hand in hand and that human mental complexity exceeds that of other species. I have taken the apparent disproportionate magnitude of human individual differences for granted and have asked what are the consequences of this condition.

I have assumed that a species whose members differ from one another in the degree that humans do is in danger of fragmentation. Perhaps this is a faulty assumption. Perhaps a group of markedly different individuals will have a smoother course than a group of similar individuals; the latter may get on one another's nerves, whereas individuals who contrast may find one another stimulating. However, I doubt it. The integrity of a group depends on uniform traditions, and the imposition or acceptance of uniformity by highly different minds seems far more problematic than the imposition or acceptance by highly similar minds.

On the assumption that humans, because of their marked difference from one another, are in danger of fragmenting, I looked for mechanisms that could counter this condition. I found four: imitation, pedagogy, a disposition to share experience, and a measure of creativity more modest than humans usually credit themselves with.

The first three of these mechanisms are either not found in other species or are found only under special conditions (imitation in human-reared chimpanzees). Each of these mechanisms may have evolved for independent reasons, yet working together they could suppress human individual differences and promote human uniformity. The differences that separate one human from another appear to be vastly greater than those that separate members of other species. Individual differences of this magnitude may be a greater threat to disunity than meets the eye.

THE EFFECT OF EXPERTS

Humans, because of massive differences in intelligence, are more affected by *experts* than any other species. The species is pulled ahead by its experts; the advantages are so clear, they scarcely need comment. But are there no disadvantages? Nonexperts lead lives determined by factors beyond their grasp. Are they confused? Or rather, how does the confusion affect them? The experts are a tiny minority. Yet they fill the lives of the majority with ever-changing alternatives. More than is true for any other species, a majority is led by a minority. Perhaps the masses of nonexperts behave irrationally as a consequence. If their lives were less affected by experts, would they behave as aberrantly?

REFERENCES

Bates, E. (1979). *The emergence of symbols: Cognition and communication in infancy.* New York: Academic Press.

Carey, S. (1995). On the origin of causal understanding. In D. Sperber, D. Premack, & A. J. Premack (Eds.), *Causal cognition: A multi-disciplinary debate.* Oxford, UK: Clarendon Press.

Edelman, G. M. (1987). *Neural Darwinism: The theory of neuronal group selection.* New York: Basic Books.

Keil, F. C. (1995). The growth of causal understandings of natural kinds. In D. Sperber, D. Premack, & A. J. Premack (Eds.), *Causal cognition: A multi-disciplinary debate.* Oxford, UK: Clarendon Press.

Lee, R., & Devore, I. (1976). *Kalahari hunter-gatherers: Studies of the Kung San and their neighbors.* Cambridge, MA: Harvard University Press.

Meltzoff, A. N., & Moore, M. K. (1983). Newborn infants imitate adult facial gestures. *Child Development, 54,* 702–709.

Premack, D. (1959). Toward empirical behavior laws: I. Positive reinforcement. *Psychological Review, 66,* 219–233.

Premack, D. (1965). Reinforcement theory. In Levine, D. (Ed.), *Nebraska Motivation Symposium.* Lincoln: University of Nebraska Press.

Premack, D. (1975). Putting a face together. *Science, 188,* 228–236.

Premack, D. (1984). Pedagogy and aesthetics as sources of culture. In M. Gazzaniga (Ed.), *Handbook of cognitive neuroscience.* New York: Plenum Press.

Premack, D. (1990). Words: What are they? and do animals have them? *Cognition, 37,* 197–212.

Premack, D. (1991). The aesthetic basis of pedagogy. In R. R. Hoffman & D. S. Palermo (Eds.), *Cognition and the symbolic processes.* Hillsdale, NJ: Erlbaum.

Premack, D., & Premack, A. J. (1994). Why animals have neither culture nor history. In T. Ingold (Ed.), *Companion encyclopedia of anthropology.* London: Routledge.

Visalberghi, F., & Fragaszy, D. M. (1990). Do monkeys ape? In S. T. Parker & K. R. Gibson (Eds.), *Language and intelligence in monkeys and apes.* New York: Cambridge University Press.

WIlson, E. O. (1975). *Sociobiology: The new synthesis.* Cambridge, MA: Belknap Press.

Chapter 13

The Minnesota Counseling Psychologist as a Broadly Trained Applied Psychologist

Howard E. A. Tinsley
Southern Illinois University

The history of psychology at the University of Minnesota involves a large cast of characters and a lengthy list of accomplishments. Lashley began his work on the localization of brain functions at Minnesota and Skinner wrote *The Behavior of Organisms*. It was at Minnesota that Festinger developed the theory of cognitive dissonance, Meehl developed construct validity theory and wrote his treatise on statistical prediction, and Paterson, Williamson, Darley, Berdie, and Hagenah created the discipline of counseling psychology; it was where Hathaway and McKinley worked on the *Minnesota Multiphasic Personality Inventory*, where Campbell worked on the *Strong Interest Inventory*, and where Lofquist and Dawis worked on the theory of work adjustment. The list of signal accomplishments by Minnesota scholars seems endless.

Borow (1990) has described the training model and development of the counseling psychology program at the University of Minnesota in an insightful and interesting treatment. Counseling psychology was not narrowly focused on training students to provide service to clients on a one-to-one basis, nor was it conceptualized as a subdiscipline of clinical psychology. Instead, counseling psychologists were trained as scholars and expert problem solvers who were prepared to function effectively in industrial/organizational and human services settings. The Minnesota counseling psychologist in the late 1960s was broadly trained as an applied psychologist with a thorough grounding in the basic science of psychology. Added to this were intervention skills that allowed them to use their scientific training effectively in attempting to solve important problems confronting society. The cornerstones of their education were the Minnesota differential/developmental philosophy and its emphasis on methodology, integration, and application. The chapters by Betz, Campbell, Rounds, and Waller, Lykken, and Tellegen in this book and my own work all bear the Minnesota stamp.

PHILOSOPHY

Differential psychology and a developmental perspective form the philosophical cornerstone of the Minnesota psychologist's education. Differential psychology might be characterized as the study of all the ways in which individuals differ. This includes not only a focus on the individual as unique, but also an examination of potential moderators of individual differences such as sex, age, social class, culture, race, and special talents (intellectual or artistic). Concern for the genesis of these differences in genetic or environmental factors is a hallmark of differential psychology, as is an emphasis on the development of new methods for analyzing these issues.

Betz's review of work on gender-related individual difference variables and Campbell's study of brigadier generals in this book illustrate the concern of differential psychologists for individual and group differences. Campbell's focus on an extraordinary group of individuals brings to mind Terman's study of genius (Terman, 1925; Terman & Oden, 1947, 1959) and Getzels and Jackson's (1962), Guilford's (1950), Roe's (1953) and Torrance's (1962) studies of creativity and eminence. Campbell's summary statistics depict the typical brigadier general, but even with so specialized a group, he often finds this generic view to be inadequate: "Averages conceal the individual richness and the enormous range of individual differences in these patterns." This also speaks for Betz's position on gender-related differences, and it articulates a central tenet of differential psychology.

Waller et al.'s (this volume) efforts to determine the extent that behavior is influenced by nature and nurture continues a line of research initiated by differential psychologists such as McNemar (1933) more than half a century ago. Minnesota psychologists have made important contributions in this quest (e.g., Gottesman, 1963; Moloney, Bouchard, & Segal, 1991). Waller et al.'s focus on the heritability of career and leisure interests, and the relation of these to personality, represents an integration of research emphases long identified with

Minnesota psychologists. Lofquist and Dawis (1978) have written extensively on work values as an important aspect of the work personality. Holland's (1985) conceptualization of career interests as an expression of personality stimulated a major shift in the way psychologists viewed vocational interests. Gottesman's (1963) early work on the heritability of personality and intelligence helped to establish Minnesota at the forefront of research on behavior genetics.

In his chapter, Rounds focuses on individual differences among occupational environments rather than people. His effort to identify groups of occupations, the relations among these groups, and the relationships of individuals to occupations continues a long and proud Minnesota intellectual history. This intellectual tradition encompasses both work done at Minnesota (Paterson and the Employment Stabilization Research Institute, Clark and the *Minnesota Vocational Interest Inventory,* Campbell and the *Strong Interest Inventory,* Lofquist and Dawis and the theory of work adjustment) and work done by Minnesota graduates (Holland and the *Self-Directed Search,* Krumboltz and social learning theory).

A major focus of Rounds' investigation is on sex differences, a traditional inquiry of differential psychologists. Rounds examines the extent to which Holland's hexagon is adequate as a model of the relations among basic interests. He concludes that the model is adequate for men, whereas I judge his data as suggesting it is inadequate. We do agree, however, that the model is inadequate for women and that the results suggest that the structural relations among occupations are different for men and women.

Rounds concludes that for men, occupations differ on a continuum from masculine to feminine, an unfortunate terminology that tends to perpetuate stereotypic views of gender-appropriate occupations. As Betz notes in her chapter, these constructs have not been defined adequately in a theoretical sense and very little progress has been made in explicating a nomological network within which they can be investigated. Further, the bipolar dimension harkens back to the single factor model, which is now discredited (see Betz, this volume). I interpret Figures 4 and 6 in Rounds' chapter to suggest the presence of instrumental-expressive and people-things dimensions. Occupations such as engineering, office practices, and agriculture require direct action to accomplish outcome-oriented objectives. In contrast, occupations such as music, art, writing, and performance activities place a premium on the ability to express oneself, with the desired objective being skillful participation in a process.

The results for women seem to vary along a dimension connoting differences in professional skill and socioeconomic level. Law, music, math, and writing require highly specialized skills and confer upon the worker a considerable level of socioeconomic status. Fewer or more easily acquired skills are needed for occupations such as those found in personal service, office practices, and domestic occupations, and a lower socioeconomic status is afforded these workers by society.

The finding that men and women's basic interests are configured differently is familiar yet important. They suggest some support for the frequently voiced view that men tend to view the world as presenting a series of problems or situations that are dealt with most effectively by a direct attempt to find solutions. Figures 4 and 6 in Rounds' chapter suggest that the basic interests expressed more frequently by men (e.g., agriculture, military activities, math) are high in this regard, whereas those they express less frequently (writing, teaching, domestic work) require expressive qualities. The observation that women tend to view the world in terms of power relationships is also supported (Rounds, this volume, Figs. 5, 7). Basic interests that are associated with less power or a lower socioeconomic status (e.g., personal service, family, domestic work, and office activities) are more often held by women.

The seeming "rightness" or face validity of these results may blind some to the fact that they raise more questions than they answer. In her chapter, Betz notes that the lack of logical definitions of the constructs of masculinity and femininity went unnoticed because scholars assumed they "knew intuitively" what constituted them. As with the initial development of the *Bem Sex-Role Inventory* and *Personal Attributes Questionnaire,* these empirically discovered gender-related differences represent atheoretical findings. I think they are important, but the lack of a theoretical context to guide their interpretation invites interpretations based on commonly held stereotypic beliefs. I echo Betz when I emphasize the need for theory to give direction to and increase the interpretability of research on gender-related differences.

The chapters by Betz and Rounds remind me of my graduate school tutelage under Lloyd Lofquist, René Dawis, and David Weiss. Under their leadership, the Work Adjustment Project was developing instruments to measure the major constructs of the theory of work adjustment. These instruments were designed for use, both in validating their theory and in facilitating the work adjustment of workers. An especially laudatory feature of the project was its applicability to blue-collar workers and workers who had mental disabilities, in addition to workers in professional and managerial occupations. Their approach stood in marked contrast to the emphasis at that time on professional and managerial occupations, most of which require a college education.

Rounds' interest in the relations among occupations and Campbell's interest (this volume) in differences among an already select group—brigadier generals—are parallel in many ways to issues I have investigated in my studies of leisure. Diane Tinsley and I have attempted to identify the attributes, benefits, and causes of leisure experience (Tinsley & Tinsley, 1986, 1988). Our inquiry focuses on the impact of leisure and work activities on the individual rather than on the externally obvious attributes of these activities. Our concern is with individuals' perceptions of their leisure and work experiences and how these perceptions influence their lives.

A study by Tinsley, Colbs, Teaff, and Kaufman (1987) illustrates the fruitfulness of investigating individual differences, even among a relatively select group of people. Using canonical analysis, we examined the relations of the psychological benefits derived from participation in 18 commonly chosen leisure activities to the personal attributes of 1,449 people who were 55 to 75 years of age. Three significant canonical variates were identified, as can be seen in Table 1. Older women (those over 65) of lower socioeconomic status with relatively low morale were most likely to seek companionship in their leisure activities. Younger women (those 55 to 65 years of age) placed greater importance on leisure activities that provided them with some form of recognition. Older men and women from higher socioeconomic backgrounds were more likely to seek leisure activities that gratified their need for power.

Minnesota counseling psychologists are interested in more than the current status of the individual. How the individual or group arrived at their current status and how they might be expected to develop in the future are other issues that enjoy their scrutiny. Identifying the relevant factors and their position in the developmental chain are special concerns illustrated in the work of Waller et al. and Campbell.

Waller et al. are interested in the relations between leisure and occupational interests, and the relations of these factors to personality. They also examine the heritability of these interests and their stability over time. Their goal is to identify the factors that influence the development of interests. They conclude that approximately 50% of the variance in vocational and leisure interests (and two-thirds of the stable variance) is attributable to genetic factors. This is comparable to earlier findings of Betsworth et al. (1994) regarding vocational interests and Tellegen, Lykken, Bouchard, Wilcox, Segal, and Rich (1988) regarding personality.

In his chapter, Campbell argues that the nature of brigadier generals results from an interaction of the person and the system in which the person operates. Selection and acceptance play a limited role, but

Table 1 Correlation of Psychological Benefits and Personal Characteristics With Canonical Variables

	Canonical Variates[a]		
Variables	I	II	III
Psychological benefits			
Affiliation	60	05	25
Cooperation	52	04	08
Nurturance	56	−12	18
Security	36	10	18
Supervision	50	34	21
Advancement	18	36	08
Reward	22	37	24
Self-esteem	13	40	09
Sentience	05	34	15
Creativity	14	30	46
Ability utilization	−05	22	43
Authority	04	−12	66
Dominance	10	−20	44
Responsibility	18	−09	38
Social service	34	04	54
Social status	19	−13	53
Achievement	18	13	29
Activity	11	18	22
Aggression	−05	−08	−09
Catharsis	28	−06	−13
Compensation	25	−28	12
Exhibition	−26	−16	00
Independence	07	−02	09
Play	16	24	08
Sex	−02	07	04
Understanding	20	28	29
Variety	11	19	11
Personal characteristics			
Gender	48	85	21
Age	80	−38	43
Socioeconomic status	−65	02	72
Morale	−30	07	26
Physical health	26	−15	11
Canonical correlation	47[b]	26[b]	23[b]
Eigenvalue	22	07	05

[a]Decimal points have been omitted.
[b]$p < 0.001$.

From "The Relationship of Age, Gender, Health, and Economic Status to the Psychological Benefits Older Persons Report From Participation in Leisure Activities," by H. E. A. Tinsley, S. L. Colbs, J. D. Teaff, and N. Kaufman, 1987, *Leisure Sciences, 9,* p. 60, Washington, DC: Taylor & Francis. Reprinted with permission. All rights reserved.

the organization shapes the individual. "It is not sufficient just to select good people," according to Campbell. "you have to put them in an environment where quality is appreciated and nurtured." Campbell speculates that our 200-year history of democracy is one of the important variables that shape the expression of these generals' possibly instinctive tendencies.

Campbell is careful to label these ideas as his own thinking, an important qualification that I would have preferred he emphasize even more. Campbell describes these generals as very dominant individuals who want to be in control and who have a strong aversion to being controlled. This description seems inconsistent with his suggestion that young officers' training occurs in a very controlled environment that strongly influences their adult personality. An equally plausible interpretation is that brigadier generals achieve their rank precisely because they are dominant, aggressive individuals who have very strong needs to be in control, and their military education has little influence on these qualities.

Campbell has studied brigadier generals in the U.S. Army, but he acknowledges that individuals of comparable rank in the air force, marine corps, and navy may differ in significant ways. Studies of generals from other branches of the service would help to illuminate his findings and establish the limits of their generalizability. Further, cross-cultural research on this issue is of worldwide significance and would make an important contribution to humankind.

Regardless of which interpretation you believe has the most merit, Campbell's focus illustrates a developmental perspective. Questions such as how these individuals came to be this way, what the social costs of their being this way are, and how and whether this situation should be modified demonstrate a clear appreciation of the importance of the developmental process.

METHODOLOGY

A concern about (some might say a fascination with) psychological measurement and its close cousins, assessment and multivariate analysis, is the methodological cornerstone of the Minnesota counseling psychologist's education. Waller et al.'s use of factor analysis followed by multidimensional scaling has the ring of a Minnesota psychologist. The fact that the multidimensional scaling algorithm is homegrown is diagnostic of the Minnesota approach. Rounds' work also reveals a high degree of multivariate eclecticism. Holland's (1985) structural hypothesis is tested using ALSCAL and SINDSCAL, and the fit of the *Strong Interest Inventory's* Basic Interest Scales and the *Jackson*

Vocational Interest Survey to the circular structure proposed by Holland is tested using nonmetric multidimensional scaling analysis.

Many Minnesota psychologists seem to believe that the path to truth must lie through multivariate space. In her chapter, Betz traces the growing complexity of models of gender-related individual differences from the first simple univariate model to the current agreement that a multivariate model is needed that includes attitudes, behaviors, information processing, and social interaction. Campbell is a well-known exception, but most of us find multivariate techniques to be indispensable. Certainly, this belief is evident in my own work (Tinsley, Bowman, & York, 1989; Tinsley et al., 1987) and in my exhortations to other researchers (Tinsley, 1984, 1990).

Rounds' chapter provides a good illustration of the kinds of contributions Minnesota counseling psychologists have been able to make over the years because of their facility with multivariate techniques. His evaluation of the adequacy of Holland's structural model in expressing the relations among vocational interests using data-ideas and people-things dimensions reveals Holland's model to be good but not optimal. Rounds' analysis of the relative fit of instruments measuring Holland's personality type to Holland's hexagon provides important information about the applicability of these instruments. His analysis of the adequacy of Holland's hexagon in explaining the domain of basic interests convincingly demonstrates the need for an octagon. These are three important findings that should be of interest to all scholars concerned with vocational interests.

My own work has made effective use of multivariate techniques at times (e.g., Tinsley et al., 1987; Tinsley et al., 1989). Hayes and Tinsley (1989) factor analyzed 33 scales measuring perceptions of and expectations about counseling, as can be seen in Table 2. Factors 1 (Expectation of Facilitative Conditions), 3 (Expectation of Counselor Expertise), and 4 (Expectation of Personal Commitment) replicated factors reported by Tinsley, Workman, and Kass (1980) in an earlier factor analysis of the Expectations About Counseling. The other three factors indicated latent dimensions pertaining to Perceptions of Counselor Attributes (Factor 2), Perceptions of Facilitative Conditions (Factor 5), and Perceptions of Counselor Effectiveness (Factor 6).

These results demonstrated conclusively the independence of these constructs. Even expectation and perception factors pertaining to somewhat similar constructs were essentially uncorrelated in the oblique rotation, that is, r (Factors 1 and 5) = $-.13$ and r (Factors 3 and 6) = $-.08$. These findings lend empirical support to the contentions of Duckro, Beal, and George (1979) and Tinsley, Bowman, and Ray (1988) that investigations that fail to distinguish adequately among these constructs are hopelessly flawed. This study has important methodological implications for scholars investigating expectations about counseling, the interpersonal influence process and help-seeking behavior.

Despite the obvious importance of a thorough grounding in psychological measurement, assessment, and multivariate techniques, the techniques must be used judiciously. I think that sometimes we play with these toys too much. In both Waller et al.'s and Rounds' chapters (this volume), the focus on the substantive issues is obscured at times, as yet another analysis or new technique is described. Some of my own work must strike readers in the same way (Trafton & Tinsley, 1989). Gelso's (1979) bubble hypothesis suggests that all research approaches have their weaknesses. This is also true of the methodological techniques often used so effectively by Minnesota psychologists. Our challenge is to use these approaches meaningfully while avoiding addiction.

INTEGRATION

The importance of integrating theory and knowledge across the arbitrary boundaries within psychology was emphasized throughout the Minnesota graduate education. This emphasis is the third cornerstone. Betz (this volume) calls for multifactor conceptions of gender-related differences that include roles, attitudes, and behaviors. Campbell's (this volume) analysis of U.S. military commanders in his chapter involves an assessment of their intelligence, personality, vocational interests, and values. Betz calls for a moratorium on instrument development and for the detailed postulation of a nomological network. Most urgently needed, according to Betz, are integrative theories. Campbell's assessment of brigadier generals across a variety of domains and his integration of this information to gain a cohesive understanding of these individuals is characteristic of the Minnesota counseling psychologist.

Waller et al. also emphasize integration, examining the relations among personality, leisure interests, and work interests. Many career theorists have regarded vocational choice as an expression of the individual's personality (Holland, 1985; Lofquist & Dawis, 1984) or self-concept (Super, 1963). Many leisure psychologists view leisure choices as a function of the individual's personality (Neulinger, 1974; Tinsley & Tinsley, 1986). Scholars such as Super (1980) and Tinsley and Tinsley (1988) regard leisure and work as two important roles that individuals assume across the life span. Waller et al.'s search for commonality among these life roles illustrates the Minnesota psychologist's emphasis on integration in the study of human behavior.

Table 2   Factor Pattern Matrix

Scale	Factor					
	1	2	3	4	5	6
Counselor Rating Form						
Expertness	−.08	.80	.04	−.10	−.04	−.07
Trustworthiness	.09	.74	−.12	−.07	.22	−.15
Attractiveness	.11	.78	−.13	.01	.07	−.13
Counselor Effectiveness Rating Scale						
Expertness	−.09	.90	.09	.03	−.04	.13
Trustworthiness	−.10	.84	.09	.05	.06	.02
Attractiveness	−.12	.72	.02	.13	.12	.06
Counselor Effectiveness Scale						
Counselor Effectiveness	.10	.76	−.18	−.03	−.13	−.14
Personal Attributes Inventory						
Negative Attitudes	.02	.67	.09	−.08	.17	.01
Counselor Evaluation Inventory						
Counseling Climate	−.08	−.03	.03	−.01	−.10	.41
Counselor Comfort	.11	−.08	−.09	.06	.01	.39
Client Satisfaction	.10	.57	−.13	−.11	.25	.31
Barrett–Lennard Relationship Inventory						
Level of Regard	−.06	.37	−.06	.04	.64	−.03
Empathetic Understanding	.03	.37	.03	.02	.59	.01
Congruence	−.02	.26	.03	−.08	.71	.03
Unconditionality of Regard	−.05	−.13	.02	−.03	.54	−.08
Willingness to Be Known	.07	.22	−.11	.01	.64	−.04

My research with Diane Tinsley on leisure reflects the value placed on integration that we learned at Minnesota. Early views of leisure and work regarded them as mutually exclusive. The residual definition of leisure, ascendant at the time we began our program of research, defined leisure as the time remaining when the work responsibilities and the maintenance activities of the individual had been accomplished. Any residual time left over was considered leisure time. Thus, leisure was defined as a nonentity, orthogonal to work, having no positive distinguishing attributes.

We began our research by focusing on the individual's psychological experience. This line of work has led to the identification of a cluster of attributes that we have tentatively labeled the leisure

Table 2   Factor Pattern Matrix (continued)

Scale	Factor					
	1	2	3	4	5	6
	Expectations About Counseling—Brief Form					
Motivation	−.13	.03	.12	.79	.05	.01
Openness	.06	.02	−.06	.91	−.03	−.02
Responsibility	.32	−.04	−.20	.69	−.05	−.11
Acceptance	.79	.00	.11	.01	.04	.17
Confrontation	.65	−.01	.19	.17	−.05	.03
Directiveness	.09	−.03	.75	.05	.04	−.10
Empathy	.12	−.03	.75	.01	.01	−.05
Genuineness	.89	.06	−.09	.02	−.11	−.11
Nurturance	.69	−.05	.25	.05	.01	−.05
Self-Disclosure	.17	.06	.56	−.04	−.03	.04
Attractiveness	.01	.01	.08	.79	−.04	.15
Expertise	.52	−.05	.44	.09	.02	−.07
Tolerance	.68	.04	.16	.10	−.09	.08
Trustworthiness	.89	−.06	.02	.07	.09	.05
Concreteness	.64	−.06	.20	.17	−.04	−.15
Immediacy	.01	−.02	−.02	.92	−.01	.01
Outcome	.16	−.04	−.10	.84	−.00	−.04

Note. Factor titles are as follows: 1 = Expectation of Facilitative Conditions, 2 = Perception of Counselor Attributes, 3 = Expectation of Counselor Expertise, 4 = Expectation of Personal Commitment, 5 = Perception of Facilitative Conditions, and 6 = Perception of Counselor Effectiveness.

The signs for all loadings on Factors 3 and 5 were reversed to facilitate the interpretation of those factors.

From "Identification of the Latent Dimensions Underlying Instruments Measuring Perceptions of and Expectations About Counseling," by T. J. Hayes and H. E. A. Tinsley, 1989, *Journal of Counseling Psychology, 36,* p. 497. Copyright © 1989 by the American Psychological Association. Reprinted with permission.

experience (Tinsley & Tinsley, 1986, 1988). As we understand it at this point, the attributes of leisure experience include:

• Feelings of freedom

• Intense concentration on or absorption in the activity at hand

• Enriched perception of objects and events

• Increased sensitivity to and intensity of emotions

• Increased sensitivity to bodily sensations

• A forgetting of self and a lessening of cognitive processing

• Decreased awareness of the passage of time

We believe that four causal conditions are prerequisite to this experience. Individuals must perceive the activity as freely chosen and engaged in because the activity itself is intrinsically enjoyable. Individuals must experience optimal stimulation (i.e., not so stimulating as to be upsetting, nor so lacking in stimulation as to be boring). Finally, a commitment to the activity is necessary (i.e., individuals must engage themselves psychologically in the activity rather than simply dallying).

We believe that experiencing leisure is absolutely essential to the individual because every individual has some needs for which leisure experience is the only source of gratification. We view leisure experience as satisfying psychological needs of the individual at all five levels of Maslow's (1970) hierarchy. The satisfaction of psychological needs has a salutary effect on mental health, physical health, and life satisfaction, as Figure 1 helps illustrate. These factors, in turn, have a beneficial effect on personal growth. Chronic deprivation of leisure experience is detrimental to the physical and mental health of the individual and results in a reduction of life satisfaction and a lack of personal growth.

Our current work is directed toward gaining a more complete and precise understanding of the attributes of leisure experience. Once these attributes have been shown to covary as an identifiable experience that occurs frequently in leisure, we plan to investigate their occurrence in other aspects of the individual's life. For example, this approach allows us to identify commonalities in the way individuals experience work and leisure. Machlowitz (1980) describes workaholics as having a neurotic adjustment to work. We have no doubt that some workaholics have a neurotic adjustment to work, but we believe that other individuals who would be labeled as workaholics by external observers are experiencing leisure during their work. That is, these individuals are so well suited to their work that the essential experiences many of us obtain in leisure are readily available to them in their work. The long hours these individuals spend at their work is not indicative of a sense of compulsion or inadequacy. Instead, these individuals find their work to be the most enjoyable and fulfilling activity they know.

APPLICATION

The final educational cornerstone of the Minnesota counseling psychologist is an appreciation of the importance of applying this knowledge to the amelioration of the problems of society. A concern for practical application is discernible in my efforts to assist counseling

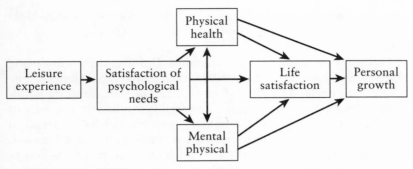

Figure 1 Causal effects of leisure experience

From "A Theory of Attributes, Benefits, and Causes of Leisure Experience," by H. E. A. Tinsley and D. J. Tinsley, 1986, *Leisure Sciences, 8*, p. 20. Reprinted with permission.

psychologists in preparing for test interpretation (Tinsley & Bradley, 1986, 1988), in my evaluations with Diane Tinsley of leisure counseling models (Tinsley & Tinsley, 1981, 1984) and explication of our own leisure counseling model (Tinsley & Tinsley, 1982).

Campbell's (this volume) rationale for use of the *Myers-Briggs Type Indicator* illustrates an informed stance about the need for practical application. I believe far too many practitioners are at the opposite extreme from Campbell—empathy run amok. Interesting-sounding assessment devices seem to be adopted on the basis of how well they fit one's preconceived notions, while little attention is given to the psychometric qualities of the instrument. Campbell's use represents the more informed position, which springs from the scientist-practitioner dialogue. Instruments having psychometric limitations may be useful when the scholar has a clearly articulated practitioner objective in mind for which an instrument with these limitations is appropriate.

Rounds' chapter (this volume) also reveals an appreciation of the distinction between statistical and practical significance. Although the ALSCAL constrained analysis accounted for 9% less variance than the unconstrained analysis, he questions the practical importance of this difference. Given the widely demonstrated heuristic benefits of Holland's model, the sacrifice of 9% of the variance in the name of practical application and useability has proven to be a good bargain over the years. Rounds' analysis of the degree to which interest inventory results fit Holland's hexagon reveals a further concern for practical application. The results suggest that Holland provided the conceptualization, but scores on the *Strong Interest Inventory* and the *Unisex Edition of ACT Interest Inventory* (UNIACT) fit his model more precisely. The *Career Assessment Inventory—Vocational,*

Career Assessment Inventory, extended, and the *Career Decision-Making Inventory* yield scores that provide relatively poor fits to the hexagon.

Psychologists seldom prove anything. Unfortunately, counseling psychologists cannot afford to wait for all answers to be known. The stronger the demand for immediate application, the greater the liability experienced by psychologists. Campbell recognizes the necessity of making recommendations for military training, but he is careful to distinguish his personal views from those findings he can document. Campbell notes that the military can impose seemingly senseless policies and practices on itself. So, too, can scholars, and one such policy is that of forever deferring attempts to address problems of practical significance until research has revealed definitive answers. I think Minnesota counseling psychologists recognize this more clearly than others.

A MINNESOTA COUNSELING PSYCHOLOGIST

These educational cornerstones serve as values that influence both my scholarly and practitioner activities. Whatever the issue confronting me, I am aware that my search for an answer inevitably takes me across the subdisciplines of psychology (e.g., personality, social psychology, geropsychology) and sometimes into disciplines such as sociology, economics, and anthropology. Constructs from disparate disciplines, multiple measures, and multivariate analyses frequently are involved, always accompanied by an awareness that the really important and interesting findings may lie in the differences among individuals and groups. Finally the questions, What does it mean? and What are the practical implications?, quickly spring to mind as the answer emerges. In short, these values direct my search for solutions to the problems confronting society. The amalgam of these influences has produced a scientist-practitioner who is personally most interested in the science of the discipline but ever mindful of the importance of applying this science to the amelioration of society's problems.

REFERENCES

Betsworth, D. G., Bouchard, T. J., Cooper, C. R., Grotevant, H. D., Hansen, J. C., Scarr, S., & Weinberg, R. A. (1994). Genetic and environmental influences on vocational interests assessed using adoptive and biological families and twins reared apart and together. *Journal of Vocational Behavior, 44*, 263–278.

Borow, H. (1990). Counseling psychology in the Minnesota tradition. *Journal of Counseling and Development, 68*, 266–275.

Duckro, P., Beal, D., & George, C. (1979). Research on the effects of disconfirmed client role expectations in psychotherapy: A critical review. *Psychological Bulletin, 86,* 260–275.

Gelso, C. J. (1979). Research in counseling: Methodological and professional issues. *The Counseling Psychologist, 8*(3), 7–35.

Getzels, J. W., & Jackson, P. W. (1962). *Creativity and intelligence.* New York: Wiley.

Gottesman, I. I. (1963). Heritability of personality. A demonstration. *Psychological Monographs, 77*(9, Whole No. 572).

Guilford, J. P. (1950). Creativity. *American Psychologist, 5,* 444–454.

Hayes, T. J., & Tinsley, H. E. A. (1989). Identification of the latent dimensions underlying instruments measuring perceptions of and expectations about counseling. *Journal of Counseling Psychology, 36,* 492–500.

Holland, J. L. (1985). *Making vocational choices* (2d ed.). Englewood Cliffs, NJ: Prentice-Hall.

Lofquist, L. H., & Dawis, R. V. (1978). Values as secondary to needs in the theory of work adjustment. *Journal of Vocational Behavior, 12,* 12–19.

Lofquist, L. H., & Dawis, R. V. (1984). Research on work adjustment and satisfaction: Implications for career counseling. In S. D. Brown & R. W. Lent, *Handbook of counseling psychology.* New York: Wiley.

Machlowitz, M. (1980). *Workaholics.* Reading, MA: Addison-Wesley.

Maslow, A. H. (1970). Motivation and personality (2d ed.). New York: Harper & Row.

McNemar, Q. (1933). Twin resemblances in motor skills, and the effect of practice thereon. *Journal of Genetic Psychology, 42,* 70–99.

Moloney, D. P., Bouchard, T. J., & Segal, N. L. (1991). A genetic and environmental analysis of the vocational interests of monozygotic and dizygotic twins reared apart. *Journal of Vocational Behavior, 39,* 76–109.

Neulinger, J. (1974). *The psychology of leisure.* Springfield, IL: C. C. Thomas.

Roe, A. (1953). A psychological study of eminent psychologists and anthropologists, and a comparison with biological and physical scientists. *Psychological Monographs, 67*(2), 1–55.

Super, D. E. (1963). Self-concepts in vocational development. In D. E. Super, R. Starishevsky, N. Matlin, & J. P. Jordaan (Ed.), *Career development: Self-concept theory.* New York: College Entrance Examination Board.

Super, D. E. (1980). A life-span, life-space approach to career development. *Journal of Vocational Behavior, 16,* 282–298.

Tellegen, A., Lykken, D. T., Bouchard, T., Wilcox, K., Segal, N., & Rich, S. (1988). Personality similarity in twins reared apart and together. *Journal of Personality and Social Psychology, 73,* 1031–1039.

Terman, L. M. (1925). *Genetic studies of genius: Vol. I, Mental and physical traits of a thousand gifted children.* Stanford, CA: Stanford University Press.

Terman, L. M., & Oden, M. (1947). *The gifted child grows up.* Stanford, CA: Stanford University Press.

Terman, L. M., & Oden, M. (1959). *The gifted group at mid-life.* Stanford, CA: Stanford University Press.

Tinsley, H. E. A. (1984). Limitations, explorations, aspirations: A confession of fallibility and a promise to strive for perfection. *Journal of Leisure Research, 16,* 93–98.

Tinsley, H. E. A. (1990). Editorial. *Journal of Vocational Behavior, 37.*

Tinsley, H. E. A., Bowman, S. L., & Ray, S. B. (1988). Manipulation of expectancies about counseling and psychotherapy: A review and analysis of expectancy manipulation strategies and results. *Journal of Counseling Psychology, 35,* 91–108.

Tinsley, H. E. A., Bowman, S. L., & York, D. C. (1989). Career Decision Scale, My Vocational Situation, Vocational Rating Scale, and Decisional Rating Scale: Do they measure the same constructs? *Journal of Counseling Psychology, 36,* 115–120.

Tinsley, H. E. A., & Bradley, R. W. (1986). Test interpretation. *Journal of Counseling and Development, 64,* 462–466.

Tinsley, H. E. A., & Bradley, R. W. (1988). Interpretation of psychometric instruments in career counseling. In J. T. Kapes & M. M. Mastie (Eds.), *A counselor's guide to career assessment instruments* (2d ed.). Washington, DC: National Career Development Association.

Tinsley, H. E. A., Colbs, S. L., Teaff, J. D., & Kaufman, N. (1987). The relationship of age, gender, health, and economic status to the psychological benefits older persons report from participation in leisure activities. *Leisure Sciences, 9,* 53–65.

Tinsley, H. E. A., & Tinsley, D. J. (1981). An analysis of leisure counseling models. *Counseling Psychologist, 9*(3), 45–53.

Tinsley, H. E. A., & Tinsley, D. J. (1982). A holistic model of leisure counseling. *Journal of Leisure Research, 14,* 100–116.

Tinsley, H. E. A., & Tinsley, D. J. (1984). Leisure counseling models. In E. T. Dowd (Ed.), *Leisure counseling: Concepts and applications.* Springfield, IL: Thomas.

Tinsley, H. E. A., & Tinsley, D. J. (1986). A theory of the attributes, benefits, and causes of leisure experience. *Leisure Science, 8,* 1–45.

Tinsley, H. E. A., & Tinsley, D. J. (1988). An expanded context for the study of career decision making, development, and maturity. In W. B. Walsh & S. H. Osipow (Eds.), *Career decision making.* Hillsdale, NJ: Erlbaum.

Tinsley, H. E. A., Workman, K. R., & Kass, R. (1980). Factor analysis of the domain of client expectancies about counseling. *Journal of Counseling Psychology, 27,* 561–570.

Torrance, E. P. (1962). *Guiding creature talent.* Englewood Cliffs, NJ: Prentice-Hall.

Trafton, R. S., & Tinsley, H. E. A. (1989). Causal predominance among work, dyadic, leisure and life satisfaction assuming a spillover model. In F. Humphrey & J. H. Humphrey (Eds.), *Recreation: Current selected research, Vol. 1.* New York: AMS Press.

Chapter 14

My Life With a Theory

John L. Holland
Professor Emeritus,
Johns Hopkins University

I had many difficulties in preparing this little talk.* I didn't like the program chairman's suggestions, and he didn't like mine. For example, he wanted a nostalgic account of counseling psychology in the 1940s versus the 1980s. That topic had formidable problems.

First, I was ambivalent about my graduate experience. I felt like quitting at the end of the second year, but I had no desirable alternative, nor could I face my father, my banker, who had already told his neighbors about his son, who was about to become a Ph.D. My wife was supportive, but she expressed no enthusiasm for my quitting, so I stayed on. Second, I retired in 1980, so I know very little about graduate life in the 1980s. So much for that topic.

The program chair's advice on style—"Be broad-brush and don't get too technical"—I could easily follow. If you are as statistically challenged as I have been for my entire career, this was welcome advice. My other handicaps include an inability to even add or subtract in a reliable fashion and a complete computer deficiency, despite numerous computer consciousness-raising efforts made by well-meaning friends.

I toyed with giving an old but polished talk—"My life with the *Self-Directed Search* (SDS)"—but I found that I was tired of talking about the SDS. I also tried to create several new talks.

For instance, "My Philosophy of Science Is Better than Yours." If you have been following the recent philosophical wars, you know that

---

*Based on a talk given at the University of Minnesota on the 40th anniversary of its counseling psychology program (Minneapolis, 1993).

logical positivism has been out for some time and almost anything else is in. These philosophical shifts have concerned me, because while my theory continues to be a fruitful enterprise, it does have some old-fashioned philosophical ideas. My personality types are arbitrary constructions without substance. My deductive logic is interesting, but it provides a misleading account of how theories are actually constructed or should be constructed.

In short, it is important to distinguish a theory's origins, that is, the discovery process, from its public testing process. I have toyed with a retraction in which I attribute my theory to my mother's ideas—that she was a bright, caring, insightful woman who told me what to write. Another idea was to have her write nasty letters to critics from her nursing home.

At any rate, Howard Kendler (1992) has written a book chapter clarifying the role of behaviorism, positivism, and psychology in everyday science. He rebuts some common misconceptions about these topics. If you are afflicted with a neobehavioristic, evidence-oriented view of science, you will enjoy this chapter. If you are afflicted with one of the new philosophies of science in which social action, imagination, or promissory notes are sometimes more important than evidence, you will find this chapter disconcerting.

I also considered abstracting a little book about research for graduate students that I have been daydreaming about. Some chapter headings will give you the flavor. They include "Getting Started," "Finding Your Style," "Coping With Critics and Controversy," "Copyrights, Lawyers, and Psychometric Burglary," "Living with the Highs and Lows (my mental health chapter), "Learning to Write," and "Publishers, Publishing, and Editorial Encounters." The problem with telling you about this book is that it has no text.

This search for a suitable topic led finally to a unifying idea: "My Experience in Developing and Revising a Typology." (I also considered lengthening these introductory comments to the point where there would be no time for a talk.)

CONTROVERSIAL AND DESTRUCTIVE TRENDS

I have received a 40-year internship that has shaped my beliefs and biases about counseling, training, practice, and research. It has also shaped my competencies—so much so I can now cope more skillfully with controversy than with support.

At any rate, I wish to comment on a few of my experiences and impressions of some controversial and destructive research trends in counseling psychology.

What are these trends?

1. *We have moved from simple data analyses that communicate to most psychologists to hyperanalytical treatments that communicate only to a sophisticated few.* Research reports often fail to report simple orienting information such as means, standard deviations, simple correlations, or proportions.

2. *There is a decline in the publication of simple empirical studies to search for initial information about neglected or unexplored problems.*

3. *This decline in empirical fishing expeditions has been accompanied by an increasing worship of theory.* Theories are two-sided tools. They can focus our vision in useful ways, but they can also blind us to new data and other more useful explanations.

4. *There is an increasing disparity between our favorite interventions and societal needs.* Years ago, clinicians used to say that "if all the psychiatrists trained in the next 50 years were available today, they couldn't take care of the people who need help." If you substitute counseling psychologists for psychiatrists, you would reach to the same conclusion today. To make matters worse, counseling psychologists are acting like psychiatrists, rushing into private practice and relegating career assistance to the bottom of the practice barrel. In contrast, there is little interest in preventive education or group interventions.

5. *The shift to private practice has been accompanied by a shift to a wide range of counseling topics as well as a host of new topics.* These topics include sports, the elderly, recreation, people of color, and women. These shifts have also been accompanied by a neglect and denigration of career interventions. This is especially unfortunate because our career interventions have a long history of positive evaluations and the need for such services by people of all ages is extensively documented. Equally important, we have a wide range of individual and group treatments that are cost effective.

This indiscriminate investment in old and new research topics is spread so thin over those in the field that little progress can be expected. For instance, there are only 2,300 counseling psychologists. About 2,000 are not engaged in research except as spectators or commentators, another 100 to 200 do an occasional piece of research, and fewer than 100 have full-time research careers. If there are only 10 major research problems or about 10 people per topic, these groups are hardly a threat to scientific ignorance.

Factors Influencing the Trends

Now I want to speculate about the environmental forces that drive these research and service trends. These influences are both benign and destructive. I will focus on destructive influences because they need exposure and because most people focus on the benign influences.

Grantism   The securing of research grants is a mixed bag. Without a grant or a rich relative, some kinds of research are simply not possible. Unfortunately, grant activities have great status among peers and administrators, leaving students with the impression that they cannot do good work unless they have a grant. At Minnesota, according to my mail, students can't even get to a convention without a grant. Apparently, they haven't heard of carpooling or writing for papers.

Focused Editorial Power   In counseling psychology, our journals are dominated by conservative beliefs about research, resulting in little risk taking. Conservative evaluations are desirable biases—otherwise, journals would contain more worthless material than they do now. These conservative biases, however, are accentuated because authors see the same club of old boys and girls no matter where they turn. Defensive editors occasionally publish analyses that show how well their consulting editors agree. They should—the editor selected them or had them certified by right thinkers. In short, the focusing of editorial power limits the range of acceptable research within a single journal, and because editors and consulting editors serve on multiple journals, authors have trouble finding a fresh, second opinion. Because authors have no union, they do nothing. To cry too much about rejections is a sign of low status. I have converted low status to high status by claiming that I have more rejections than most people have acceptances. Not only that, but poor journals reject my work as frequently as good journals.

Destructive Training   Most graduate training in research is devoted to how to collect and process ideal data (representative of something and preferably with a large N) through statistical sieves so that a defensible report emerges. Or research training focuses on the evaluation of information, so good ideas prevail and bad ones are suppressed. This kind of training is of major importance, for it distinguishes a scientific discipline from a cult, among other groups.

The problem with this aspect of training is that the processes of problem finding, speculation, and theorizing are neglected. Students usually leave graduate work with a few well-developed technical muscles, but with many underdeveloped problem-finding skills, along with little experience or confidence in their speculations or theorizing.

Graduate schools cannot be finishing schools with endless curricula, but they do neglect the subjective side of science. At the same time, it is easy to see how students come to believe that useful inventories, scales, and theories come only from careful, explicit research activities rather than from multiple sources. Careful research is one source. For instance, the *Strong Interest Inventory* came from considerable empirical thrashing around by Strong and others. The *Kuder Occupational Interest Survey* came from a factor analysis. The *Self-Directed Search* came from looking at multiple factor analyses, a primitive theory, reading Strong's book, looking at correlational matrices, and so on. Incidentally, the use of six rather than some other number of types was cemented in the theory when a psychiatrist, whose hobby was numerology, told me that "six was a good number." That did it.

Conservative Views of Journals   Journals and funding agencies reinforce many of our training biases, because they are usually populated by people with conservative views of science. Put another way, journals and funding agencies covet scientific respectability, which translates as "don't fund or publish deviant or fragile projects." Decision making about such projects is difficult because it is often hard to see the difference between a creative idea and a psychotic one, yet it is important to keep these gates open to some innovative work.

Finally, over the last 40 years, my impression is that there has been a marked decline in open discussion and writing about controversial topics. Research and writing about ethnic minorities, women, the elderly, people with physical disabilities, and so on has become balkanized: Women talk to women, white males talk to white males, and so on, so there is little constructive feedback. Different groups have acquired some inaccurate, in-and-out group beliefs about one another, but because there is little open discussion, some crazy ideas receive no corrective feedback or simply no response. A kind of political correctness cloud seems to hang over some topics and despite the public appearance of concern and sensitivity, many (how many?) simply no longer voice an opinion.

A similar division or void exists between the developmentalists and the structurally oriented career researchers. They have avoided any constructive interaction for more than 40 years. The only interaction occurs in journals in which one side implies that the other view of careers is simplistic, evidence deficient, or some other scientific slur.

POSSIBLE REMEDIES

I have some ideas for softening these destructive trends and influences. These remedies are arranged in order of their increasing difficulty to achieve. For some problems, I have no useful solutions.

First, our focused editorial power could easily be decentralized or dispersed by asking people to serve on a single journal. As it stands, many serve two or more journals. We have editors for a single journal who also serve as consulting editors for other journals. We can't do anything about book publishers and funding agencies.

Limiting people to serving on a single journal would also create more opportunity for minorities, women, as well as the young and the old. I also forgot—it may also be wise to limit editors to serving on one journal per lifetime. This idea may represent overkill.

To get things started, we need someone who does not intend to publish research, run for office in the American Psychological Association (APA), or need tenure, and has some engrossing hobbies and a supportive social group. A report would be required that documents the overlap among the relevant journals. A computer, however, is not required; three-by-five-inch cards will do. Publication could be achieved by submitting a minority report at an APA Division 17 business meeting. The rejection of the report could then be used to attract attention to a convention program with a purpose that is disguised with a deceptive title such as "Improving the Research Climate."

How to cope with grantism, model gazing, theory worship, and the decline in empirical fishing expeditions poses a very complex array of problems, as they require an understanding of the developing self interacting with a cultural environment that is undergoing dramatic shifts. At any rate, that's what some of our colleagues might say. I see these problems differently.

It might be helpful to encourage more people to perform research without grants. Data processing is no longer a substantial expense, except for a very atypical project, but data collection can be an expensive barrier. One solution is to find a school, a company, a religious institution, or a group that will trade consulting services for access to research participants. Another strategy is to provide psychological or educational materials in exchange for access. Data entry work for small samples ($N < 250$) can be performed by the preteen children of faculty members. They are less expensive to employ than graduate students, and they worry more about making errors than about a project's scientific merit. The only problem I have encountered was in one instance when I raised a student's hourly rate because of good performance. Her mother complained that her daughter's allowance had lost influence. Another time, I used psychiatric patients to do item analyses—they are also more efficient than graduate students.

I have been doing small-scale research for the last 18 years. The out-of-pocket costs to me have always been small. I barter to secure data, consultation, data processing, and typing. Currently, reprints are my largest single expense.

I am not saying that my way is the best or only way to get research done. I am saying that more people should consider using their social skills, ingenuity, and professional capital to do research. At first, this strategy may seem like a lot of work and a waste of time, but compare a few research and sales visits to likely sources with the time spent in preparing grant proposals that often fail. In the do-it-yourself strategy, you can take great risks (empirical or theoretical fishing); in a grant proposal, you have to work hard to create the impression that your proposal is important and infallible.

Another funding strategy is to knuckle under and get grants while at the same time engaging in cheap, empirical or theoretical fishing expeditions to learn what you can. This is, of course, what most grant-addicted researchers do, but it is a stressful life for many and tends to focus one's work on safe designs of popular topics.

I have no promising ideas for improving research training. When I read some of the imaginative articles written by psychologists who believe evidence is a dirty word, I think we need more of the same old traditional training that I have been knocking.

I also have no promising ideas for more open and constructive discussions about research and social problems. If psychologists can't organize their professional concerns in a single institution, it is unlikely that they can have more constructive and open discussions. Psychologists cannot escape American culture: We issue credit cards; we now have a stylish corporate logo; and we have a flourishing cadre of professional politicians—even one in the House of Representatives. Being cool has become more important than being frank.

SO WHAT?

I don't have a big windup for my ideas, but I do have a few cautions in thinking about my remarks:

- They represent my impressions of what's going on. At no time did any data appear.

- As one of my friends said: Beware of mature (old) people bearing intellectual gifts.

- I ignored the positive qualities of journal editors, traditional research training, and other benevolent influences.

Finally, if you feel the urge to respond, let me rest at the cocktail hour, and wait until you can pay your own way to the next celebration. There will always be opportunities for speakers who can give rather than receive.

REFERENCE

Kendler, H. H. (1992). Ethics in science: A psychological perspective. In W. M. Kurtines, M. Azmitia, & J. L. Gewirtz (Eds.), *The role of values in psychology* (pp. 131–160). New York: Wiley.

Contributors

Nancy E. Betz, Ph.D., is professor of psychology at Ohio State University. Since joining the university in 1976, she has coauthored two books, *The Career Psychology of Women* and *Tests and Assessment,* and 70 articles and chapters focused on such topics as the career development of women, applications of self-efficacy theory to career development, the underrepresentation of women and minorities in the sciences and engineering, and psychological assessment. Dr. Betz served as editor of the *Journal of Vocational Behavior* from 1984 to 1990 and has also served on the editorial boards of the *Journal of Counseling Psychology,* the *Journal of Vocational Behavior,* the *Journal of Career Assessment,* and *Psychology of Women Quarterly.* She is a fellow of the American Psychological Association and American Psychological Society and a past recipient of the American Psychological Association's John Holland Award for Outstanding Achievement in Career and Personality Research.

David P. Campbell joined the faculty of the University of Minnesota after receiving his Ph.D. in psychology from the university. While there, he coauthored the *Strong-Campbell Interest Inventory.* In 1973, he became a visiting fellow at the Center for Creative Leadership in Greensboro, North Carolina, and, shortly thereafter, joined the center as executive vice president. In 1981, he was appointed as the first Smith Richardson Senior Fellow. Dr. Campbell has recently published a new psychological test battery, the *Campbell Development Surveys.* His honors include the E. K. Strong, Jr., Gold Medal for Excellence in Psychological Testing Research.

René V. Dawis received his Ph.D. from the University of Minnesota, where his mentor was Donald G. Paterson. After a year as assistant professor at the University of the Philippines, he returned to Minnesota to head up the Work Adjustment Project. There he teamed up with Lloyd H. Lofquist and David J. Weiss to do research in vocational rehabilitation and produce, among other things, the theory of work adjustment. In 1963, he joined the faculty of the University of Minnesota's Industrial Relations Department and, in 1968, transferred to the Psychology Department, where he remains today. His research interests continue to be in vocational psychology.

Susan E. Embretson is professor of psychology at the University of Kansas, where she has been since completing her Ph.D. in 1973 from the University of Minnesota. She has served as president of the American Psychological Association's Division of Measurement, Evaluation, and Statistics and associate editor for *Psychometrika* and the *Journal of Educational and Behavioral Statistics*. Her major research interest is interfacing psychometric theory with cognitive psychology. She has published numerous articles, edited *Test Design: Developments in Psychology and Psychometrics,* and coauthored *Cognitive and Psychometric Analysis of Analogical Problem Solving.*

Robert R. Golden received his Ph.D. from the University of Minnesota, where his mentor was Paul E. Meehl. His main research interest is in pursuing the potential of taxometrics and its application to the study of behavioral syndromes such as dementia, autism, and cerebral palsy. He is currently a member of the faculty in the Department of Neurology at Albert Einstein College of Medicine.

John L. Holland, Ph.D., has been a researcher-practitioner and research supervisor and teacher for 40 years. He is best known for the *Self-Directed Search,* a leading interest inventory. His hobbies include art and music. Dr. Holland is considering a return from retirement so that he can influence change in the field of career practice and research.

James J. Jenkins, Ph.D., is distinguished research professor of psychology at the University of South Florida. He received his Ph.D. from the University of Minnesota and served on the faculty there from 1950 to 1982. He was the first director of the Center for Research in Human Learning at the university. His research has been concerned with individual differences, memory, cognition, and, most recently, speech perception. He has authored or edited seven books and more than 150 articles.

David Lubinski, Ph.D., is associate professor of psychology at Iowa State University and director of its Psychometrics and Applied Individual Differences Division. He codirects the university's Study of

Mathematically Precocious Youth (SMPY), a 50-year longitudinal study of intellectually gifted participants now in its third decade. His research interests are aimed at identifying different "types" of intellectually gifted adolescents (e.g., the mathematically, spatially, and/or verbally gifted) and finding optimal ways to facilitate their educational and vocational development. His expertise are especially concentrated in the area of assessing individual differences in human behavior.

David T. Lykken, Ph.D., is professor of psychology at the University of Minnesota. He is a past president of the Society for Psychophysiological Research. He began doing research in 1970 and has collaborated with T. J. Bouchard, Jr., on the Minnesota Study of Twins Reared Apart since 1979. Dr. Lykken is the author of *A Tremor in the Blood: Uses and Abuses of the Lie Detector* and, most recently, *The Antisocial Personalities*. A third book, *The American Crime Factory,* is thus far unpublished.

Mary J. Mayer, M.A., was a member of Merrill Roff's development of abnormal psychology research team at the University of Minnesota, where she devised and applied methods for life history research. Since then, she has worked as a researcher, editor, and consultant in a variety of areas, including opinion measurement, medicine, and law. Her current research interest is the psychological and legal aspects of peer harassment among public school students.

Paul E. Meehl, Ph.D., is regents' emeritus professor of psychology and emeritus member of the Minnesota Center for Philosophy of Science at the University of Minnesota. He is a clinical psychologist and was a practicing psychotherapist for more than a half century. He has done research in animal behavior, learning theory, psychometrics, interview assessment, clinical prediction, and forensic psychology. A past president of the American Psychological Association, he has received its Distinguished Contributor Award and its Award for Distinguished Professional Contributions to Knowledge, the Bruno Klopfer Award in Personality Assessment, the American Psychological Foundation's Gold Medal Award for Life Achievement in the Application of Psychology, and the Society for Research in Psychopathology's Joseph P. Zubin Award for Distinguished Contributions in Psychopathology, among others. In 1987, he was elected to the National Academy of Sciences. He is a William James Fellow of the American Psychological Society. He is currently working on new taxometric methods for classification and genetics of psychopathology, the elaboration of his widely recognized theory of schizophrenia, and the development of cliometric metatheory for appraising scientific theories.

Linda Polka received her Ph.D. from the University of South Florida. She is assistant professor in the School of Communication Sciences and Disorders at McGill University in Montreal. Her research program has focused on speech perception with special emphasis on understanding the interaction between developmental changes and language experience. Most recently, her work has dealt with infants; she is currently conducting cross-language studies of speech perception with German infants. Her teaching interests include speech science and clinical audiology.

David Premack received his Ph.D. from the University of Minnesota in 1955 and is currently a visiting member of CREA Ecole Polytechnique in Paris. He has been a Guggenheim Fellow, and a fellow at the Institute for Advanced Thought in the Behavioral Sciences at Stanford University; in Wissenschaftskollege, Berlin; at the Van Leer Jerusalem Institute; and the Japan Society for Promotion of Science. He was awarded the Francis Craik Research Award from St. John's College, Cambridge, and the Fyssen Foundation International Research Prize. His recent work concerns the phylogenetic and ontogenetic bases of human social competence. He is the author of *Intelligence in Ape and Man, Mind of an Ape,* and *Gavagai! Or the Future History of the Animal Language Controversy.*

James Rounds, Ph.D., is associate professor of educational psychology and director of clinical training and division chair for the Counseling Psychology Program at the University of Illinois at Urbana-Champaign. He is also a clinical and research associate at the Department of Psychology, Roswell Memorial Park Institute in Buffalo, New York. His research program concentrates on investigating the interactions of people and environments at work and on the structure of vocational interests.

Winifred Strange, Ph.D., is professor of communication sciences and disorders at the University of South Florida. She received her doctoral degree in psychology from the University of Minnesota in 1972 and was a member of the Center for Research in Human Learning at the university until 1982, when she joined the University of South Florida. She was coauthor and editor of *Speech and Language in the Laboratory, School, and Clinic.* She is a fellow of the American Psychological Association and the Acoustical Society of America. Her research is concerned with the acoustic dynamics involved in the perception of vowels in American English and with cross-language speech perception. She is currently engaged in research with colleagues in

Japan and Germany and recently edited a state-of-the-art book, *Cross-Language Speech Perception.*

Stanley R. Strong, Ph.D., is a professor of psychology at Virginia Commonwealth University, where he is director of graduate studies and the Counseling Psychology Program. He has focused his career on the study of social influence and interpersonal processes in counseling and psychotherapy. In addition to numerous articles and chapters, he has coauthored the book *Change Through Interaction: The Social Psychological Processes of Counseling and Psychotherapy.* He recently received the Leona Tyler Award from the American Psychological Association's Division of Counseling Psychology for outstanding career contribution's to counseling psychology.

Auke Tellegen, Ph.D., is a professor in the Department of Psychology at the University of Minnesota. His current interests include the identification and study of basic dimensions of mood and personality, including emotional temperament, approached both as scientific constructs and as natural language or "folk" constructs. He has published work on the substance and methods of assessing personality and mood. He participated in the recent restandardization of the *Minnesota Multiphasic Personality Inventory* and is author of the *Multidimensional Personality Questionnaire.*

Howard E. A. Tinsley, Ph.D., is professor of psychology and director of the graduate training program in counseling psychology at Southern Illinois University at Carbondale and a professor at WLRA International Centre of Excellence at Leeuwarden, the Netherlands. He is a diplomate of the American Board of Vocational Experts. Dr. Tinsley was formerly assistant professor at the University of Oregon. He is editor of the *Journal of Vocational Behavior,* a guest editor for the *Journal of Counseling Psychology,* and a former member of the Editorial Advisory Board of the Test Corporation of America. He has served as a member of the editorial board for eight prominent psychological journals and manuscript reviewer for 20 journals. He has authored more than 120 publications dealing with counseling psychology, psychological measurement, and leisure; he has also contributed chapters to 16 books. He is a recipient of the research award of the American Rehabilitation Counseling Association and the Allen V. Sapora Research Award for research excellence in leisure psychology.

The late **Leona E. Tyler** received her Ph.D. in psychology from the University of Minnesota in 1941 under the direction of Donald G.

Paterson. Since that time, she spent her entire professional career at the University of Oregon, Eugene. Dr. Tyler's editions of *The Psychology of Human Differences* and *The Work of the Counselor* are considered classics in the field of psychology. A past president of the American Psychological Association, she is one of the most widely cited and respected counseling psychologists of this century.

Niels G. Waller, Ph.D., is associate professor in the Department of psychology at the University of California at Davis. Director of the California Twin Registry, his research focuses on the genetic and environmental influences on psychopathology, personality and attitudes, quantitative genetic modeling, modern psychometric theory, and, most recently, taxometric methods. He serves on the editorial boards of the *Journal of Personality* and *Psychological Assessment.*

David J. Weiss, Ph.D., is professor of psychology at the University of Minnesota and director of the Psychometric Methods Program in the Department of Psychology. From 1959 through 1970, he was a researcher with the Work Adjustment Project at the University of Minnesota and was its project director from 1963 through 1970. Several instruments developed in this project are still in use today. Beginning in 1970, Dr. Weiss began a program of research on computerized adaptive testing, which was supported by a number of agencies of the Department of Defense until 1985. This research program laid the groundwork for many current implementations of computerized adaptive testing and trained many of its leading researchers. In 1976, he founded the international research journal *Applied Psychological Measurement,* which he has edited since its inception in 1977.

Index

Abelson, R. P., 41
ability tests, 4, 5, 7, 12
  and brigadier general profiles,
    148–150, 151
  See also intelligence tests
Ackerman, P. L., 27–28
ACT Interest Inventory. See
  *American College Testing Interest
  Inventory—Unisex Edition*
Adams, J. S., 281
adaptive tests, 7, 74
  advantages, 67, 76
  concepts, 63–65
  defined, 16
  and IRT, 65–66
  self-referenced tests, 72–73
  See also computerized adaptive tests
affirmative action, 5
Aguilar, M. C., 321
Aiken, C., 287
Aldenderfer, M. S., 97
Algina, J., 52
Alley, W. E., 234, 237
Allport, G. W., 11
Alzheimer's disease, 94, 99, 104
  See also clinical dementia
*American College Testing Interest
  Inventory—Unisex Edition*
  (UNIACT),
  correlations between interests and
    personality, 249–250
  and RIASEC interest types, 193, 197,
    204–207, 209–210, 353
American College Testing Program,
    193, 203
  See also *American College Testing
    Interest Inventory—Unisex Edition*
Amirkhan, J., 278
Anchin, J. C., 269–270
Anderson, J., ix

Anderson, S. N., 125
Andrich, D., 54–55, 77
androgyny,
  in gender schema theory, 128
  measurement, 122–124, 127
  models, 124–126
Annual Review of Psychology, 17
appropriateness measurement,
  defined, 62–63
  See also person fit
Arabie, P., 192–193, 201, 203–204,
    209, 222, 247
Arkin, R. M., 278
Army War College (Carlisle Barracks),
    157
artificial intelligence, 41
  See also computers and testing
Arvey, R. D., xi
Aslin, R. N., 313, 317
assessment centers, 6–7
Assessment Systems Corporation, 66
Athanasou, J. A., 194
attitudes, gender-related, 133–137
Attitudes Toward the Male Role Scale,
    136
Attitudes Toward Males in Society, 136
Attitudes Toward Women Scale (AWS),
    134, 135
AWS. *See Attitudes Toward Women
  Scale*

Bailey, K. G., 263–264
Bakan, D., 126
Baker, F. B., 53–54, 61, 65
Bar, R., 207
Barak, A., 207
Bartholomew, D. J., 97
basal level in test administration, 64
basic interests,
  Cole's studies of, 210–219

371

basic interests, *continued*
  comparison of conceptual levels of
    generality, 184–190
  Holland's order of, 219–227
  similarity and order of categories, 224–227
Bates, E., 335
Baucom, D. H., 290–291
Bavalas, A., 277
Beach, S. R., 290–291
Beal, B., 348
Bechtoldt, H., 19–20
Becker, B. J., 120
Bee, H., 123
Beere, C., 126–127, 132, 134–137
Beere, D. B., 134
behavior,
  and brigadier general profiles,
    150, 152, 153–154
  classification, 266–268
  determinants, 269–292
  gender-related, 132–133, 136–137
  as resource exchange, 263–265
Behavior of Organisms, The (Skinner), 341
Bejar, I. I., 54, 56, 62
Bem, S. L., 122–124, 126–128, 130
Bem Sex-Role Inventory (BSRI), 288, 344
  and androgyny models, 124
  correlation with EPAQ, 126
  correlation with PAQ, 130–131
  item selection for, 122–123
  in tests of gender-related traits,
    126–130
  validity, 137
Benbow, C. P., 120
Benet, V., 257
Bennett, S. K., 135
Ben-Yehuda, A., 207–208
Berger, R., 279
Bernstein, S., 128
Best, C. T., 307–310, 314–317, 320, 322
Betsworth, H., 345
Betz, N. E., xvi, xviii, 117, 132, 135, 342
bias,
  in MAXCOV-HITMAX procedure,
    86–87
  in research, 360, 361
  and tests, 4, 5–6
  See also errors
Billings, A., 279
Binet, A., 63
Blashfield, R. K., 96–97
Blessed, G., 99, 104
Blumstein, P., 277, 279, 284
Bock, R. D., 44, 53

Bodenhausen, G. V., 279
Bolton, B., 180
Bond, N. A., 178–188, 234, 237
Borgen, F. H., 209–211, 227, 233
Borow, H., 341
Bouchard, T. J., xi, 234, 250, 254–255,
    342, 345
Bowman, S. L., 347–348
Bradley, R. W., 353
Brannon, E., 136
Brannon Masculinity Scale, 136
Bray, D. W., 7
Brayne, C., 105
Brennan, R. L., 69
brigadier general profiles, 145–147
  aggressive adventurer in, 167, 172–174
  behavior assessment ratings for,
    150, 152, 153–154
  cognitive ability test for, 148–150, 151
  individual selection vs. systems
    development, 167, 170–171
  military retention of leaders, 171–172
  psychological inventories for, 152,
    155–167, 168–169
  samples and demographic data,
    147–148, 149
Broderick, P. C., 135
Broen, P. A., 298
Brookings, J. B., 180
Broverman, D., 123
Broverman, I. K., 123
Brown, D. J., 67
Brown, S. S., 134–135
BSRI. See *Bem Sex-Role Inventory*
Bull, P. E., 195
Bunker, B. B., 287
Burisch, M., 178
Burnham, D. K., 318
Buss, D. M., 257, 284, 287
Butcher, J. N., 124–126
Buttafuoco, P. M., 207

CAI. See *Career Assessment Inventory*
calculus assumption,
  defined, 190
*California Occupational Preference
    System* (COPS), 207–208
California Psychological Inventory
    (CPI), 121, 286–287
  and brigadier general profiles,
    152, 155–157, 158, 167
Calloway, P., 105
Campbell, D. P., xvi, xviii, 118, 183, 193,
    195–196, 203, 210–211, 215–217, 221

Campbell, J. P., 51
Campbell, M., 98
Career Assessment Inventory (CAI),
  and RIASEC interest types, 193, 197,
    204–207, 210, 353–354
Career Decision-Making System (CDM),
  and RIASEC interest types, 193,
    197–198, 204–207, 210, 353–354
careers,
  gender-related roles in, 131–132,
    136–137
  See also occupational interests;
    vocational interests
Carey, S., 332
Carlsmith, J. M., 278
Carlson, E. B., 81
Carlson, J. E., 55
Carpenter, P., 30
Carroll, J. B., xi, 17–18
Carroll, J. D., 193, 201, 203–204
Carroll, T. D., 317
Carson, R. C., 273
Carter, H. D., 253
CAT. *See* computerized adaptive tests
Cattell, J. M., xxi
Cattell, R. B., xi, 184
caution indexes,
  defined, 62–63
  See also person fit
CDM. See *Career Decision-Making
  System*
ceiling level in test administration, 64
Center for Creative Leadership, 146
change,
  measurement of, 50, 68–73
  in relationships, 290
  in vocations, 268, 280
cheating, 63
Chertkoff, J. M., 277, 286–287
children, 279
  disposition to share experience,
    335–336
  learning by imitation and
    pedagogy, 332–335
  speech perception by, 313–315, 322
  speech sound discrimination by,
    298, 304–306, 316, 317
  test of diversity of, 331, 337
Chirico, B. M., 269–270
choices,
  measurement of, 7–9, 11
  of vocations, 256
Christensen, P. R., 178–188, 234, 237
Clark, K. E., 210–211

classical test theory (CTT),
  comparison with IRT, 58, 59, 62, 63
  defined, 49
  differentiating between and within
    individuals, 73, 75
  equating, 56
  problems with, 50–52, 68–69, 73, 75–76
  SEMs in, 51–52, 58, 62, 73, 75
Cleveland, W. S., 88
clinical dementia,
  discovery of dementia taxon, 104–107
  tests for taxonicity of traits, 95,
    99–104, 112
Clogg, C. C., 97
cognitive ability tests. *See* ability
  tests; cognitive tests
cognitive component analysis, 18
cognitive correlate analysis, 18
cognitive design system, 17–18, 45–46
  construct validity and cognitive
    psychology, 19–23
  evaluation of test properties, 25–26,
    41–45
  nature of, 23–25
  stages, 25–26
    features in task domain, 27–28
    goals of measurement, 27
    item banking, 25–26, 45
    item distributions, 38–41
    item generation, 41
    model development, 28–37
    model evaluation, 37–38
    test assembling, 45
    validation, 45
cognitive model, 25–26
  development, 28–37
  evaluation, 37–38
cognitive psychology, 18
  and validity of cognitive design
    system, 19–23
cognitive tests,
  design system for, 19–46
  revision of, 23–24
  theoretical status, 17–18
Cohen, D. B., xi
Cohen, L. H., 126
Cohen, R. S., 132–133
Colbs, S. L., 345, 348
Cole, N. S., 190, 193–194,
  210–219, 223
Colletti, G., 128
competencies measurement, 7
complementarity,
  defined, 273

computerized adaptive tests (CAT), 66–68
  differentiating between and within
    individuals, 73–75
  longitudinal measurement, 68–73
  See also adaptive tests; computers
    and testing
computers and testing, 5–7, 41
  See also computerized adaptive tests
conformity through learning,
    332–336, 338
Connor, J. M., 128
consistency tests,
  and taxonicity of traits, 97–98
  and validity of latent class model,
    99–100
Constantinople, A., 120–122, 130
constructs,
  traits vs., 9–10
construct validity,
  of BSRI and PAQ, 137
  of cognitive design system, 15–16, 17–46
  See also validity
Cook, L. L., 109
Cooley, W. W., 190–192
Cooper, C. R., 345
Cooper, F. S., 299–304
Cooper, L. A., 30
COPS. See *California Occupational
  Preference System*
correlation,
  between interests and personality,
    233–257
  historical development of, xiii–xiv
  *See also under individual tests and
    procedures*
Costa, P. T., Jr., 243
Cottle, W. C., 183, 201
counseling. *See* counseling psychologist
counseling psychologists, 341–342
  application of test results, 3–7, 74–75,
    256–257, 352–354
  integration of theory and knowledge,
    349–352
  methodology, 347–349
  philosophy, 342–347
  research trends, 358–363
covariance, nuisance. *See* nuisance
  covariance
Cowan, G., 277, 284
Coxon, A. P. M., 204
CPI. See *California Psychological
  Inventory*
Crabtree, P. D., 194
Cramp, L., 226

Crane, M., 128
creativity,
  in diversity, 336–338
  in research, 360, 361
criterion-referenced tests, 7, 72
Crites, J. O., 180, 224
Crocker, L., 52
Cronbach, L. J., xiii, 18–19, 50, 137, 320
Cruer, D., 126
CTT. *See* classical test theory
Cudeck, R., 192

Darley, J. G., 224
Darwin, C. R., 1
DAT. See *Differential Aptitude Tests*
David, L., 136
Davis, J. M., 97
Davison, M. L., 192, 205, 245, 248
Dawis, R. V., xi, 178, 180, 182–188, 192,
    205, 233–234, 237, 343–344, 349
Day, N. E., 97
Deaux, K., 119–120, 127–128, 137–138
De Gruijter, D. N. M., 59
Delattre, P., 298
DeSalvo, J., 279
DeSarbo, W. S., 193, 201, 203–204
Desire to Work Scale, 132
Devore, I., 331
DeVries, H., 269–270, 273, 277–278,
    282, 284–285, 288–289
*Diagnostic and Statistical Manual
  of Mental Orders* (DSM–III), 106
Dictionary of Holland Occupational Codes
  (Gottfredson & Holland), 225
Differential Aptitude Tests (DAT), 28, 30
  cognitive theory application, 20–23
  comparison of cognitive design
    system, 35, 37–41
Dillon, R. F., 18
Dimitrovsky, L., 126
direction measurement, 7–9
disabilities, people with, 7, 344
discriminability of speech sounds,
  defined, 299
  See also speech perception
Dittmann, A. T., 277, 291
Dittmann, S., 310–311, 317, 320
diversity,
  control of, 329
    conformity through learning,
      332–336, 338
    creativity, 336–338
    disposition to share experience,
      335–336, 338

diversity, *continued*
  effect of experts, 338–339
  imitation and pedagogy,
    332–336, 338
  power, abuse of, 331–332, 338
  threat of diversity, 330–331, 338
  evolution theory, 1–2, 331–332, 335
  frameworks for, 9–11
  freedom and tolerance, xxi–xxii
  measuring, 2–3, 4 (*see also*
    measurement)
  in personality, 7–9
  possibilities approach, 8–9, 11–12
  test application, 3–7, 74–75, 256–257,
    352–354
  See also individual differences tests
Dorus, E., 97
Doughtie, E. B., 192, 194
Doyle, J. J., 136
Dozier, J. L., 147
Drasgow, F., 63, 76
Dreyer, N. A., 134–135
Drinkard, J., 277, 284
Droege, R. C., 182–187
Duckro, P., 348
Dvorak, B. J., 4

Eagly, A. H., 119–120, 287
Eastes, S., 210
Eaves, L. J., 110
Edelman, G. M., 331
education,
  of brigadier generals, 148, 170,
    172–174
  creativity in, 336–337
  See also Minnesota, University of;
    training
Edwards, V. J., 127–130
Eefting, W., 314–315
Egan, D. E., 18
Eimas, P., 304–305, 313
Ekstrom, R. B., 181
Elliott, R., ix
Elton, C. F., 196
Embretson, S. E., xv, 15, 18, 20, 22,
  25, 28, 30, 32, 35, 42
English as a second language. *See*
  speech perception
entry point in test administration, 65
EPAQ. See *Extended Personal
  Attributes Questionnaire*
Ericsson, K. A., 46
errors, xxi
  in androgyny models, 124

errors, *continued*
  in speech production and perception,
    306–307, 312
  in taxonicity conjecture and its
    tests, 82, 102
  See also bias; sampling errors;
    standard error of measurement
ETS catalog of reference tests, 181
Everitt, B. S., 97
Eversoll, D. B., 134
experience,
  disposition to sharing of, 335–336
  role in speech perception and
    production, 307–313, 320–321
expertise, 338–339
*Extended Personal Attributes
  Questionnaire* (EPAQ), 126
Eyde, L. D., 132
Eysenck Personality Questionnaire, 284

Falbo, T., 284
Falcone, H. T., 128
Farbman, I., 277, 291
Farney, D. L., 257
Faunce, P. S., 135
Federico, P. A., 18
Federman, E. J., 269–270
feedback in training, 318–319
Feingold, A., 119
Feldt, L. S., 69
femininity,
  and androgyny, 122–126
  concepts, 128–129
  measurement problems, 120–130
  relationship to other variables, 130–131
  See also gender-related differences; women
Femininity (Fe) scale, 121
Feng, C., 30
Fincham, F. D., 290–291
FIRO–B,
  and brigadier general profiles,
    152, 160–163, 164
Fischer, G., 25, 42–43
Fitzgerald, L. F., 132, 135, 208, 245
Flege, J. E., 314–315, 320
Fleischer, R. A., 277, 286–287
Fleishman, E. A., 181
Fleiss, J. L., 96
folk concepts,
  defined, 155
Folkes, V. S., 278
Folsom, C. H., Jr., 194
Forsyth, D. R., 279
Fouad, N. A., 192

Frable, D. E. S., 126, 128, 134–135
Fragaszy, D. M., 333
frameworks,
　cognitive design system, 19–46
　cognitive test development, 17–18
　diversity, 9–11
Freedman, D., 135
Freeman, D. C., 298
Freeman, K., 100
French, J. W., 181
Fujimura, O., 299–304, 308, 320
Furby, L., 50

Gable, R. K., 136
Gaelick, L., 279
Galton, F., xiii
Gangestad, S., 81
GATB. See *General Aptitude Test Battery*
Gati, I., 192, 207–209
Gelso, C. J., 349
gender,
　identity, 128–130
　ideology, 134–135
　as organizing principle, 127–128
gender-related differences, 138
　characteristics, 130–131
　historical background, 119–120
　in interpersonal behavior,
　　287–288 (*see also* relationships)
　models
　　recent, 126–130
　　single-factor, 120–122
　　two-factor, 122–126
　in roles, behaviors, and attitudes,
　　44, 131–137
　in vocational interests, 210–223
　See also women
Gender Role Conflict Scales (GRCS–I), 136
Gender Role Conflict Scales (GRCS–II), 136
gender schema theory, 127–128, 130
General Aptitude Test Battery (GATB), 4
general interests,
　category order and similarity, 224–227
　conceptual levels of generality
　　compared to, 184–190
　Gati's structure, 208–209
　Holland's RIASEC structure,
　　190–200, 203–207, 208,
　　209–210, 224–227
　Prediger's structure, 201–203
　Roe's structure, 207–208, 209–210,
　　224–227
generalized MAXCOV,
　estimating nuisance covariances, 87–92

generalized MAXCOV, *continued*
　robustness, 85–87
　validity, 82–84
George, C., 348
Gergen, K. J., 272, 279, 282, 285
Getzel, J. W., 342
Ghiselli, E. E., 51
Gialluca, K. A., 62
Gibbons, R. D., 97
Gilbert, J. H. V., 313–314
Gintner, G., 277
Golden, R. R., xvi, 16, 81, 85, 93,
　　97–100, 105, 110
Gomes, M., 284
Goodenough, F., ix
Goodman, L. A., 97, 246–247
Goto, H., 306–307
Gottesman, I. I., 342–343
Gottfredson, G. D., 194, 205, 225
Gough, H., 121
Graduate Record Examination, 66
grantism for research, 360, 362, 363
Grayson, D. A., 110
Greenhaus, J. H., 132
Grisanti, C., 136
Gross, A. E., 277
Grotevant, H., 253, 345
group behavior,
　CTT results of examinees, 50–52, 73
　influences, 263–292
　See also interpersonal influence theory
growth measurement, 50, 68–73
Gruszkos, J., 272, 282, 285
Guerney, B., Jr., 282
Guilford, J. P., 178–188, 234, 237, 342
*Guilford-Zimmerman Temperament
　Survey,* 121
Gulliksen, H., 49, 68–69
Gurland, B. J., 98

Haberman, S. J., 97
Hales, L. W., 194
Halverson, C. F., 127
Hambleton, R. K., 53, 60, 65, 109
Hand, D. F., 97
Handelsman, M. M., 278
Haney, W., 5
Hansen, J. C., 180, 192, 195–196, 203,
　　205, 211, 216–217, 221, 253–255,
　　345
Hanson, G. R., 193, 197, 210, 212
Hare-Mustin, R. T., 135
Harmon, L. W., 210
Harrington, D. M., 125

Harrington, T. F., 197–198, 203
Hartigan, J. A., 97
Haskins Laboratories (New Haven),
    cross-language studies, 299, 300, 307
Hasselblad, V., 97
Hastie, R., 284
Hastorf, A. H., 277
Hathaway, S., ix
Hawk, J., 182–187
Hawks, B. K., 287–288
Hayes, T. J., 348
Hedges, L. V., 120
Heller, J. F., 279
Helmreich, R. L., 122–127, 133–134,
    137–138
Helms, B. J., 136
Hennessy, B. L., 317
Henry, N. W., 97
heritability of interests, 250–254, 255
Higgins, D. S., 284
Hills, H. I., 267–270, 273, 277–278,
    282, 284–285, 288–289
Holahan, C. K., 126
Holdsworth, R., 226
Holland, J. E., 194
Holland, J. L., x, xvii, xix, 177–227,
    233–234, 240, 243, 245, 249, 343,
    347, 349
Holtzworth-Munroe, A., 284, 290
Holzman, P., 98
homosexuality, 120
Hoover, H. D., 56
hostility toward tests, 5–6, 15
Howard, J. A., 277, 284
Hoyt, D. P., 132
Hubert, L., 192, 201, 208–210, 222, 245
human individual differences. *See*
    diversity
Humphrey, K. K., 313–314
Humphreys, L. G., x, 120
Hunt, E. B., 18–19
Hyde, J. S., 119

ICL. See *Interpersonal Check List*
identity, gender, 128–130
idiographic research, defined, 11
idiothetic theory of personality, 11
IMI. See *Impact Message Inventory*
imitation, learning by, 332–333, 338
Impact Message Inventory (IMI),
    269–270, 288
Index of Sex Role Orientation, 134
Indiana University,
    Speech Research Laboratory, 312

individual differences. *See* diversity
individual differences tests,
    background and challenges, xv, xxii, 1–12
    and brigadier general profiles, xvi–
        xvii, 118, 145–175
    cognitive design system, xv, 15–16, 17–46
    and control of human diversity, xviii,
        327, 329–339
    gender-related variables, xvi, 117,
        119–138
    generalized MAXCOV equation, xv–
        xvi, 81–91
    indicators of taxonicity of latent traits,
        xv, xvi, 16, 93–112
    interests and personality correlations,
        xvii, 118, 233–257
    interpersonal influence theory, xvii–
        xviii, 261, 263–292
    measurement with IRT and CAT, xv,
        16, 49–76
    Minnesota training for psychologists,
        xviii–xix, 327, 341–354
    research trends, xix, 327–328, 357–363
    speech perception, xviii, 261–262,
        297–322
    vocational interests, xvii, 118, 177–227
    See also diversity
Ingram, R. E., 126
Instone, D., 287
instrumental values, defined, 9
intelligence tests, 12
    as adaptive tests, 63–65
    and bias, 5–6
    diversity in scores of, 2–3, 6–7
    See also ability tests
interdependence in relationships,
    273–275, 287, 291–292
    factors affecting, 275–283
interests. *See specific types*
internal calculus,
    defined, 129
Interpersonal Adjective Scale, 284
Interpersonal Check List (ICL),
    284–286, 288
*Interpersonal Communication Rating
    Scale,* 269–270, 279, 288
interpersonal influence theory,
    classification of behavior, 266–268
    individual differences, 269, 274–275,
        283–292
    the other's behavior, 269–273
    relationship dependence, 273–283,
        287, 291–292
    resource exchange, 263–265

Introduction to Type (Myers), 159
IRT. *See* item response theory
item characteristic curve theory. *See* item
    response theory
item response theory (IRT),
    and adaptive tests, 65–68
    and CAT, 66–68
    characteristics of models, 55–59
    cognitive processing as merging with,
        75–76
    comparison of CTT and, 58, 59, 62, 63
    defined, 52
    differentiating between and within
        individuals using CAT and, 73–75
    estimating individual trait levels, 59–61
    family of mathematical models, 42–45,
        52–59, 75–76
    longitudinal measurement using CAT
        and, 68–73
    person fit and individual SEMs,
        62–63, 66–67, 71–76
items,
    definitions
        item difficulty, 50
        item discrimination, 50
        item information, 56
        local independence, 57, 60
    evaluation of content, 17–18
    generation, 25–26, 38, 41
    selection, 111
        in adaptive tests, 64, 65, 67
        for BSRI, 122–123
        in CAT, 66–68
        in cognitive design system, 37–38
    item-solving process, 22–23, 30–41

Jacklin, C. N., 119, 128
Jackson, D. N., 182–188, 211–215,
    223–227
Jackson, P. W., 342
Jackson Vocational Interest Survey (JVIS),
    and RIASEC interest types, 182,
        183–184, 211–215, 218–224,
        346–347
Jacobsen, P. R., 281
Jacobson, N. S., 284, 290
James, S. A., 134–135
James, W., ix
Jamieson, D. G., 315, 317, 319
Jannarone, R. J., 25
Jansen, P. G. W., 55
Jenkins, J. J., xviii, 261–262, 299–304,
    308, 315, 320
Johansson, C. B., 195, 197, 203, 210, 253

Johnson, B. R., 126
Johnson, D. J., 279
Johnson, J. A., 284
Johnson, R. W., 196, 210
Jones, E. E., 266–267, 277
Jones, R. E., 98
Jones, R. G., 277
Journal of Applied Psychology, ix, 193
Journal of Counseling Psychology, 193
Journal of Occupational Psychology, 193
*Journal of Personality and Social
    Psychology,* 137
Journal of Vocational Behavior, 193
Jung, C. G., 9
Jusczyk, P. W., 313
Just, M., 18, 30
JVIS. See *Jackson Vocational Interest
    Survey*

Kahgee, S. L., 98
Kalin, R., 134
Karten, S. J., 287
Kass, R., 348
Katzman, R., 105–106
Kaufman, N., 345, 348
Keeling, B., 195
Keil, F. C., 332
Kelley, H. H., 278
Kelly, G. S., 9–10
Kelly, L., 253
Kendler, H. H., 358
Kennedy, C. E., 132
Kiesler, C. A., 279
Kiesler, D. J., 269–270, 273
Kiley, G. L., 63
Kilmartin, C. T., 269–270, 273, 277–278,
    282, 284–285, 288–289
King, D. W., 134
King, L. K., 134
Kingsbury, G. G., 65, 72, 74
Kite, M. E., 128
Kite, W. R., 277
Klein, R. E., 313
Klos, D., 190
Knapp, L., 180, 207–208
Knapp, R. R., 180, 207–208
Knaub, P. K., 134
KOIS. See *Kuder Occupational Interest
    Survey*
Kolakowski, D. D., 44, 46
Kolditz, T. A., 278
Kolen, M. J., 56
Korfine, L., 81
Kruskal, J. B., 245–247

Kuder, F. G., 178, 180–188, 203,
    210–211, 226
Kuder Occupational Interest Survey
    (KOIS), 361
    and RIASEC interest types, 182, 183,
        210–211
Kuder Preference Record, 226
Kuhl, P., 313
Kurtzberg, D., 98
Kyle, E. M., 269–270

LaForge, R., 284
Lahav, G., 207
Lalonde, C. E., 313
Lamb, R. R., 193, 197, 249
Lamiell, J. T., 11
Landauer, T. K., 278
Lange, K., 98
language. *See* linguistics
Lanier, K., 269–270, 273, 277–278,
    282, 284–285, 288–289
Laskey, R. E., 313
latent traits,
    and criteria of taxonicity, 95–98
    discovery of dementia taxon, 104–107
    kinds, 94–95, 96
    models, 42–45, 107–111, 112
    quasi-taxonic threshold traits, 95
    research implications, 93–94, 111–112
    taxonicity of clinical dementia traits,
        99–104
    See also item response theory
latent trait test theory. *See* item response
    theory
Lauterbach, K., 284
Lawler, E. E., , 281
Lazarsfeld, P. F., 97
leadership, 281, 282
    See also brigadier general profiles
learning,
    by imitation, 332–333, 338
    by pedagogy, 332–336, 338
    See also education; training
Leary, T., 285
Lee, R., 331
legal issues of tests, 5, 18
leisure interests,
    attributes of leisure experiences,
        350–352, 353
    correlations with personality, 233–257
    of older women, 345, 346
Leisure Time Interest Inventory (LTI),
    235, 237, 250
Lenney, E., 126–127

Lenzenweger, M. F., 81
Lepper, M. R., 278
Levine, M. V., 63, 76
Levy, D. L., 97
Lewis, C., 55
Lewis, E. C., 132
Lewis, J., 18–19
Lewis, L., 120, 128
Lewyckyj, R., 193
Liberman, A. M., 299–304, 308, 320
Lighter, J., 134
Lindskold, S., 277
linguistics,
    evolution of language, 335–336
    and speech perception, 297–322
linking,
    defined, 55–56
    in longitudinal measurement, 69–70, 71
Linn, M. C., 119
Linn, R. L., 63
Lively, S. E., 307, 312, 319
Llewellyn, L. G., 277, 291
LLTM. *See* logistic latent trait model
local independence of test items, 57, 60
Lofquist, L. H., xiv, 188, 233, 328,
    343–344, 349
Logan, J. S., 307, 312, 319
logistic latent trait model (LLTM), 42–45
Lohnes, P. R., 190–192
Lord, F. M., 53, 109
LTI. See *Leisure Time Interest Inventory*
Lubinski, D., 121, 124–126, 128, 184
Lunneborg, C., 18–19, 192, 194,
    207–208, 223
Lunneborg, P. W., 180, 192, 194,
    207–208, 223, 226–227
Lykken, D. T., xi, xvii–xviii, 118, 181,189,
    192, 218, 234, 254–255, 342, 345
Lyons, D. W., 20
Lyson, T. A., 134–135

MacArthur, D., 145–146
MacCallum, R., 245
Maccoby, E. E., 119–120, 127
MacGavin, L., 277, 284
Machlowitz, M., 352
MacKain, K. S., 307–310, 314, 320
Major, B., 119–120, 127, 287
Major, L. L., 137
Making Vocational Choices (Holland), 210
Makov, J. E., 97
malingering, 63
Markus, H., 128
Marshall, G., 145

Martin, C. L., 127
Martin, J. R., 65, 67
masculinity,
  and androgyny, 122–126
  concepts, 128–129
  measurement problems, 120–130
  relationship to other variables, 130–131
  See also gender-related differences
Masculinity (M) scale, 121
Maslow, A. H., 352
Masters, G. N., 54, 109
Matlin, M., 120
Matthews, M. D., 234, 237
Matthysee, S., 98
MAXCOV-HITMAX procedure,
  estimating nuisance covariances, 87–92
  and generalized MAXCOV, 82–84
  idealization problems, 81–82
  robustness, 82, 85–87
maximum likelihood estimation, 60–61
Maxwell, S., 17–18
Mayer, M. J., xvi, 16
Mayr, E., 1
MBTI. See _Myers-Briggs Type Indicator_
McBride, J. R., 65, 67
McCarton, C. M., 98
McClaskey, C. L., 317
McCrae, R. R., 243
McGaw, B., 25
McGillicuddy, N. B., 283
McGue, M., 234, 250
McHugh, M. C., 119
McKinley, R. L., 55
McLaughlin, M. E., 63, 76
McNemar, Q., 342
McRoberts, G. W., 315–316
measurement, 2–3, 4, 15
  of androgyny, 122–126
  of attitudes and gender, 133–137
  of behavior and gender, 132–133, 136–137
  between and among individuals, 73–75
  CAT use in, 63–76
  of change, 50, 68–73
  of choices and direction, 7–9, 11
  of diversity in different species, 330
  goals, 25–27
  IRT use in, 52–63, 65–76
  longitudinal, 68–73
  of masculinity and femininity, 120–131
  of occupational roles and gender, 131–132, 136–137
  peaked indicators in, xv, xvi, 16, 93–112

measurement, _continued_
  of personality, 4, 9–11, 12, 235
  of traits, 3, 5, 6, 12
  of values, 8–9, 11
  See also specific measurement tools;
    standard error of measurement
Measurement and Evaluation in
  Counseling and Development, 193
Meehl, P. E., ix–x, xvi, 16, 18–19, 81–83,
    85, 90, 93–94, 97–98, 100, 110,
    137, 184, 188
Megargee, E. I., 286–287
Meir, E. I., 207–208
Meltzer, H. Y., 97
Meltzoff, A. N., 333
Mendelian latent structure analysis
  model, 98
mental tests. _See_ intelligence tests;
  psychological tests
Metzler, J., 30
Meyer, C. W., III, 269–270, 273,
    277–278, 282, 284–285, 288–289
Meyer, E., 194
Mezydlo, L., 135
Mezzich, J. E., 97
Micceri, T., 311
Miles, C. C., 121
Miller, H. R., 98
Minnesota, University of,
  cross-language study of listeners, 299
  Employment Stabilization Research
    Institute, 4, 343
  history of research at, ix–xi, xiv
  philosophical focus, 167
  pursuit of truth at, 329–330
  training cornerstones for
    psychologists, 341–353
_Minnesota Multiphasic Personality
  Inventory_ (MMPI), ix, 98, 341
  gender discrimination items, 100, 121
  profiles from, 5
Minnesota Twins Registry, and interests
  study, 233–257
Minnesota Vocational Interest Inventory
  (MVII), 210–211, 343
minority groups,
  African-American leaders, 148
  in military academies, 171
  nonnative English speakers and
    accents, 297–322
  women leaders, 148, 149 (_see also_
    women)
  workers with disabilities, 7, 344
Miranda, S., 311

Mislevy, R., 25
Mitchell, T., 279
Miyawaki, K., 299–304, 308, 320
MLTM. *See* multi-component latent trait model
MMPI. See *Minnesota Multiphasic Personality Inventory*
Mochizuki, M., 307
model fit,
  and item response pattern information, 62–63, 76
  of RIASEC interests model, 203–207, 208, 209–210
models,
  androgyny models, 124–126
  Best's model of assimilation, 315–317, 322
  cognitive design system model, 25–26, 28–38
  of dimensional traits, 107–109, 112
  gender-related differences models, 120–130
  Guttman scaling model, 55
  of interests, 177–227
  IRT family of, 42–45, 52–59, 75–76
  latent class models, 98, 99–100
  latent trait models, 42–45, 107–112
  Likert scaling model, 55
  Rasch model, 42–44, 53
  of speech perception, 315–322
  Thurstonian scaling model, 55
  See also specific models
Mokken, R. J., 55
Moloney, D. P., 342
Montague, W. E., 18
Moore, M. K., 333
Moore, R. J., 136
Morosan, D. E., 315, 317, 319
Morrow, G. D., 279
Moses, J. L., 7
motivation and learning, 333–334
MPQ. See *Multidimensional Personality Questionnaire*
Mueller, W. J., 291
multi-component latent trait model (MLTM), 42–45
Multidimensional Personality Questionnaire (MPQ), 235, 240, 242–245, 248, 255
Muraki, E., 54–55
Murray, H. A., 10
MVII. See *Minnesota Vocational Interest Inventory*
Myers, I. B., 159

Myers-Briggs Type Indicator (MBTI), 9, 353
  for brigadier general profiles, 152, 157, 159
National Defense University (Washington, D.C.), 157
Nelson, B. N., 269–270, 273, 277–278, 282, 284–285, 288–289
Neufeld, R. W. J., 81
Neulinger, J., 349
Nevill, D. E., 132
Nichols, D. S., 98
Nichols, R. C., 253
Nicholson, I. R., 81
nomothetic research, defined, 11
norm-referenced tests, 7, 72
Norvell, N., 279
Novick, M. R., 109
nuisance covariance,
  estimating, 87–92
  and generalized MAXCOV, 82–84
  and MAXCOV-HITMAX procedure, 81–82, 85–87
number-correct score theory. *See* classical test theory
Nutall, S. B., 279–280, 285, 287–288
Nyquist, L. V., 286–287

occupational interests,
  correlations with personality, 240, 242–250
  heritability and stability, 250–254, 255
  results and discussion, 254–257
  structure of, 237–240
  See also vocational interests
Occupational Interests Inventory, 234–235, 237, 250
Oden, M., 342
O'Gorman, J., 194
O'Heron, C. A., 129–130, 132, 134
O'Neil, J. M., 136
Orford, J., 273
Orlofsky, J. L., 129–130, 132–133
O'Shea, A. J., 197–198, 203
Ostrow, D. G., 97

Pachella, R. G., 29
Pallak, M. S., 279
Pandey, G. N., 97
PAQ. See *Personal Attributes Questionnaire*
parallel tests, defined, 68–69
Paterson, D. G., ix, xiv
Payne, T. J., 128

peaked indicators,
  analysis of, 110–111
  defined, 61, 94, 107, 110
  See also taxonicity
Pearlman, M., 59
Pearson, K., xiii–xv
pedagogy, learning by, 332–336, 338
Pedhazur, E., 128
Pellegrino, J. W., 18, 20
Peplau, L. A., 284
perception of speech. *See* speech
  perception
Perey, A. J., 317
Perkins, M. J., 269–270
Perry, R., 98
Personal Attributes Questionnaire (PAQ),
  123, 344
  and androgyny models, 124
  correlation with BSRI, 130–131
  correlation with SRBS, 133
  in tests of gender-related concepts,
    126–127, 128
  validity, 137
personality, 233–234
  correlation with interests, 240,
    242–250, 254–257
  defined, 10
  diversity in, 7–9
  measurement, 4, 9–11, 12, 235
person fit,
  defined, 62–63
  and SEM in IRT, 62–63, 66–67, 71–76
  and vocations, 256–257
Petersen, A. C., 119
Peterson, N. S., 56
Peterson, R. A., 210
Pisoni, D. B., 307, 312–313, 317, 319
Pittman, T. S., 266–267
placement, xiv
Pleck, J. H., 135–136
Polek, D., 287
Polka, L., xviii, 261–262, 321
Popper, K. R., 98
possibilities study of diversity, 11–12
power, abuse of, 331–332, 338
precision,
  defined, 56
prediction,
  of cognitive measurement, 17, 38
  and correlation, xiii–xiv
Prediger, D. J., xvii, 188, 192–193,
    196–197, 201–203, 209–210, 218,
    249
preequating, defined, 56

Premack, A. J., 333
Premack, D., xviii, 332–335, 337
Price, L. A., 181
privacy, right to, 5–6
problem-solving abilities,
  of brigadier generals, 150, 152,
    153–154
processing, cognitive,
  and IRT, 75–76
  in spatial aptitude tests, 22–23, 30–41
  profiles, 3–5
  See also brigadier general profiles
Pruitt, D. G., 283
Pruitt, J., 321
Pruzansky, S., 193
psychographs, 3–5
psychological tests,
  for brigadier general profiles, 152,
    155–167, 168–169
  historical development, xiv, 2–3
  See also specific tests or types of tests
psychology, disciplines, xiii–xiv,
    15–16
Psychology of Women Quarterly, The,
  137
Putnam, S. W., 81

Quaintance, M. K., 181
questionnaires, 4
  See also individual questionnaires

Ramak (Hebrew interest inventory),
    207–208
Ramsden, M. W., 132–133
Rand, L., 132
random errors. *See* sampling errors
Rasch, G., 53, 109
Rausch, H. L., 277, 291
Ray, S. B., 348
Reckase, M. D., 55
rehabilitation services, 7
reinforcement theory, 331–332
Reise, S. P., 53, 63, 76, 285
relationships,
  classification of behavior, 266–268
  dependence, 273–283, 287, 291–292
  individual differences, 269, 274–275,
    283–292
  the other's behavior in, 269–273
  resource exchange in, 263–265
  structure, 265
reliability,
  in CTT, 51–52
  of interests, 250–254, 255

Repp, B., 304
research,
  bias, 360, 361
  face validity, 344
  trends, 357–363
  types, 11
  at University of Minnesota, ix–xi, xiv
RIASEC interests model, 177–178
  fit of, 203–207, 208, 209–210
  order of, 219–227
  structure of, 190–200, 203–207, 208,
    209–210
  studies using, 178–180, 210–219
Rich, S., 234, 254–255, 345
Richards, J. M., 190, 193–194
Rindskopf, D., 97
Rindskopf, W., 97
Roberts, C. A., 253
Roe, A., xvii, 177–227, 234, 249, 342
Roff, M., ix
Rokeach, M., 9, 11
roles, gender-related, 131–137
Roos, P. E., 126
Rose, H. A., 196
Rosenberg, S., 202–203
Rosenkrantz, P. S., 123
Roth, D. L., 25
Roth, M., 99, 104
Rounds, J., xvii–xviii, 118, 180,
    182–188, 192, 196, 205, 207,
    209–210, 234, 237, 245
Rusbult, C. E., 279

Salience Inventory, 132
Samejima, F., 54, 62
sampling errors,
  and estimating nuisance covariances,
    87–88
  in generalized MAXCOV, 82–83,
    86–87
  reducing, 88–92
  in tests for dementia taxon, 102
Sanders, E. K., 298
Sawin, L. L., 127
Scarr, S., 253, 345
scenes, traits vs., 10–11
Schank, R. C., 41
Scheibelchner, H., 25
Schneider, L. M., 25
Schussel, R. H., 193, 197
Schwartz, P., 277, 279, 284
scientific theory, x
SCII. *See Strong-Campbell Interest
    Inventory*

scores,
  for adaptive tests, 65
  in CTT, 50–51
  of intelligence tests, 2–3
  of interest inventories, 7–9
  interpretation of, 2–3, 6–7, 19–20
  of personality tests, 4
  and right to privacy, 5–6
  See also item response theory
script theory, 10–11
SDS. See *Self-Directed Search*
second-language learning. *See* speech
    perception
Sedlak, A., 202–203
Segal, N., 234, 254–255, 342, 345
selection,
  ability testing vs. personality testing
    for, 12
  differentiating between and among
    individuals for, 73
  individual selection vs. systems
    development, 167, 170–171
  as purpose for testing, xiv, 3–7
Self-Directed Search (SDS), 343, 361
  and RIASEC interest types, 193, 195,
    203, 204–207, 209–210
self-esteem, 4, 5–6
SEM. *See* standard error of
    measurement (SEM)
sex differences, 331, 334–335
  See also gender-related differences
Sex-Role Behavior Scale (SRBS), 132–133
Sex-Role Egalitarianism Scale, 134
Sex-Role Identity Scale, 129
Sex-Role Ideology Scale (SRIS), 134
Sex Roles (journal), 137
Sex-Role Stereotype Questionnaire, 123
Shalhever, R., 207
Shankweiler, D. P., 299–304
Shannon, J., 282
Sheldon, A., 306–307
Sheldon, W. H., 9
Shepard, R. N., 30, 247
Shipley Institute of Living Scale (SILS),
    148–150, 151
Shubsachs, A. P., 188
Siladi, M., 128
SILS. See *Shipley Institute of Living Scale*
Simon, H. A., 46
Simon, S., 126
Simpson, A., 276–277
Singer, J., 126
Sithole, N. M., 315–316
Skinner, B. F., ix, 341

Slevin, K. F., 135
Smith, A. F. M., 97
Smith, M. B., 8
Smith, T. W., 278
Sneath, P. H. A., 97
Snow, R. E., 18
Snyder, C. R., 278
Snyder, M., 81
Sokal, R. R., 97
Solomon, H., 97
Spada, H., 25
spatial aptitude tests,
   application of cognitive theory to,
      20–23
   cognitive design system for tasks in,
      25–45
   processes for item solving, 22–23,
      30–37
Spearman, C., xiii, xv
speech perception, 297–299, 300
   cross-language studies, 299–307,
      315–322
   perceptual categories, 307–315
   production as related to, 306–307,
      315, 320
Spence, J. T., 120, 122–128, 130–131,
      133–134, 137–138, 286–287
SRBS. See *Sex-Role Behavior Scale*
SRIS. *Sex-Role Ideology Scale*
Stafford, I. P., 135
Stafford, R. E., 253
standard error of measurement (SEM),
   in adaptive tests, 66
   in CTT, 51–52, 58, 62, 73, 75
   in IRT, 57–59, 62–63, 66–67, 71–76
Stange, W., 298
Stapp, J., 122–124, 133–134
Stegelmann, W., 25
stereotyping, 131, 133
Sternberg, R. J., 18–19, 43
Stocco, J. L., 253–254
Stocking, M. L., 59
Stone, M. H., 63
Storms, M. D., 128–129
Strandmark, N. L., 63
Strange, W., xviii, 261–262, 299–304,
      306–308, 310–311, 314, 317,
      319–321
Streeter, L. A., 313
Streiner, P. L., 98
Strickland, D., 269–270, 273, 277–278,
      282, 284–285, 288–289
Strong, E. K., Jr., 8, 178, 201, 205, 211,
      218, 224, 226, 253

Strong, S. R., xvii–xviii, 261, 267–270,
      273, 276–278, 282, 284–285,
      288–289
Strong-Campbell Interest Inventory,
   (SCII), 183, 341, 343, 361
   and brigadier general profiles, 152,
      163, 165–167, 168, 169
   and RIASEC interest types, 193, 196,
      203–207, 209–212, 215–224,
      346–347, 353
Strong Vocational Interest Blank (SVIB),
      121
   and RIASEC interest types, 182, 183,
      203, 204–207, 209–211
   women and occupations, 131–132
Strube, M. J., 81
Studdert-Kennedy, M., 299–304
Suczek, R., 284
Super, D. E., 132, 180, 224, 349
Sutton, M. A., 178–188, 234, 237
SVIB. See *Strong Vocational Interest
   Blank*
Swaminathan, H., 53, 60, 65
Swanson, J. L., 253–254
Swanson, L., 59
Swensen, C. H., 291
Sympson, J. B., 76
Syrdal-Laskey, A., 313
systems development,
   individual selection vs.,
      167, 170–171

Tactics of Manipulation questionnaire,
      284
Takane, Y., 193
Tanner, M. A., 97
TAT. See *Thematic Apperception Test*
Tatsuoka, K. K., 63
taxonicity, 16
   criteria, 95–98
   definitions, 94–95
   and pseudotaxonicity, 107–111, 112
   research implications, 111–112
   of traits of clinical dementia, 95,
      99–107, 112
Taylor, M. G., 272, 282, 285
Taylor, S. E., 128
Taylor, T. J., 277, 291
Teaff, J. D., 345, 348
technology. *See* computerized adaptive
   tests; computers and testing
Tees, R. C., 313–314, 317–320
Tellegen, A., xi, xvii–xviii, 93, 118, 121,
      124–126, 128, 181, 184, 189, 192,

Tellegen, A., *continued*
218, 234, 245, 254–255, 257, 285,
342, 345
Teresi, J. A., 98
Terman, L. L., 121
Terman, L. M., 342
terminal values,
defined, 9
Terry, R., 105–106
Tetenbaum, T., 128, 134
thema,
defined, 10
Thematic Apperception Test (TAT),
269
Thibaut, J. W., 278
Thissen, D., 75
Thompson, E. H., 136
Thompson, T., 184
Thorndike, E. L., 15
Thornton, A., 135
Thurstone, L. L., 178, 201, 226
Tilby, P., 134
Tinsley, D. J., 135, 345, 349, 351, 353
Tinsley, H. E. A., xviii–xix, 345,
347–349, 351, 353
Titterington, D. M., 97
Tokyo, University of, 299
Tomkins, S. S., 10–11
Tomlinson, B. E., 99, 104
Torrance, E. P., 342
Trabin, T. E., 63
Tracey, T. J., 210
Trafton, R. S., 349
training,
feedback in, 318–319
learning by imitation and pedagogy,
332–336, 338
for research, 360–361, 363
role in speech perception and
production, 307–313, 317, 321,
322
See also education
traits,
constructs vs., 9–10
measurement, 3, 5, 6, 12
scenes vs., 10–11
See also latent traits
Travis, A., 134
true and error score theory. *See* classical
test theory
Tuck, B. F., 195
Tukey, J. W., 253
Tyler, L. E., ix, xv, xxii, 5, 7–8, 10–11,
15–16

Underbakke, M., 311, 319–320
Unger, R., 120
UNIACT. See *American College Testing
Interest Inventory—Unisex Edition*
U.S. Air Force Academy
(Colorado Springs), 170–171
U.S. Department of Labor, 183
U.S. Employment Service, 4, 183
*U.S. Employment Service Interest
Inventory* (USES), 183
U.S. military,
academies, 170–171
as bureaucracy, 171–172
effect of education and democracy on,
172–174
retention of leaders in, 171–172, 174
See also brigadier general profiles
U.S. Military Academy (West Point),
170–171
U.S. Naval Academy (Annapolis),
170–171
USES. See *U.S. Employment Service
Interest Inventory*

Vail, D., 37
Vale, C. D., 55, 66, 69
validity, 29
of androgyny models, 125
of BSRI and PAQ, 137
of cognitive measurement, 17
face validity of research, 344
of generalized MAXCOV, 82–84
of latent class model for dementia
taxon, 99–104
See also construct validity
values,
measurement of, 8–9, 11
in relationships, 275–278, 290
Vandenberg, S. G., 253
Vaughan, H. G., Jr., 98
Verbrugge, R. R., 299–304, 308, 320
Verette, J. A., 278
Verhelst, N., 25
Vetter, L., 132
VII. See *Vocational Interest Inventory*
Visalberghi, F., 333
Vocational Interest Inventory (VII),
207–208
vocational interests,
catalog of interest factors, 181–184,
185–187
conceptual levels of generality, 184–190
structure of interests, 177–181,
224–227

vocational interests, *continued*
    basic interests, 210–224
    general interests, 190–210
    See also occupational interests
Vocational Preference Inventory (VPI),
    and RIASEC interest types, 190,
    193, 194, 203, 204–207, 209–210,
    225–226
vocational psychology,
    application of test results, 3–4, 256–257
    gender-related roles in occupations,
    131–132, 136–137
Vogel, S. R., 123
VPI. *See Vocational Preference Inventory*
Wakefield, J. A., 192, 194
Waller, N. G., xi, xvii–xviii, 53, 81, 118,
    181, 189, 192, 218, 257, 285, 342
warm-up effect, 63
Washington, G., 145
Waxman, M., 22, 28, 30, 32, 35
Weinberg, R., 253, 345
Weiner, B., 278
Weinrach, S. G., 199
Weiss, D. J., xv, 16, 62–67, 72, 74, 344
Welton, G. L., 283
Werker, J. F., 313–314, 317–320
Wetzel, D., 25
Whitely, S. E., 25, 42
Whitley, B. E., Jr., 119
Whitney, D. R., 190, 193–194
Wigington, J. H., 196
Wilcox, K., 234, 254–255, 345
Wilkinson, L., 211, 245

Williams, L., 314
Wilson, E. O, 332
Wingersky, M. S., 56
Wingrove, C. R., 135
Wish, M., 245
Wishnov, B., 279
Wisnicki, K. S., 126
women,
    in leadership, 148, 149
    leisure interests of, 345, 346
    in military, 170, 171, 175
    and relationship dependence, 279
    vocational interests, 210–223
    See also femininity; gender-related
    differences
Wood, W., 287
Woods, N. F., 134–135
Workman, K. R., 348
Wright, B. D., 63, 109
Wrightsman, L. S., 136
Wyer, R. S., Jr., 279

Yonce, L. J., 81, 85, 90, 98
York, D. C., 347
Young, F. W., 193, 204
Young, M. A., 97

Zanna, M., 279
Zedeck, S., 51
Zevon, M. A., 192, 207, 209, 245
Zubin, J., 96
Zuckerman, D., 135
Zytowski, D. G., 203, 210